A BIOPSYCHOSOCIAL APPROACH TO HEALTH

RACHEL C. SUMNER

A BIOPSYCHOSOCIAL APPROACH TO HEALTH

FROM CELL TO SOCIETY

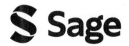

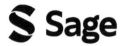

1 Oliver's Yard
55 City Road
London EC1Y 1SP

2455 Teller Road
Thousand Oaks
California 91320

Unit No 323-333, Third Floor, F-Block
International Trade Tower Nehru Place
New Delhi – 110 019

8 Marina View Suite 43-053
Asia Square Tower 1
Singapore 018960

Editor: Janka Romero
Assistant editor: Emma Yuan
Production editor: Rabia Barkatulla
Copyeditor: Bryan Campbell
Proofreader: Leigh Smithson
Indexer: Adam Pozner
Marketing manager: Fauzia Eastwood
Cover design: Wendy Scott
Typeset by: KnowledgeWorks Global Ltd
Printed in the UK

Library of Congress Control Number: 2022949370

British Library Cataloguing in Publication data

A catalogue record for this book is available from the British Library

ISBN 9781529791242
ISBN 9781529791235 (pbk)

At Sage we take sustainability seriously. Most of our products are printed in the UK using responsibly sourced papers and boards. When we print overseas we ensure sustainable papers are used as measured by the Paper Chain Project grading system. We undertake an annual audit to monitor our sustainability.

For Ruby. May your heart always speak softly with kindness for all things, and roar like a hurricane for justice, fairness, and the pursuit of truth.

TABLE OF CONTENTS

ABOUT THE AUTHOR

Dr Rachel C. Sumner is a psychobiologist and chartered psychologist with the British Psychological Society Division of Health Psychology. She is a senior research fellow in the Health and Human Performance Global Academy at Cardiff Metropolitan University. Rachel researches areas that consider how our lived environment impacts our health and wellbeing, using a variety of methods and outcomes to try and make sense of the very complicated procedures that make our health a function of our lived experience. She is an interdisciplinary researcher who has made her career in collecting knowledge from various fields and trying to bring it together to make sense of the ways in which our health can be made better or worse through our everyday contexts. She was previously the course director for the Master of Science Health Psychology programme at the University of Gloucestershire, from which this book has been adapted. This book was developed from a module she created that was written to give health psychology trainees a comprehensive understanding of health from its very smallest indices (our cells) right up to its largest measure (our societies). Taking both critical social and community aspects of health provides a comprehensive and inclusive means of accounting for the incredible intricacies of health at the individual and population levels. It is hoped that this book will provide a broad and integrated starting point for those interested in health psychology, whether they are psychologists, public health practitioners, in medicine, or in medical areas of the social sciences.

NOTES ON THIS BOOK

This book was written by someone who is probably best described as a jack of all trades but a master of none. Essentially, I am someone with an over-commitment problem who wants to know everything about everything. As an interdisciplinary health researcher who always secretly wanted to be a 'real' doctor, but never had the stomach for it, I have ventured into psychology bringing with me my love for biology and crowbarring it into just about everything I can think of. The intersection of biology and psychology continues to fascinate me, and I hope you will acquire some of that fascination too as you read through these pages. I very much hope this book will be of interest and of use to a variety of students, from those in my own discipline (health psychology), to those in the disciplines I always wanted to be in (medicine and nursing), and to broader health practitioners. I have recently had pause to reflect on my career whilst writing this book, trying to summarise a theme or an underlying thread for the work I have done over the last few years. For me, there is one unifying factor to all of the research I have done, and that is my passion for wanting to right the injustices of the world, which is something I think that every researcher in health has the power to do. At its heart, I hope you will find the spirit of social justice strongly shining through these pages. Those who learn have a responsibility to use that knowledge wisely and for the greater good, and there can be no greater good than seeking to protect and support your fellow beings on this little planet.

A commitment to being anti-racist

As a white woman, I can barely even begin to understand the depths to which racism injures, undermines, and degrades people's lives. I do, however, seek to understand this as well as I can and to serve as an agent for change. That is what being anti-racist is about, and being anti-racist is a commitment I hold very dear. It is simply not enough to be 'against' racism or to dislike it – we must make constant and deliberate movement against it. I encourage you all to be agents for change against all social injustices, from racism to any of the other very harmful -isms our societies put forth. I would argue that it is your responsibility – and I hope by the end of this book you will agree with me (if you don't already).

From a perspective of health, I have some understanding as to how racism harms, and it is mentioned at various points throughout this book. In my understanding of life and the world, I am still learning and always will be. In discussions with my editorial team, I was introduced to (mostly through my terrible efforts of copy-editing) a critical debate about the way in which categories of 'race' are written, that at that stage I was not aware of. The debate centres on whether they should be treated as proper nouns (i.e., with an uppercase beginning) or not.[1] On the one hand, the argument for capitalising the word (e.g., Black or White) serves as a reminder that these are socially derived categorisations, and whilst they are false and arbitrary, the very fact they have been made has served as a function of control, subjugation, harm, and denigration for a very long time and this should be respected and acknowledged. The converse of this argument is that categories should not be written with capitals (e.g., black or white), understanding that these categories are socially derived and are illegitimate as groupings of peoples. For this text I have chosen to write any racialised groupings (which I seldom refer to) in their lowercase forms. This may not be the 'right' choice for all, but given that I am focusing on health throughout this book, and health aspects of racialised groups are associated with their social treatment rather than some underlying unifying biological aspect that these very diverse groups of peoples may share in their racialised categories, I felt at the time this was the right choice to make. I welcome feedback on this warmly.

Human-based knowledge

I am very passionate about animal welfare, and whilst I do understand that animal-based research has its place in scientific knowledge, I personally feel that if we want to talk about people then we should talk about people. As such, I always commit to using human-based research in my teaching and in my own research. In this book, all of the research I will be discussing comes from humans unless there is no way that research can be done with humans for ethical reasons. It is very rarely the case, but it can happen. When I have had to refer to animal research I will say so, because I think it is important to remember that research based on animals can only be at best extrapolated to humans, and is always a best guess with regard to how reliable it may

---

1 For a more comprehensive overview of the debate, please do take a look at Kwame Anthony Appiah's article that discusses this in more detail: www.theatlantic.com/ideas/archive/2020/06/time-to-capitalize-blackand-white/613159/

be in humans. Importantly, I think we all can do and be better to the other species that we share this planet with, and one of the ways we can do that is to consume products (including research!) that do not compromise our ethical standards towards them. All those on this earth who have less power and capability to speak deserve the highest protections we can give them.

Questions and activities

There will be key question boxes throughout the book to give you the opportunity to discuss, reflect on, and consolidate the information I've tried very hard to (accessibly) cram into your heads. Do use them. I have always found I've learned best with others, so talk with others to help your learning too.

I have also provided further reading and resources at the end of each chapter to help to expand your knowledge. Some of these resources are academic, some are not. Some are written, some are videos. The point is to provide you with next steps to expand on what you have learned, to help underline key debates, or in some cases to link chapters together.

Warnings

These stop points are interjections to alert you to the potential pseudoscience that often gets discussed in public arenas. The term 'pseudoscience' I define as claims that are emerging and still experimental, as yet scientifically inconclusive, lacking evidence and factually baseless. It is the sometimes well-meaning, often misleading, and potentially dangerous way that fancy technical terms and concepts are used to legitimise or otherwise add weight to an idea, a concept, or (as is most frequently the case) a product. I won't put the fault squarely with those that peddle it – us scientists have a lot to answer for as well. We don't communicate our work well. We write our articles so obscurely and with such complex and dense language that most people can't even work out what the article is about from the title, let alone anything else. It is no wonder that those who seek to profit from health and wellbeing can do so with impunity whilst scientists do the bare minimum to accessibly explain their knowledge. We must do better. The point of these warning points is to draw your attention to topics and areas of interest that are frequently misused, misunderstood, or mis-sold. I want to draw your attention to these for two reasons: 1) these issues are commonly misunderstood, and 2) these issues are commonly poorly communicated. Handling these issues requires care in order to ensure that knowledge is made accessible to all, but also so that common misconceptions are addressed fairly and with respect.

ACKNOWLEDGEMENTS

The development of this work was ultimately borne out of the very frequently magic conversations I had with colleagues during my days at the University of Gloucestershire. To Dai Jones in particular, I extend my sincere thanks for his enthusiasm and constant sage advice. I also thank my colleague Elaine Walklet for her contribution on the particular module from which this book is drawn, and for taking up the mantle of leading this beautiful course once I moved on to Cardiff Metropolitan University.

I also owe my thanks to two other outstanding colleagues who supported the development of this book. I am very grateful to Dr Daniel Stones for his contribution to the lecture (and subsequent chapter) around psychobiology, specifically bringing in his wonderful expertise on cancer. His ability to communicate something so complex to students with no prior biomedical or cell science training was amazing to witness. I am also hugely grateful to Dr Samantha Dockray for her excellent support of this work (and of others in my career!), and for her contribution to constructing and refining the chapter on the life course. She is a true inspiration as an academic and as a person.

Of particular note, I extend my sincere thanks to my first cohort of students from this MSc in Health Psychology: Abbey, Ben, Beth, Jo D, Jo H, Michelle, and Rachel. I couldn't have picked a more incredible group of people with whom to start this adventure. Thank you for taking the chance on this new course, for jumping in with both feet, and for being excellent companions on that wonderful journey.

This work was made possible by the support and opportunities provided by many people in my life, on whose shoulders I have stood. Academically, Prof Diane Crone, Prof Stephen Gallagher, Prof David James, Prof Yori Gidron – your kindness, support, and belief will stay with me forever, and will be paid forward by me to future academic generations for the rest of my career.

I am also grateful to many colleagues around me who have supported my development in many ways: Dr B., Elaine K., Simon, Steve, Rhiannon, Professor Anne, David S., Katerina, Aisling, Sandra, Orla.

To my PhD supervisees, Samantha, Natasha, Sarah, Gemma, and Elaine, who have taught me more than I have probably ever imparted on them, thank you for your unending patience with my chronic inability to manage my diary and for the privilege of allowing me to guide your respective rising stars.

I owe thanks also to Donna Goddard, Emma Yuan, and Esmé Carter at SAGE whose patience, kindness, support, and excellent feedback made this work possible.

Personally, to my family, Clair, Gordon, Ben, and Christina – you have always cheered me on no matter what mad venture I have set myself on, and my success is in no small part down to your love and support. Thank you for being my steer and for helping me every step of the way in my sometimes-questionable path through life.

To my wonderful friends and fellow adventurers of the world (GB, DB, LOR, KA, SM, RS, RL, CJ), thank you for being my context. Your belief and support have meant the world to me, although I am not very good at showing it (I am, as always, a work in progress). To our dear LB, whom we sorely miss, thank you for being an early adopter of believing in my potential as an academic. I would say you'd never believe I'd written a book, but deep down I know you would because you were just wonderful like that. We miss you, but you shine through us all.

Finally, to my dear four-legged research and teaching assistant, Martin, whose constant unconditional love and esteem has only ever been contradicted by the occasional loud snoring through my online lectures during pandemic lockdown teaching, thank you. You are – and always will be – a very good boy.

'You have to act as if it were possible to radically transform the world.

And you have to do it all the time.'

Angela Davis

1
THE CELL

INTRODUCTION

The aim of this chapter is to introduce you to some aspects of cell biology, to provide a foundation for understanding how psychological factors can impact the very tiniest mechanics of our bodies. First, you will start thinking about cellular activity and why it is important for psychologists to consider it. Then, we will have a look at some of the ways in which we can view health, and factors that influence health. Finally, we will look at two key aspects of cell biology to illustrate how cellular-level thinking is important for understanding the complex and intertwined ways that our lived experiences and social worlds can influence our health.

Learning Outcomes

- Understand the contribution of cellular factors on everyday physical functioning.
- Have an appreciation of the intersecting influences of human health on the cellular level.
- Be able to explain some of the key cellular processes that have lifelong impacts on health.
- Evaluate the influence of a variety of factors on cellular health with a critical lens.

WHAT DOES PSYCHOLOGY HAVE TO DO WITH CELLS?

This is probably the question that goes through most students' heads when they sit down to a lecture expecting psychology but getting biology. The answer that I hope most readers will conclude by the end of this chapter is: everything! To be a health psychologist, it's important to understand health – and to understand health, there is a need to understand biology. Before we can understand how psychological factors or psychological experiences can impact our health, we need to develop our knowledge of the specific mechanics of what makes health – and that means biology.

Our cells dictate all the larger structural and systems-level processes that our bodies undertake. If we think about our bodies as buildings, our cells are literally the bricks that hold them up and make them a structure. If they do not function, or if they start to experience problems, then the whole structure is vulnerable. Continuing the house metaphor, when we look at systems in Chapter 2, this will be like considering our internal plumbing and electrical systems – ensuring that the facilities of the house are fully functional. These are also hugely important, but if your bricks are crumbling then whether or not your bathroom tap leaks is probably the least of your worries.

We also need to consider that the very organ that underpins psychological processes – the brain – is also made of cells. Even though we don't fully understand the complexities of the brain yet, every single thing we do, feel, think, or experience is processed at the cellular level. These tiny cells – our neurons – talk to each other to create our psychological experiences, but they also send and receive information from the body all the time. So, everything we do, everything we are, and everything we experience is processed by cells; but even more than that – everything we do, everything we are, and everything we experience is also generated by cellular activity. This means that psychology has *everything* to do with cells, and health psychology even more so – as beyond the cells of the nervous system, we are now considering the cells of all other systems in the body.

THE BIOPSYCHOSOCIAL MODEL AND THE HEALTH ONION

Much of the premise of this book is centred on the biopsychosocial model of health. In short, this model considers health to be a product not simply of biological factors, but also of social and psychological experiences and conditions (see Figure 1.1). Before the biopsychosocial model, we had the medical model. The medical model principally understood health as being a biological situation – that it could be cured or treated with drugs or surgery, and that health was simply an absence of disease. This all sounds very straightforward and common sense, but anyone who has had an illness that could not be treated by medicine will tell you it's not that simple. The biopsychosocial model, on the other hand, asserts that biological factors are simply just a part of what constitutes our health, and that our broader personal and social influences are equally important in dictating our wellbeing. It is the understanding that whilst things like genetics and individual immune responses are critical to our health, they are not the total sum. Psychological factors such as our personality, our mental health, and our thoughts and attitudes can be just as important in dictating our health and wellness. Similarly, social factors such as our interpersonal relationships, our socioeconomic status, and our social support also impact our health and wellbeing. Of course, these social factors

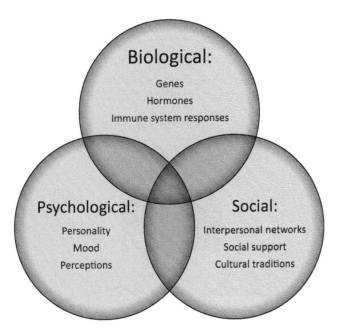

Figure 1.1   The biopsychosocial model

are also dependent on our personal factors, such as our gender identity, ethnicity, and racial identity, where our interpersonal relationships can be dependent on the social norms of our culture (both positive and negative) with regard to these factors. These interlinking factors are critical to understanding health as a whole, and the fact that they interlink means that if we don't consider them all, we are failing to truly make sense of what health means. Not only this, but each of the levels of health discussed in this book (the cell, the system, the person) can be influenced by each of these factors as well; so, it is very important to keep in mind.

Beyond the intersecting influences of our lived experiences and our physical selves, we can organise factors that influence our health in a hierarchy as well. Perhaps the best and most useful depiction of the layers of health influence was produced by Dahlgren and Whitehead (1991) in a report for the World Health Organization to illustrate the influence of policy on individual health. Sometimes referred to as the health rainbow, or the health onion, this model (see Figure 1.2) shows the various layers of factors in our lives that have the potential to impact our health. The very centre concerns those individual-level factors, things like our age, our physical functioning, and our ability to cope with challenge. The second layer considers our individual lifestyle factors. These will be considerations such as our diet and our level of physical activity. Above this, we have social and community networks: our social support, how connected we are to others, and both the quality and quantity of our social infrastructures. Next are our living and working conditions. Here, there are more specific factors to

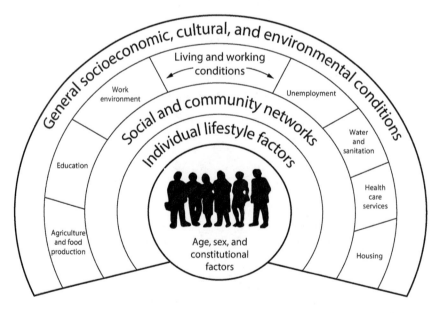

Figure 1.2   The Health Rainbow (or Health Onion), based on Dahlgren and Whitehead 1991

Source: Public Health England, *Health profile for England:* 2017, www.gov.uk/government/publications/health-profile-for-england/chapter-6-social-determinants-of-health

consider: our work, education, the availability of food resources, the availability of water and sanitation, the quality and accessibility of our health service systems, and the quality and context of our housing. At the uppermost layer sit any final considerations regarding our socio-economic, cultural, and environmental conditions. Each of these layers has important influences on our health and wellbeing, but they can also influence each other as well, and in either direction. The model was originally created to provide a framework for policymakers to consider how policy impacts individual health, with the idea that the further into the core of the onion you go, the less ability external factors have to determine that individual's health. However, what I hope you will get from this book is that there is virtually nothing about our health that cannot be influenced by our social context, even those things at the very core. What is important to consider here is that there is no hierarchy with regard to how important any of these layers are to individual health, nor how profoundly the impact of decisions in each of those levels (beyond the central level where 'decisions' are not objectively made by the individual) affects the person's health and wellbeing. If we attempt to bring both the biopsychosocial model and the health onion together, it should be easy enough to see that there are biopsychosocial factors at each level of the onion, and onion levels in each circle of the biopsychosocial model. Before we move on to understanding some of the ways that cell machinery can be impacted by psychological factors, have a look at the following questions and work through the various aspects of the models discussed to see how many answers you can come up with. Don't worry if you end up with a lot of very complicated and intertwining answers – that means you're doing it right!

Key Questions

- Thinking about the biopsychosocial model, how do you think someone's job impacts their health?
- Thinking about the experience of **stress**, what aspects and layers of the health onion would impact health via the experience of stress?

OXIDATIVE STRESS

Basic Cell Function

The vast majority of cells in your body, whilst having different purposes and responsibilities, undergo similar functional changes as part of their day-to-day operation.

One of these functions is **respiration**. Your cells, just as you as an organism, require molecular components to use as fuel to support their mechanics. They gain fuel by a process referred to as **catabolism**, which basically means the breaking down of larger molecules to release energy. A bit like when we chew an apple to absorb its energy (its nutrients and molecules), our cells break down nutrients and molecules (mostly **amino acids** and sugars) to absorb their energy. These processes don't just serve to provide fuel, the whole cycle also culminates in the production of waste particles as well – again, much like eating an apple. It is a metabolic process, serving to power the day-to-day functioning of our cells, and to keep our whole bodies ticking over. The process in which our cells break down these molecules is by using oxygen: reduction-oxidation or **redox**.

Redox is the process of electron transfer from one molecule (specifically, a **chemical species**) to another. When an atom (the reducing agent) loses electrons, this is referred to as **oxidation**, and when an atom (the oxidising agent) gains electrons it is referred to as reduction (because its oxidation state has been reduced). Essentially, this swapping over of electrons allows the breaking down of molecular structures to be used as fuel. These reactions happen constantly in cells all over your body, millions of times a day. As a result of some of this electron hopping, molecules referred to as **reactive oxygen species** (ROS) are created. These ROS are sometimes referred to as **free radicals**, and are unstable atoms. An oxygen molecule (O_2) is two oxygen atoms in a chain, allowing the electrons to be paired, or balanced, providing stability. When the molecule is split for redox, however, the atoms are now singular with just one electron, rendering them unstable. If atoms are unstable, this means they can react very quickly with other atoms in order to achieve their required stability. These more unstable versions of oxygen molecules are a normal part of healthy cell functioning, but if they are not effectively detoxified by other cellular processes, then this can result in **oxidative stress.** We can also have increased ROS from external processes as well as healthy cellular action. External factors that cause this (referred to as *pro-oxidants*) are many, but include tobacco smoke, pollution, radiation (including UV radiation from the sun), pesticides, and other chemicals like drugs. There is also some evidence to suggest that psychological stress may play a part in oxidative stress, particularly anticipatory stress (Aschbacher et al., 2013). Ultimately, the more free radicals there are clattering around in our bodies, the more risk there is of something going wrong in our cellular processes, as these unstable molecules seek out stability and will obtain it through any means. This can be in the form of damage to our DNA and vital proteins in our body that can cause malfunctioning of cells, or even conformational changes to cells. In order to counteract this, we turn to molecules referred to as **antioxidants**.

Warning

You may have heard of antioxidants before, for example in adverts for face creams or breakfast cereals, particularly in Western countries. They are discussed in health and wellness marketing far more than they are understood unfortunately. I'm sure many of you will have read this section several times by now trying to understand what these new and fancy concepts mean (I certainly did when I was trying to get to grips with this stuff!). Science is not very good at being accessible, and we get very hung up on our long words and technical jargon. These obscure and opaque terms are a marketer's dream. Stick 'source of antioxidants' on a packet of fruit or some beauty potion and you are sure to add that air of knowledge and gravitas (and high-end price tag) behind it.

Antioxidants are an important component found in many foods. Certain vitamins and other basic nutritional components are required as part of our 'healthy and balanced diet' simply because they are antioxidants. Micronutrients such as vitamin E (tocopherol), vitamin C (ascorbic acid), pre-vitamin A (beta carotene), and vitamin A (retinol) are all antioxidants that help to balance the accumulation of ROS in the tissues in our bodies. Other trace elements such as selenium, magnesium, copper, zinc, and manganese all provide electrons to restabilise free radicals. So, we can see that nutrition is clearly important for helping to counteract the potentially harmful effects of the redox process, and one of the simplest ways to understand how this could be harmful to health is in the case of poor nutrition or malnutrition. With the insufficient intake of suitable antioxidant components, the redox process can leave us without adequate resources to redress this balance, leaving us in a state of oxidative stress. Therefore, oxidative stress can be a product of external damaging factors (such as toxins or radiation), and also because we are not taking in sufficient dietary antioxidants, or both.

Oxidative Stress and Health

Once free radicals have been created, and are not neutralised by antioxidants, they can interact with other free radicals in the body. There are a lot of variables associated with how much of a problem this may become, but suffice it to say that the more free radicals there are, the more problematic it can be for health. There are a huge number of health conditions (both physical and mental health) that are thought to be related to ROS or oxidative stress, and there are likely many more that we have not established a link with as yet. One of the key ways in which oxidative stress is thought to lead to poor health is via damage to DNA, which is important in the development of cancer, heart disease, and neurodegenerative diseases. If the DNA of a cell is damaged, this can cause a variety of problems – the cell may fail to repair itself, it may be encoded incorrectly when it replicates, or it may fail to function properly altogether. Oxidative stress, therefore, is an excellent example of how health can be altered at the very basic cellular level, which makes it an important thing to consider for anyone interested in how our lifestyles or behaviours affect our wellbeing. Before we even think about considering larger systems-level changes that can occur, understanding that tiny changes to cells can initiate larger process changes that result in potentially very serious health concerns is very important.

There are several different cellular mechanisms that, if disrupted due to **DNA damage**, can cause health issues. It will depend on what type of cell is undergoing the DNA damage, and what purpose that cell serves in the grander scheme of regulating the organism, as to what potential health outcomes may occur. Damage to certain types of immune cells, for example those that suppress the development of tumours, may be one of the ways in which oxidative stress can lead to the development of cancer. Alternatively, the damage to DNA of a tissue cell that causes a significant mutation may also lead to the development of cancer if that specific mutation allows favourable replication of itself (either in increased growth or better survival, for example) that is able to evade the immune system. To this end, DNA damage can occur that interferes with genetic transcription and replication, thereby making the cell less likely to work effectively and/or replicate itself properly. This latter aspect is particularly important as we are constantly renewing our cellular stock through mitosis – from muscle cells to bone cells to skin cells, they all need to be effectively replicated to ensure that we have enough of what we need. Some of these mechanisms, particularly those that are related to behaviour and lifestyle, are not irreversible. For example, cigarette smoking is known to cause oxidative stress in the cells of lung tissue, but after smoking cessation this damage can be mostly reversed. We have in-built repairs for DNA that can undo some of this harm, which means that there are potentially routes out of DNA damage due to oxidative stress. This is why ceasing harmful behaviours is often not just to prevent further damage, but can also promote healing.

Psychological Stress and Oxidative Stress

Beyond those environmental factors that influence pro- and anti-oxidation (diet, pollution, etc.), there are also psychological and behavioural factors that influence oxidative stress. The most well understood of these is stress. Stress is both a psychological factor and a physiological state. It is so because our bodies were designed to react physiologically in times of danger to fight or run away, so we cannot have one without the other. Psychological stress is very easy to understand: the argument with your close friend, the breaking down of a relationship, the loss of employment, or even the flat tyre that causes you to be late to a meeting. Physiological stress occurs with psychological stress (and is a direct consequence of psychological stress) but can also occur on its own. A good example of physiological stress is exercise. Exercise in its acute sense is physiologically stressful. It sets off a chain of physiological processes intended to support the body in exertion – and that is exactly what happens with psychological stress too, because our bodies are designed to react to psychological stress by initiating high intensity action (see Chapters 2 and 6 for more detail). As an event, exercise sets off physiological patterns that we may consider 'bad' – the suppression of some aspects of immunity, the massive release of sugars into the bloodstream, the increase of oxidative metabolism. These are all necessary functions that help us to mobilise our bodies in times of need. However, as a behaviour that is prolonged over time, exercise improves many physiological processes that are good for us – such as regulating our blood pressure and resting heart rate and promoting the balance and good function of our hormonal systems. The same is true for its ability to allow our bodies to adapt to bursts of increased oxidative metabolism, actually lowering oxidative stress in the long run. Our bodies are built on habit, and our systems adapt to these habits accordingly. Just like when the New Year rolls in and we decide to take up jogging when we are normally quite sedentary – that first jog will feel harmful, stressful, and very difficult. Provided we don't give up by 2nd January, given time our bodies adapt to these behaviours to work more efficiently with what we're doing. In the case of exercise, our bodies learn to adapt between high- and low-active states very well, we burn up a lot of our stress hormones, and generally we get things working in the way our bodies were designed to work, rather than the way our bodies have adapted to work in our modern lifestyles. So that is how exercise as a one-time event and exercise as a regular habit can be quite different. Keep these distinctions in mind, because we will be talking about stress a lot in this book.

You might be tempted at this point to consider what has just been said about exercise and question why repeated psychological stress doesn't give you the same regulatory benefits. This is because the actual mechanics of exercise resolve and rebalance all those things that throw our body into that stressed state. In the absence of physical exertion to burn up all those mobilised fats and sugars, our bodies don't know when stress ends. Our bodies were made to deal with the following simple algorithm:

see bear → initiate stress response → start to run/fight → use up mobilised energy and hormones → return to equilibrium

The problem nowadays is that we have the following algorithm:

see looming deadline → initiate stress response → continue stress response → ?

So, without some sort of 'resolution' to burn up or utilise the physiological reaction to these psychological stressors, they just sort of hang there. This is one of the reasons why exercise is so hugely beneficial. Imagine instead the following algorithm, and how it may differ:

see looming deadline → initiate stress response → go for a run → use up mobilised energy and hormones → return to equilibrium

Physical activity provides an appropriate physiological resolution to stress. We will be talking more about this in future chapters.

For psychological stress and its link to oxidative stress, first consider what I've said above about how modern lives (and their stressors) in the UK, for example, are not behaviourally countered by their designed actions. We don't tend to physically fight or run away from an exam, a traffic jam, or an argument with a loved one. Well, we can do, but it's not really appropriate. Instead, we remain seated at our desks, motionless in our cars, or lounging on our sofas. The internal processes that prepare us for action – regardless of the nature of the stressor – need to be used, and if they're not used this can cause havoc. We will be discussing this more in later chapters, but for now remember that it's a bit like if we were to stretch a rubber band: if we let the rubber band loose, it will ping off, return to normal size, and remain elastic; if we either leave it stretched and do nothing, or even occasionally stretch it a little more, the rubber band will lose its elasticity and the band will fray. Our bodies don't tend to break with cumulative unresolved stress, but our ability to adapt to times of stress reduces, and some of our systems can eventually end up with excess wear and tear. The redox process is no different.

Stress can accelerate the redox process whilst it initiates the variety of cellular processes required for the physiological response. Remember that the redox process is part of normal cellular function, so anything that requires a mass mobilisation of systems or processes in the body will accelerate the redox process, and potentially increase the levels of reactive oxygen species that we know to cause DNA damage. Even if we have an excellent diet that is rich in all the nutritional components to neutralise them, they are generally available at a steady state within the body and are not mobilised in line with their potentially increased need. In fact, during psychological stress, one of the first things to be de-prioritised by the body is our digestion. Who needs to break down that sandwich if you're facing off with a sabre tooth tiger? So, in times of stress, we may also be absorbing less of the nutrients we need to offset this explosion of redox activity. Double whammy. If this happens from time to time, we can probably adapt to it reasonably well. Our bodies are designed to be balanced in the face of adversity after all. However, if we experience repeated or prolonged stress then this is another example of active oxidative stress–this time not through the intake of environmental (**exogenous**) toxins, but through the toxic build-up of internal (**endogenous**) toxins.

Telomeres

Telomeres are the shoelace tip-like ends to your chromosomes (see Figure 1.3). Just like the ends of your shoelaces, they are there to protect your chromosomes from becoming ratty and fraying. Now, your chromosomes obviously don't go through the same type of wear and tear as your shoelaces, but they do experience wear and tear as they are replicated over and over again. The telomeres at each end shorten a tiny bit each time your chromosomes are reproduced, and this shortening works a bit like a countdown clock. The majority of cells in your body (excluding your neurons) were not made to last the entire 80 to 90 years of your lifespan. Our cells are constantly replicating and renewing to ensure that we are operating with the fastest and most efficient machinery we can. Each time our chromosomes replicate, the telomeres get a tiny bit smaller until one day they are at their smallest size, and that cell then stops dividing or dies. This all sounds very sad, but it is the best way to ensure that we are operating with well-functioning parts.

So, what do telomeres have to do with psychology? As it turns out, quite a bit. Telomere length can be impacted by the DNA damage that results from oxidative stress. There has been a great deal of work done to understand more about this from Professor Thomas von Zglinicki and his colleagues. So much work has been done, in fact, and the connection between oxidative stress and telomere length has become so well understood, that telomere length can now be considered a biomarker for understanding levels of oxidative stress (Von Zglinicki, 2002). The precise mechanisms behind the capacity for oxidative stress to shorten telomeres are quite complex (see Houben et al., 2008 for a good overview), but it is largely down to the way that oxidative stress damages DNA components, specifically guanine, which makes up a large portion of telomeres. We also know that antioxidants are protective against telomere shortening, which is another good reason why we should all try and eat more healthily. So effectively all those psychological factors that are associated with oxidative stress (such as health behaviours as well as things like stress) also have an impact on telomere length.

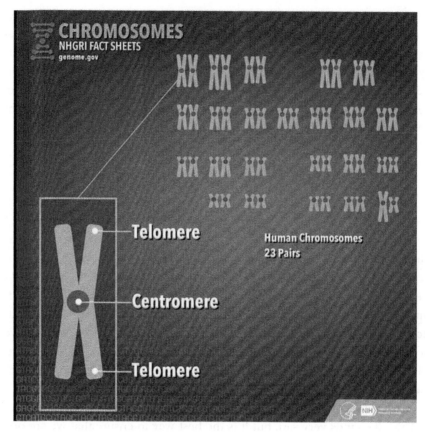

Figure 1.3

Source: National Human Genome Research Institute, reprinted under CC By 2.0 license

You may be asking yourself at this stage why higher cellular turnover would be a problem. Surely it must be better if we have snazzy new cells working all the time than relying on older, more tired cells. Actually, we know that certain conditions that are characterised by mutations in telomerase (the enzyme responsible for regulating the length of telomeres) are associated with an overall shorter lifespan. Remember also that telomeres, being present on your chromosomes, are important for the vast majority of the cells in your body,[1] including your immune cells. If your immune cells are

---

1 It is important to note here that our red blood cells do not contain DNA, and therefore do not include telomeres. White blood cells, by comparison, do have chromosomes and therefore have telomeres.

dying prematurely, there may be issues in ensuring you have enough stock of these cells to keep you healthy. So, telomere length can impact a huge number of regulatory processes (as well as defence processes) in our bodies when it comes to health. The quicker we wear our cells out, the less likely we are to have the appropriate amount available to serve the purposes for which they exist. The reduced telomere length in certain types of white blood cells has been shown to be associated with a variety of markers of cardiovascular health, including the development of atherosclerosis (a condition characterised by the accumulated deposition of fats, cholesterol, and other debris in the arteries), hypertension (a condition of having chronically high blood pressure), and myocardial infarction (heart attacks). Whilst some of the data on telomere length and health outcomes can vary (mostly due to the smaller number and diversity of participants in studies, and the complicated processes behind establishing telomere length), some physical health outcomes have stronger associations than others. There is support for telomere length being associated with certain types of gastric cancers as well as with diabetes and even Alzheimer's Disease (Smith et al., 2019). However, it is important to remember that telomere length itself is associated with a wide variety of health factors that we know relate to these types of health outcomes via different mechanisms, so whilst telomere length (and the impact that psychological and behavioural factors can have on it) is an important consideration, it is just one piece of a very complex puzzle.

EPIGENETICS

Another important cellular factor in health is **epigenetics**. Epigenetics as a field of study has absolutely exploded in recent years with advances in technology making research more feasible than ever. As an area of study, epigenetics is vast, and whilst we have discovered so much, there is still so much more left to understand. There are people who dedicate their whole careers to understanding epigenetics, so it is somewhat beyond the scope of a health psychology textbook, and there is some further reading at the end of the chapter for those keen to dig in. That said, it is important to understand that these changes can occur, and what this may lead to in health terms. Having a basic understanding of epigenetics is important because we know now that things are a lot more complicated than nature versus nurture (or the genes versus environment) debate when it comes to behaviour and when it comes to health. For a very long time there was a debate about which was a more compelling predictor of behaviour or health outcomes, with a sort of final settlement being that whilst genetics are important to lay the groundwork, the environment provides a profound impact on human outcomes as well. This was initially understood in the context of the way that our environment shapes our development and behaviour (more on this later), but with the dawn of epigenetics we have also discovered that our environment can modify the expression of our genes, in what we term a *gene × environment interaction.*

The Basics of (Epi)genetics

Our instruction manual is our genes. This is the code with which our entire biological make-up is written, and it is written with the use of four bases: Adenine (A), Cytosine (C), Guanine (G), and Thymine (T). Your genetic code is essentially the order in which these four bases pair up along a double helix, which we refer to as DNA (**D**eoxyribo**N**ucleic **A**cid). This double helix is so jam-packed with information, with 21,000 protein-coding bases in our genome and over 3 billion individual bases, that if they were laid out on the ground it would be around the same height (if not taller) than you, at 1.8 metres in length. In data terms, our genome packs in almost 3.5 GB of data into something 32,000 times smaller than the width of a human hair. We've already talked about DNA quite a bit with reference to oxidative stress and telomere damage, but that was mostly with reference to DNA damage. Epigenetics considers DNA in its normal functioning state, but when changes are made to it. In fact, that's what the term means: *epi*, meaning to add on or be in addition to. Epigenetic changes occur from the cell-making amendments to the function of the genetic code, impacting the transcription and translation (*protein synthesis*) of it, and ultimately altering its expression. These changes are not to be confused with mutations – epigenetic changes are not fundamental changes to the genetic code, more the way the code functions, and they can be reversed. There are a few different ways that epigenetics work (for a good overview see Zhang et al., 2020), but basically these processes serve to switch our genes 'on' or 'off'. It is also important to remember that epigenetic changes are completely natural – our cells are designed to be able to make these modifications in response to our environment. It's part of how we grow and develop, in fact these epigenetic changes are responsible for creating you in the form you are now. When we are just a small cluster of stem cells, epigenetic changes allow these basic building-block cells to differentiate to their new jobs and functions. That's what makes a bone cell a bone cell, and a neuron a neuron. The rate at which epigenetic changes occur during your lifetime changes as well, with decreasing amounts of on/off changes occurring as we grow older.

Stress and Epigenetics

One of the best known and well characterised examples of epigenetics comes from stress, particularly in early development and childhood. Trauma in early childhood can create all sorts of problems for the developing human (more to be discussed later in Chapter 4). Not only can it impact the way that the brain develops, which subsequently then has a knock-on effect to bodily systems, it can also create epigenetic changes. Adverse childhood experiences (sometimes referred to as ACEs) are so profoundly impactful on health across the lifespan that many scholars believe they should be accounted for in all health research, or we will never truly understand the root causes of what does or does not change our health and wellness. Deprivation in childhood, which constitutes all sorts of environmental and psychosocial stressors such as malnutrition, stress from over-crowding, less environmental and psychosocial enrichment, exposure to pollution, and inadequate access to healthcare, has been shown to produce epigenetic changes that influence the immune and endocrine systems in adulthood (Danese & McEwen, 2012). Some of this may come from the impact of under/over development in certain neuronal systems as well, but much of it is also epigenetic (Kundakovic & Champagne, 2015; Teicher & Samson, 2016). The colossal level of cellular proliferation and differentiation that happens during foetal development and early life means that this is a time during which we are most sensitive to epigenetic changes (Champagne, 2010). *In utero* exposure to a variety of environmental factors (both uterine environment, and *ex vivo* environment) such as exposure to diesel fumes, mercury, and certain types of drugs have an ability to alter the genes that encode for Brain-Derived Neurotrophic Factor (BDNF) along with some key **antibodies** and immune cells (Anway et al., 2005; Champagne, 2010). In adulthood, stress is similarly strongly associated with epigenetic changes. However, as we discovered earlier, epigenetic changes tend to happen less over the life course, so those stressors that occur earlier on in life have the potential to create the most severe and most long-lasting epigenetic changes.

The Dutch Hunger Winter

One of the most clear and stark examples of epigenetic changes due to environmental influence comes from the Netherlands in the latter part of the Second World War. In the autumn of 1944, just as the Nazi front was in retreat from most of the country, they were able to retain their hold on one corner of the Netherlands. The control of the area was under threat from the allied forces, and from a surging counterforce of the exiled Dutch government, so in order to retain control over this portion of the country, the Nazis imposed a food embargo, in an attempt to starve them into submission over what turned out to be a particularly harsh and frozen winter. During this time, they also destroyed some of the rail infrastructure and flooded agricultural land, meaning that internal stocks of food were depleted, and external replenishment was all but impossible. Over 20,000 citizens died before the liberation of the region in 1945, and those that survived suffered long-term health effects of severe malnourishment. However, once the region was liberated, the healthcare systems (and importantly their records) were recouped quickly, and those who had been subject to this period of starvation and survived were able to become part of an extraordinary opportunity to observe and track the results of the event.

Very quickly after the liberation of the region, researchers from the US and UK flew into the Netherlands to learn more about what could be done with the medical record data. They were particularly interested to see what may happen to the children of pregnant women who had survived this experience, as this would allow the opportunity to observe how maternal nutrition may impact birth outcomes and child health. It was immediately apparent through examination of birth records that those children who were born to mothers who carried them during this period were born with significantly low birth weight. This isn't really too surprising considering that the mothers were starving, and since then a reliable relationship between gestational nutrition status and birth weight has been consistently observed. Perhaps more interesting were the observations that would be made over the decades to come. Once many more decades of data became available it became apparent that this early development malnutrition had impacts across the life course, and these impacts depended on when during their gestation they had experienced this malnutrition. Those conceived during the famine (i.e., where the parent was starving in early pregnancy) had an increased risk of obesity and related health conditions (Tobi et al., 2014). They found these were related to epigenetic changes in the genes that control metabolism, presumably to prime the foetus for hard times to come. Those born during the famine (i.e., their parent suffered starvation in later pregnancy) did not appear to have the same associated health outcomes. This suggests epigenetic changes across generations are most likely to happen with strong environmental influences in early gestation. These effects lasted into the grandchildren's generation as well (Veenendaal et al., 2013).

Transgenerational Epigenetics

The previous example of epigenetics describes what can happen *in utero* to a developing foetus when the pregnant parent is exposed to hard times, which can have lifelong health impacts. But what of the capacity to inherit these changes? The grandchildren of those starved parents also appear to have been impacted by that time, but is that because these epigenetic changes were inherited, or was it something about the uterine environment of the second generation that caused the observed outcomes for the third? There are many examples of natural disasters or social circumstances that could constitute excellent points of study for understanding more about transgenerational epigenetics, but one of the real problems we have with this type of work is trying to understand what are true epigenetic changes, and what may be socially inherited behaviours or traits. Studying DNA is very expensive, and so attempting to understand changes that are truly evident in our DNA on any large scale is very rarely done. More work to understand the epigenetic inheritance (versus social inheritance) has been carried out in animals, which I will not go into here.

The vast amount of work to come out of the meticulous records of the Netherlands after the period of famine are not the only accounts of transgenerational environmental impact. Further European[2] work to make sense of epigenetic changes in response to environmental conditions has come from the study of very thorough (and long-established) data from generations of individuals from a rather remote area of Sweden, called Överkalix. The data from this region have been collected in quite some detail since the 1800s on both the human population and (amongst other things) the quality of the harvests each year. Researchers interested in understanding the longer-term impacts of nutritional status during development have found that not only does it have the potential to impact two subsequent generations, but also this is more likely to be carried down in a sex-specific way. Paternal grandfathers' food supply was associated with mortality risk of grandsons only, and paternal grandmothers' food supply only associated with mortality of granddaughters (Pembrey et al., 2006). This is important because the demonstration of heritability through the male line removes the potential for conflation with changes in response to uterine environment. Rather, they are inherited epigenetic changes.

Epigenetics and Cancer

Some cancers have behavioural links that can be explained by mechanistic changes in the body (e.g., higher levels of exercise result in less fat deposits, which then

---

2 Much of the transgenerational epigenetic work has been carried out using examples of European collective trauma, mostly due to the availability of sufficiently rich data to document and make sense of patterns over time. Collective trauma is not of course limited to European nations, so it is worthwhile bearing in mind that these findings – whilst very interesting – are just one part of a larger story we do not yet fully understand.

means less peripheral inflammation that may be a risk factor), but others have less obvious links. It is thought that inherited gene mutations may account for 5–10% of cases of cancer, but we also know exposure to environmental factors plays a huge role too (more on cancer in Chapter 5). Cancer cells are essentially normal cells gone bad: anything and everything can change in the cell from its DNA to its various RNAs and proteins. We're still trying to work out the chicken/egg scenario with epigenetics and cancer, because it is likely that tumours may develop because of epigenetic changes, and that they also may cause epigenetic changes. Some specific epigenetic changes that tumours may cause are in switching off tumour suppressing genes in cells – meaning cancer has the ability to disable the safety protocols embedded in our cells. Epigenetic changes also likely add to direct cell damage and diminished internal defence capabilities from environmental exposure (e.g., pollution, cigarette smoke).

The process of tumour development is essentially one of genetic micro-evolution, so epigenetics, which are changes to gene expression, are intimately entwined in cancer pathology. Cancer development relies on a balance of two types of genes: oncogenes (or cancer-promoting genes) and tumour suppressor genes. Cancer cells themselves tend to exhibit reductions in methylation, which is one of the processes by which epigenetic changes occur. This basically means that genes that should be active (particularly tumour suppressor genes) may become less active or completely inactive due to the lower level of methylation present, allowing the abnormally fast growth of cancer cells. On the reverse of this, cancer cells also exhibit an unbinding of DNA wrapping proteins called histones (another mechanism for epigenetic change), which has the potential to suppress gene activity, therefore allowing oncogenes (or cancer-promoting genes) to accelerate their activity. Whilst these processes have been well-established in cancer pathology, there is still some debate as to whether these are more, less, or as important as the genetic mutation processes involved in tumour growth. To complete the connections between these various factors, it is also known that oxidative stress plays a role in the epigenetic changes associated with the development of cancers. Oxidative stress can impact each of the processes that are responsible for epigenetic regulation, including methylation and the regulation of histone.

Intergenerational Trauma

Intergenerational trauma is the transgenerational experience of significant trauma that has psychological, behavioural, and physiological impacts throughout generations. Whilst trauma can potentially be subjective, there are obviously some larger scale events that most will recognise to be traumatic. War and conflict are situations that are universally traumatic and comprise a variety of traumatic influences on the people caught within. Perhaps most directly, you have the very real and imminent threat to life and health by being a potential casualty of war and being a subject of violence. Alongside this, you are living in a nation or area that is destabilised. Perhaps there is no clean water supply, perhaps your food supply has been threatened, maybe the destruction and violence are causing disease to spread. Further afield, the whole infrastructure of your society is also beginning to crumble. Essential services are having funds diverted to sustain the fighting, critical infrastructures such as healthcare and transport are either not working or are worked beyond their ability to function. Socially, those around you are scared; you may be able to find support and solidarity from some, but everyone is in survival mode. There is stress and trauma almost everywhere you look, regardless of your position or privilege in the conflict.

Key Questions

- What sorts of events do you think may cause intergenerational trauma?
  - o Can you think of specific events, or perhaps types of events?
  - o Remember that trauma can be both physical and psychological.
- Through what mechanisms do you think these traumatic events may impact subsequent generations?
  - o Think back to the health onion – how many layers do you think may be impacted by these types of traumatic event?

One of the common outcomes to understand the impact of widespread trauma is the impact it may have on the most vulnerable: the children that are being born at the time. Just as we saw with the Dutch famine, children born into heavy conflict are born smaller and lighter, and sadly the rate of infant mortality is often higher. When someone is pregnant, their stress hormones (along with many other circulating chemicals) are shared with the foetus. The placenta is an excellent barrier for many potential toxins and **pathogens**, but hormones and other circulating signalling molecules are able to cross over.

Outcomes after the Holocaust have also given us much to learn in terms of how trauma may reverberate down the family lines. Here, it is sometimes difficult to understand what elements of the hugely significant trauma experienced by survivors may be passed down. When something so culturally and personally malicious as genocide occurs, it quite rightly leaves those persecuted traumatised, but it also has another insidious influence via the impact of prejudice and hatred. Experiencing traumatic events when those events are not about who you are is one thing, but when you are the victim of trauma because you and your people are hated by others, this speaks to your very sense of self and self-worth. Given this deeply personal attack on your identity, it could be easy to understand how this trauma may be transmitted to other generations behaviourally or socially. On the other hand, someone who has been a victim of such persecution may do all they can to end the cycle of violence with the next generation, ensuring they do not suffer the same injustices, and may shield them from the worst of humanity that they have experienced. The impact on individuals of the same traumatic event can be varied and wide-ranging, and so the threads of intergenerational trauma are very hard to disentangle.

Some work that has been carried out making sense of the intergenerational fallout of the Holocaust has offered some insight into these pathways. Maternal (but not paternal) exposure to the Holocaust has been associated with cardiovascular health outcomes, as well as measures of perceived physical and emotional health in the second generation (Flory et al., 2011). This finding does not particularly do much to disentangle the biological from the psychological from the social; however, a large population-based study has shown that Holocaust survivors do not transmit psychological health outcomes to their children, which would suggest a potentially stronger biological thread (Levav et al., 2007). Further work on survivors of genocidal conflict, including the Holocaust, have also found that genes that encode for glucocorticoid (stress hormones) and serotonin receptors have had paternally transmitted epigenetic changes as a result of parental trauma, leaving future generations more vulnerable to the physical and mental health effects of stress and emotional distress (Bowers & Yehuda, 2016). Taken together, it would support the view that trauma can be both transmitted to the next generations as well as inherited, with evidence so far up to the third generation. As researchers who have been following up the descendants of the Holocaust continue their work, we will get a better understanding of how long the shockwaves of social and cultural injustice persist.

Learning Outcomes Summary

- Understand the contribution of cellular factors on everyday physical functioning.

We have covered a broad and introductory overview to understanding both oxidative stress and epigenetics, and how they contribute to health outcomes.

- Have an appreciation of the intersecting influences of human health on the cellular level.

Through examining various personal and social factors we have been able to see that changes at the cellular level can be effected in a variety of different ways, and that they may combine to influence health.

- Be able to explain some of the key cellular processes that have lifelong impacts on health.

We have explored how oxidation works to understand what oxidative stress is, and how these molecular changes impact cell function.
We have learned that our genes are not the final decision makers in our lives, and that our environments (and the environments of our parents and grandparents) can impact the way our genes work.

- Evaluate the influence of a variety of factors on cellular health with a critical lens.

We have looked at a variety of different potential explanations for some of the findings discussed.
You can explore these further by engaging with the key questions throughout the chapter.

FURTHER READING AND RESOURCES

There are some excellent TED Ed videos illustrating epigenetics and DNA damage available:

What is epigenetics? – Carlos Guerrero-Bosagna: https://ed.ted.com/lessons/how-the-choices-you-make-can-affect-your-genes-carlos-guerrero-bosagna
What happens when your DNA is damaged? – Monica Menesini: https://ed.ted.com/lessons/what-happens-when-your-dna-is-damaged-monica-menesini is provided by the National Institutes of Health here: https://medlineplus.gov/genetics/understanding/basics/dna/

Blackburn, E. H. (1991). Structure and function of telomeres. *Nature, 350*(6319), 569–73. This is a great starter on telomeres. Elizabeth Blackburn is one of the biggest names in telomere research, so she is a good name to look up if you are interested in diving further into this.

Crews, D., Gillette, R., Miller-Crews, I., Gore, A. C., & Skinner, M. K. (2014). Nature, nurture and epigenetics. *Molecular and Cellular Endocrinology, 398*(1–2), 42–52.

A great paper that helps make sense of the difference between nature/nurture and epigenetics.

Phillips, T. (2008). The role of methylation in gene expression. *Nature Education, 1*(1), 116. For those really wanting to get stuck into the harder science perspectives associated with epigenetics, this paper will set you off down a very interesting rabbit hole!

Sies, H. (1991). Oxidative stress: From basic research to clinical application. *The American Journal of Medicine, 91*(3), S31–S38.
This paper provides a very comprehensive overview of oxidative stress. Whilst it was published quite early in what would become an entire field of science, it gives a good foundational approach to getting to grips with this important cellular health factor.

Weinhold, B. (2006). Epigenetics: The science of change. *Environmental Health Perspectives, 114*(3), A160–A167. CID: https://doi.org/10.1289/ehp.114-a160
A very accessible overview of the field of epigenetics.

REFERENCES

Anway, M. D., Cupp, A. S., Uzumcu, M., & Skinner, M. K. (2005). Epigenetic transgenerational actions of endocrine disruptors and male fertility. *Science, 308*(5727), 1466–9.

Aschbacher, K., O'Donovan, A., Wolkowitz, O. M., Dhabhar, F. S., Su, Y., & Epel, E. (2013). Good stress, bad stress and oxidative stress: Insights from anticipatory cortisol reactivity. *Psychoneuroendocrinology, 38*(9), 1698–708. https://doi.org/https://doi.org/10.1016/j.psyneuen.2013.02.004

Bowers, M. E., & Yehuda, R. (2016). Intergenerational transmission of stress in humans. *Neuropsychopharmacology, 41*(1), 232–44. https://doi.org/10.1038/npp.2015.247

Champagne, F. A. (2010). Epigenetic influence of social experiences across the lifespan. *Developmental Psychobiology, 52*(4), 299–311.

Dahlgren, G., & Whitehead, M. (1991). *Policies and strategies to promote social equity in health*. Institute for Future Studies, Stockholm.

Danese, A., & McEwen, B. S. (2012). Adverse childhood experiences, allostasis, allostatic load, and age-related disease. *Physiology & Behavior, 106*(1), 29–39.

Flory, J. D., Bierer, L. M., & Yehuda, R. (2011). Maternal exposure to the holocaust and health complaints in offspring. *Disease Markers, 30*(2, 3), 133–9.

Houben, J. M., Moonen, H. J., van Schooten, F. J., & Hageman, G. J. (2008). Telomere length assessment: Biomarker of chronic oxidative stress? *Free Radical Biology and Medicine, 44*(3), 235–46. https://doi.org/10.1016/j.freeradbiomed.2007.10.001

Kundakovic, M., & Champagne, F. A. (2015). Early-life experience, epigenetics, and the developing brain. *Neuropsychopharmacology, 40*(1), 141–53. https://www.nature.com/articles/npp2014140

Levav, I., Levinson, D., Radomislensky, I., Shemesh, A. A., & Kohn, R. (2007). Psychopathology and other health dimensions among the offspring of Holocaust survivors: Results from the Israel National Health Survey. *Israel Journal of Psychiatry and Related Sciences, 44*(2), 144.

Pembrey, M. E., Bygren, L. O., Kaati, G., Edvinsson, S., Northstone, K., Sjöström, M., & Golding, J. (2006). Sex-specific, male-line transgenerational responses in humans. *European Journal of Human Genetics, 14*(2), 159–66. https://www.nature.com/articles/5201538

Smith, L., Luchini, C., Demurtas, J., Soysal, P., Stubbs, B., Hamer, M., Nottegar, A., Lawlor, R. T., Lopez-Sanchez, G. F., Firth, J., Koyanagi, A., Roberts, J., Willeit, P., Waldhoer, T., Loosemore, M., Abbs, A. D., Johnstone, J., Yang, L., & Veronese, N. (2019). Telomere length and health outcomes: An umbrella review of systematic reviews and meta-analyses of observational studies. *Ageing Research Reviews, 51*, 1–10. https://doi.org/10.1016/j.arr.2019.02.003

Teicher, M. H., & Samson, J. A. (2016). Annual research review: Enduring neurobiological effects of childhood abuse and neglect. *Journal of Child Psychology and Psychiatry, 57*(3), 241–66. www.ncbi.nlm.nih.gov/pmc/articles/PMC4760853/pdf/nihms741660.pdf

Tobi, E. W., Goeman, J. J., Monajemi, R., Gu, H., Putter, H., Zhang, Y., Slieker, R. C., Stok, A. P., Thijssen, P. E., Müller, F., van Zwet, E. W., Bock, C., Meissner, A., Lumey, L. H., Eline Slagboom, P., & Heijmans, B. T. (2014). DNA methylation signatures link prenatal famine exposure to growth and metabolism. *Nature Communications, 5*(1), 5592. https://doi.org/10.1038/ncomms6592

Veenendaal, M. V., Painter, R. C., de Rooij, S. R., Bossuyt, P. M., van der Post, J. A., Gluckman, P. D., Hanson, M. A., & Roseboom, T. J. (2013). Transgenerational effects of prenatal exposure to the 1944–45 Dutch famine. *BJOG: An International Journal of Obstetrics & Gynaecology, 120*(5), 548–54.

Von Zglinicki, T. (2002). Oxidative stress shortens telomeres. *Trends in Biochemical Sciences, 27*(7), 339–44.

Zhang, L., Lu, Q., & Chang, C. (2020). Epigenetics in health and disease. *Epigenetics in Allergy and Autoimmunity, 1253*, 3–55.

2
THE PERSON

INTRODUCTION

The aim of this chapter is to introduce you to some of the systems of the body to give you a crash course on the intricate and interconnected infrastructure you carry around with you every day. Some systems will be covered in good depth, others will be introduced to give you a working overview of what they are and their importance in every day physical functioning. We will look at each system with the specific focus of understanding how psychological, social, and behavioural factors influence their day-to-day operation.

Learning Outcomes

- Understand some of the key systems in place in the human body and how they are regulated.
- Have an appreciation of the intersecting influences of human health at the systems level.
- Be able to explain some of the key psychological factors that have implications for health at the system and person level.
- Evaluate the influence of a variety of factors on individual health with a critical lens.

WHAT DOES PSYCHOLOGY HAVE TO DO WITH SYSTEMS?

We saw in the last chapter how psychological factors can influence various operations of cellular health, and how these, in turn, relate to overall health and wellbeing at the person level. Just as cellular-level functioning is important in determining person-level health, looking at our systems and how psychological factors influence their operation is just as important. If the cells are the building blocks of our bodies, they are there to create the organs and systems that operate to support the person. As people, we are essentially a walking, talking network of interconnected systems. We have a huge number of different types of cells that operate independently, like our blood and immune cells, but we also have a vast number of cells that make up structures like our organs, tissues, and muscles. These larger structures, like our organs, tissues, and muscles, can be considered and understood as independent components, but more often than not, they are parts of larger, interconnected, and complex systems that operate within strict parameters during good health, and operate beyond these parameters in poor health. Many of these systems share similar real estate within the body, so we have multi-purpose tissues and connections, meaning that when certain structures or even systems start to operate beyond their parameters, this can have a knock-on effect on many other systems in the body. We also have some very highly specialised structures and pathways that are used exclusively for a key purpose, and even in those cases their malfunction or dysfunction will often cause further malfunction or dysfunction to other systems also. There is a balance required within our bodies to ensure that all is working as it should, and when you gain an appreciation for how finely tuned this balance is, I hope you will be as amazed at its beauty and complexity as I have been as I have continued to learn about it.

Our bodies are made up of lots of different types of tissues: skin, bone, organs, muscles, and tissues that create connections and pathways, to name just a few. Our bodies are also made up of lots of systems, each with either one or several 'jobs' to do in regulating our health and wellbeing. When we think about our health, or – rather – if we think about our ill health, we tend to think about what structures and roles may be malfunctioning. When trying to vocalise the status of our health, we talk about whether certain systems are performing as they should (e.g., 'I need to pee more often than normal'), or what specific sites of our bodies may be experiencing odd sensations or behaviours (e.g., 'I can feel my heart racing'). We rarely see a doctor when something is wrong to simply state that we feel 'not quite right', there is very commonly an attempt to make sense of what it is specifically that is going wrong in terms of comparing our current status to what was previously our normal functioning. So, whether you realise it or not, you probably already have an understanding of systems in your body purely on the basis that you have been able to observe its regular (and irregular) functioning over the course of your life. With this in mind, try the following exercise before you start reading more about your systems.

Key Questions

- What factors about a human as a network of systems are important to understand in health psychology?
- What systems in the body are impacted by psychological or social issues?

A CRASH COURSE ON YOUR SYSTEMS

This chapter is going to talk you through some of the key systems in the body to give you a feel for how all this works. Bear in mind that this particular subject, the systems of the body, could make an entire book in itself, so this chapter is aimed at being an introduction to various systems and the biopsychosocial factors that can influence the way that they work, which will, in turn, influence the overall health of the person.

The Nervous System

If you have a background in psychology, then this system is one that you probably know most about. The nervous system is a super-system made up of other subdivisions of networks around the body. This is a good place to start regardless of your background because the nervous system is more or less the apex of control in terms of the other systems in your body. All of your systems are interconnected throughout your body, but they are all also plugged into your nervous system, because your nervous system effectively works as the electrics for your entire body to communicate. For us to move, talk, and navigate our social and physical environments, our brains and bodies must talk to each other all the time. It is important to remember that because of this, anything that happens to change the way that your brain is working will also have a descending impact on other tissues and systems in your body (whether you notice it or not). In short, what happens in your brain doesn't stay in your brain, it can (and very frequently does!) have an impact elsewhere in the body.

Central and Peripheral Subdivisions

To get to grips with this, we will start off simply by considering the nervous system at its most basic level: the **central nervous system** (CNS) and the **peripheral nervous system**. The central nervous system is essentially the boss and is made up of your brain and your spinal cord. Your brain is a large mass of neurons (the specialised cells of your nervous system), other supporting cells (such as glia), and fat. It, and all other neural tissue, is made up of neurons and other supporting cells. Neurons are specific to the nervous system and have a very specific structure (or **morphology**) that is unique to this system. Your brain is made up of several sub-structures and systems, so not even your brain is one 'thing' in itself. Within your brain you also have some hormonal tissues (referred to as **neuroendocrine** tissues: *neuro* – being of the brain/nervous system; **endocrine** – being of the hormonal system). Your brain and spinal cord operate as your control centre and communication mast (although our spinal cords also do quite a bit more than just relay information). Your peripheral nervous system is the collective term for pretty much all other neural tissue in your body. This peripheral nervous system runs throughout your entire body, allowing you to move, sense, and regulate the processes and functions of your body, and is mostly accessed by the brain via your spinal cord. There are a few exceptions to this, where you have nerves (i.e., long cables of neurons) that come directly from your brain: the *cranial nerves*. You have twelve pairs of cranial nerves, and these are nerves that make more sense to come directly from the brain rather than through your spinal cord. Your optic nerves are a good example of this. It is far easier for information to be passed straight from eye to brain than it is from eye to spinal cord to brain.

When considering all the rest of your neural network map that is the peripheral nervous system, we also group divisions of this large network according to their destination and function. We have groups that deal with our internal organs (*visceral*) and those that deal with the organs and structures associated with our senses (*somatic*). With these groups, we also have further subdivisions associated with the function of these pathways: movement (*motor*) and sensation (*sensory*). Motor pathways are described as being *efferent* as they lead from the brain to the periphery, whereas sensory pathways are *afferent* as they lead from the periphery to the brain. Consider the next two grossly over-simplified examples. We can have two pathways with our hearts (visceral): a visceral motor pathway to make it beat (efferent; from our brains), and a visceral sensory pathway that provides our sensation of our heart beating (afferent; from our hearts). Similarly, we can have two pathways that lead to our tongues (sensory): a somatic motor pathway to allow the tongue to move (efferent), and a somatic sensory (or *somatosensory*) pathway that allows us to taste (afferent). One of these subdivisions, the *visceral motor* subdivision, also has another pair of pathways within, and this is the **autonomic nervous system**.

The Autonomic Nervous System (ANS)

We will consider the autonomic nervous system (ANS) throughout this book because it is a central piece of psychobiological infrastructure that is very much involved in the multiple ways in which psychological (and social, and neurological) factors can influence the physical workings of our bodies. The ANS is responsible for a pattern of behaviour throughout the body in reaction to certain stimuli, and is initiated without needing specific conscious direction (think of *autonomic* as *automatic*). The most well-known of these is the **sympathetic nervous system** (SNS, yes another 'system' and another acronym), which is responsible for our *fight-or-flight* response (sometimes also referred to as the *fight, flight, or freeze* response). This response is a pattern of finely tuned internal behaviours that have been keeping our species (and the many tens of thousands of vertebrate species on the planet) alive for the 530-odd million years they have been around. We talked a bit about the stress response in Chapter 1, and we will talk about it a lot throughout the book. The opposing force to the SNS is the **parasympathetic nervous system** (PNS), sometimes referred to as our *rest-and-digest* response. The PNS has for a long time played second fiddle to the SNS, with a lot of people thinking it is just the antithesis of the fight-or-flight response, there to calm all things down after we have been terrified by a bear or a disappointed manager, but the PNS has responsibilities of its own to take care of too, which we will talk about throughout the book.

Essentially these two systems initiate patterns of behaviour in the body that have opposing actions (see Figure 2.1). There are some quite straightforward ones, and some less so. If we consider the fight-or-flight pathway, the sympathetic, this pattern of

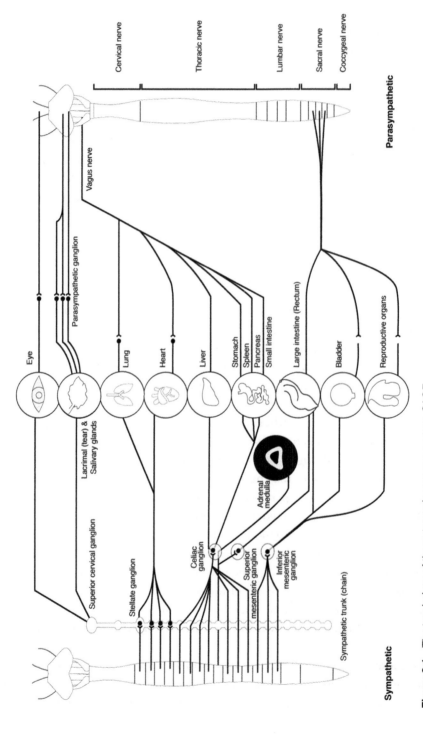

Figure 2.1   The two halves of the autonomic nervous system. SAGE

Source: Boore et al. (2016), *Essentials of Anatomy and Physiology for Nursing Practice*, Sage

internal behaviour is geared entirely to our survival in a threatening situation. We need our muscles to work harder and faster, and potentially for longer than we might normally require, so the SNS fires up the heart to beat faster, to increase blood pressure, to dump energy into the bloodstream, and to facilitate higher oxygenation by dilating the airways and increasing the respiration rate. Our senses need to be heightened to evade whatever it is that is trying to eat us, so our pupils dilate, and our brains are flooded with the same increased energy that our muscles are. At the same time, in order to pay for all of this overtime being carried out by the cardiovascular system, other 'non-essential' systems and processes are slowed down. There is basically nothing in your body that is non-essential, but in the context of fleeing for your life, there are things that are less important. There is no point in digesting your breakfast if that costs you the opportunity to survive a deadly fight. So, in order to pay for all this overtime, our SNS also does a lot of slowing or shutting down of other functions. Our saliva production is decreased; our digestive system is slowed down (and sometimes our bodies just get rid of whatever is on board to expedite this); our sex hormones are told to stand down; our pancreas is slowed down; if we happen to be growing bones or repairing tissue, those processes are slowed down; and sometimes – particularly if they're full and the situation is scary enough – our bladders relax and empty.

Some of these latter processes can be seen to be writ large in the health conditions of those who suffer long-term stress. People with stressful lives can suffer a variety of digestive problems such as irritable bowel syndrome (IBS), or develop disorders of the upper gastric system such as peptic ulcers or gastro-oesophageal reflux. Menstrual periods can become heavily disrupted and irregular. Chronic stress can also cause problems with insulin regulation, leading to disorders like diabetes. If we are growing bones or repairing tissue, repeated stress can cause these processes to slow down a great deal, leading to longer healing times and sometimes to stunted growth in the very young. If we did not have an opposing force (i.e., the parasympathetic) then stress would be fatal to us all, so the PNS is very important indeed to undo this pattern of biological behaviour. Pretty much everything the SNS has done, the PNS will undo, but it will require some triggers to allow it to kick into action. It is not enough that we can realise that the stressor has gone, or understand that we are no longer in imminent danger; there are physical processes that are required to initiate this climb down of the fight-or-flight response. The most obvious of these is the fighting or fleeing. We use up the energy rapidly mobilised in our bodies to fight or run away, and in doing so, our PNS will engage to restore standard operating protocols. However, as we found in Chapter 1, there is little about our modern lives that is attuned to this ancient survival system. We don't fight an overdue bill, and we don't run a mile in the opposite direction of a workplace quarrel. What we tend to do more of is sit, which is the exact opposite of what this system was designed to do. The problem is not that our physiology hasn't caught up to our modern sedentary lifestyles yet, but because sedentary living is not what we were designed to do. If we are not using up all this mobilised energy, it doesn't just disappear. It festers. Our bloodstream is filled with fats and sugars to help us exert ourselves, and if we don't do the thing, the fats and sugars keep going around and around, and eventually deposit in our vasculature (i.e., the vast network of our blood vessels) like silt on a riverbed. So, as we saw in Chapter 1, exercise is not just an important health behaviour for keeping us fit and healthy, it is also a vital activity to counteract the impact of stress and the damage it can do to our bodies.

The Gut-Brain Axis

Another nervous system that is worth a mention is the **enteric nervous system** (ENS). This network of neural tissue localised in your gut is technically part of your parasympathetic subdivision, but is really a 'system' in its own right. This nervous system operates in a similar way to the rest of your nervous system, but – critically– can operate entirely on its own without input from the brain if necessary. In fact, not only can it operate on its own, it can actually tell the brain what to do as well. There is a direct (and bidirectional) gut-to-brain pathway hardwired through the **vagus nerve**, but about 90% of the direction of travel is from the gut to the brain, not the other way around. The ENS contains more neurons than our spinal cords, making it a significant piece of neural hardware. We often think of **neurotransmitters** such as dopamine and serotonin as being brain-related chemicals, but would it surprise you to know that more than 90% of your body's serotonin and about 50% of its dopamine is found in the gut? Not only this, but the bacteria in your gut produce these neurotransmitters too! These neurotransmitters are largely there to help with gut motility (that is the squishing of your gut to move digesting food along – or *peristalsis*). The micro-organisms in the gut and living in and on the rest of your body (mostly bacteria) outnumber your own body's cells 10 to 1, meaning that we are more bacteria than human. The neural circuits of the ENS control motor function, local blood flow, mucosal functions, and can modulate both immune and endocrine operations. Your gut even has its own blood–brain barrier as well, protecting your delicate neurons from potentially dangerous pathogens and molecules.

The **gut–brain axis** is important in the context of health because over 70% of your body's immune system is focused on the gastro-intestinal tract. There is a very good reason for this, as we rely on the ingestion of food to provide us with the nutrients required in order to function. As we need to eat, we are also potentially opening ourselves up to infection or infestation with every bite we take. If our guts were not properly protected and armed, we would be vulnerable to any of the infinitesimally huge number of microbes, pathogens, toxins, and parasites that can exist on or in our food. The other very important part of our gut is our **microbiome**, that colony of microbes and bacteria that exist in our guts and all around our bodies that outnumber our own cells. We are only just beginning to understand the critical importance of our microbiome, but what we do know so far is truly astonishing. The microbiome can 'talk' to your ENS *and* your CNS as well as creating your important neurotransmitters. The things we eat and the behaviours we engage with can all impact the microbiome, which can then in turn impact our brains. Increased peripheral inflammation in response to stress, poor diet (such as a typical Western diet high in carbohydrates and saturated fats), or illness are good examples of the intricate ways in which our various systems talk to and influence each other via the gut–brain axis. So much so, that the interplay between the immune system, microbiome, and brain are now considered to be important factors in a wide variety of illnesses in the brain and the body, including Parkinson's Disease, depression, and various types of cancer.

Warning

Your second warning in this book comes from the wonderful world of probiotics. Many have latched onto the idea of probiotics as being 'essential' and also potentially panaceas of health that can reverse the awful effects of many progressive diseases and disorders. The truth is the consensus is not yet in. Whilst supplementing your diet with probiotics is unlikely to be harmful, it is also important to remember that their benefit is not yet conclusive. Remember that probiotics are readily available in a variety of very common foods across the world, and do not need to have expensive packaging and a heavy price tag.

With the growing knowledge around the microbiome has come increasing research on how to attain a more favourable balance of bacteria that is supportive of good overall health. This has been regarding not only physical health but also mental health, with the interest in what have been termed **psychobiotics** – or probiotic supplementation that can support or improve good mental health. The research into psychobiotics has been conflicting, with almost as many studies suggesting there is no link between probiotic supplementation and mental health as there are that suggest there is one. Another area of microbiome supplementation that has had more definitive support is the potential for faecal transplants (yes, that's right) to support the gut microenvironment in those that are struggling with specific gut-related health conditions, and other non-gut-related conditions also. The multi drug resistant 'superbug' *Clostridium difficile* (C. Difficile, or sometimes just C Diff) can be suppressed effectively in some people, and there is some evidence to suggest that a faecal transplant from such a person to another that cannot mount a successful response has been effective in combatting the bacterial infection

(Drekonja et al., 2015; Shogbesan et al., 2018). Other conditions that have been identified as potential candidates for faecal transplant have been obesity and metabolic syndrome (with some mixed findings, e.g., Proença et al., 2020; Zhang et al., 2019) and inflammatory bowel diseases (again with mixed findings, e.g., Caldeira et al., 2020; Colman & Rubin, 2014), and are beginning to be explored in conditions like multiple sclerosis (Boziki et al., 2020; Ghezzi et al., 2021).

Key Questions

- What aspects of our lives impact our nervous system(s)?
  - o Think about the health onion!
- What consequences do you think these impacts have for our health and wellbeing over time?
  - o Are there times in our lives when these impacts may be more - or less - important?

The Cardiovascular System

The **cardiovascular system** comprises a central organ (the heart) and a vast network of blood vessels (**vasculature**) that run throughout the body, allowing blood to circulate to everywhere it is needed. You have around 60,000 miles (100,000 kilometres) of blood vessels around your body, ranging from large-capacity arteries to delicate and fine capillaries (see Figure 2.2). You have about five litres of blood in your body, and your heart pumps this around your whole body in less than a minute in its approximate 100,000 beats per day.

Your heart works as what is termed a *demand pump*, in that it can alter its pace by adjusting to the demand put upon it. The general pace of your heart is set by the **sinoatrial node** (SAN), a structure made up of pacemaker cells that zaps your heart into beating. The SAN receives input directly from the medulla oblongata in the brain with both sympathetic (from the *sympathetic trunk*) and parasympathetic (from the *vagus nerve*) input, providing executive control for the brain. However, the pressure of the beat (**cardiac output**) must be able to vary according to demand, or it may take time for our hearts to catch up with what our brains (or the rest of our bodies) are doing. Your breathing rate is an example of this, and in fact this is a top tip for exam stress or any other type of performance jitters – breathe out very slowly, this will help engage parasympathetic input to the heart, slowing it down. Your heart is powered by a balance between the sympathetic and parasympathetic inputs. General resting heartrate is enabled by parasympathetic control from the brain via the vagus nerve.

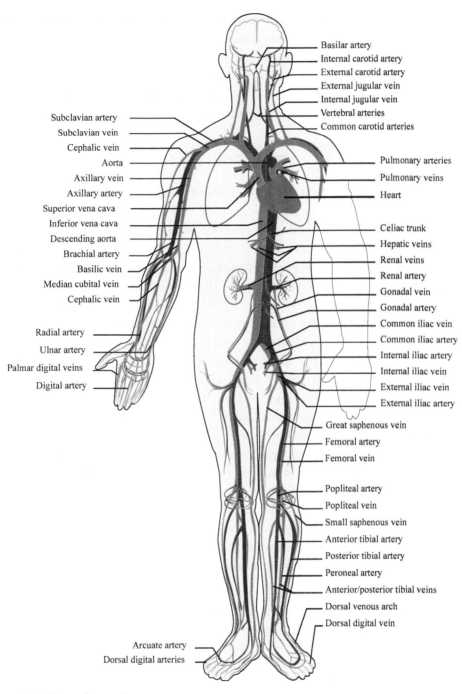

Figure 2.2 The cardiovascular system

When your heart rate needs to increase, parasympathetic output is decreased to allow the sympathetic to take control. The communication between the heart and the brain (in the medulla oblongata) is bidirectional, so when the heart demand pump kicks in, this information is also sent up to the brain to alter the balance of sympathetic/ parasympathetic tone. Your heart rate is not just adjusted by demands or by electrical input, it is also altered by hormones like adrenaline (also referred to as epinephrine[1]).

Blood Pressure

There is a lot of talk in the field of health of **blood pressure**. It is an important marker for current health as well as a prognostic marker for future health risk. Having high blood pressure is considered both a specific condition in itself (that can be treatable), and a risk factor for subsequent cardiovascular disease (we will talk more about this in Chapter 10). Blood pressure is effectively the pressure at which blood is whizzing around your vasculature. It is determined by the strength of your heartbeat (the cardiac output, or how much blood is ejected from the squishing of your heart) and your **peripheral resistance** (or your vascular tone – how spongey or hard the walls of your blood vessels are). Think about a hose on a tap: how much you open the tap will dictate the pressure of the water to some extent, but that pressure can also be changed by squeezing or relaxing the hose. As much as your heart is dictated by SNS and PNS outflow, your blood pressure is also impacted by these opposing forces, and this is partly because these two control your heart. The SNS and PNS don't just have some dictation over the frequency of your heartbeat, but also over the force of it. They also can alter your vascular tone (squeeze or release the hosepipe), which also affects blood pressure. This is all because your heart and your blood pressure are important fight-or-flight gear. Your heart needs to pump faster, and your body needs to get more blood around it, so having both your heart and your vasculature receive commands from the ANS assists in this process. It is not just the fight-or-flight response that alters your blood pressure, however; your whole cardiovascular system is altered by the ANS in response to a variety of homeostatic sensing, such as thermosensitivity (temperature),

---

1 Adrenaline and epinephrine actually mean the same thing, but come from two different languages. They both mean something close to 'in addition to the kidneys' in Latin and Greek, respectively. *Ad renal* or *epi neph* mean exactly the same thing. You will see both terms in academic literature, so it's good to know they are the same thing. Similarly, noradrenaline and norepinephrine are the same thing as well. Why 'in addition to the kidneys'? Your adrenal glands are situated just above your kidneys, so it is a very literal term for these pieces of endocrine tissue.

barosensitivity (pressure), and glucosensitivity (blood sugar). These are all important to keep us ticking over at just the right level according to our environment and our activity in that environment.

Blood pressure is measured in the very old-fashioned mmHg, which is milligrams of mercury. This harks back to the age before the automatic blood pressure monitors you will probably have seen or had used on you before, and was essentially a hand-pumped cuff attached to a large tube that contained mercury. This measurement is used in a variety of difference scientific fields to understand pressure, and whilst we generally don't use mercury in sphygmomanometers (blood pressure meters) anymore, the mmHg term is still used. Blood pressure is expressed in one number 'over' another, e.g., 120/90. These two numbers denote different aspects of blood pressure, the *systolic* and the *diastolic*. **Systolic blood pressure** (SBP) is the pressure of blood at your heart's squish (*systole*), when your heart is pushing blood out of it, and **diastolic blood pressure** (DBP) is the pressure of blood at your heart's relaxation (*diastole*), when the heart muscles relax to allow it to refill. Blood pressure can tell us a lot about someone's health, and is monitored closely during medical interventions such as during operations or over time when a patient is prescribed medication that may have side-effects that can cause complications for the cardiovascular system (such as hormonal therapies like the combined oral contraceptive pill, or drugs to remedy migraines). A 'healthy' range for adult blood pressure is considered to be between 90/60mmHg and 120/80mmHg. A clinical diagnosis of **hypertension** (high blood pressure) is made when it exceeds 140/90mmHg, and a clinical diagnosis of **hypotension** (low blood pressure) is made when it is under 90/60mmHg. Both of these conditions would normally require some sort of medication to adjust the blood pressure back into a healthy range, and these medications act on either the SNS or the PNS to make these changes.

Cardio- and Cerebro vascular Diseases

As we saw previously, our cardiovascular systems are highly affected by stress, because they are an important part of the fight-or-flight response. It is not only stress, however, that can impact the good functioning of this system. Our diets, the behaviours we engage in (e.g., consumption of tobacco or alcohol, how much we exercise, how sedentary we are, or how much we sleep), and medications we require to support our health can all have an impact on our cardiovascular system. The fats and sugars that whizz around our blood vessels in response to stress can also be there in excess in response to the things we eat, particularly if they are not counteracted (or used up) by strenuous activity, which can also lead to the deposition of plaques within our blood vessels. Over time, these deposits build up, narrowing our blood vessels and making it harder for our blood to get around and do what it needs to do, a condition called *atherosclerosis* (more on this in Chapter 10). We can also have chunks of it break off and start zipping around our blood vessels until it gets to one too narrow to pass and causes a blockage. If we are very unlucky, one of these blockages can occur in the blood vessels that supply the heart, causing *coronary heart disease*, leaving us vulnerable to experiencing a heart attack (**myocardial infarction** – infarction meaning the death of vital tissue as a result of deprivation of oxygen). Generally speaking, vascular problems are caused by one or perhaps a combination of four actions: *stenosis* (the narrowing of the internal capacity of the vessel, commonly through internal depositions), *thrombosis* (the formation of clots, which can be caused by diet, medications, and aging), *embolism* (the blockage of the blood vessel by a clot, or a breakaway piece of plaque), and **haemorrhage** (the bursting of a blood vessel, usually due to excess pressure and/or the weakening of the vessel wall). All of these disorders are clumped under the term **cardiovascular disease** (CVD), and CVDs are usually caused by multiple factors. If such a blockage occurs in a blood vessel feeding the brain, this is termed **cerebrovascular disease,** which can result in a stroke, which is where damage to the brain occurs due to a lack of blood supply. We can also have clots that affect other parts of our bodies, causing problems for whichever tissue the blood vessel is feeding. **Pulmonary vascular disease** is a similarly broad umbrella term for problems that affect the vasculature of the lungs. Clots in the blood vessels that feed the lungs can result in what is termed **pulmonary embolism**, which is a rupture of the blood vessels that feed the lungs. We can also have clots and ruptures in other blood vessels that will cause varying levels of damage depending on what the blood vessel is there to feed. Essentially, the more important or critical the tissue that is being fed, the more catastrophic and complicated the damage can be. So, the cardiovascular system is critically important to keeping us going, and problems with our blood supply can cause all manner of very serious conditions almost anywhere in our bodies – so it is very important we take care of it all, and understand what factors are associated with its healthy functioning.

Key Questions

- What aspects of our lives impact our cardiovascular system?
  - Think about the health onion!
- What consequences do you think these impacts have for our health and wellbeing over time?
  - Are there certain diseases or conditions that may be more responsive to psychological/social/environmental influence?

The Lymphatic System

Very closely aligned to your vascular system is your lymphatic system. The **lymphatic system** is a network of vessels (**capillaries**), similar to those of your vascular system, and nodes throughout your body. Some of your vital organs feed into the lymphatic system as well, and so the lymphatic system is a bit of a cross-purpose network to support the transport of cells, nutrients, and molecules across and between systems. It is a part of the physical infrastructure of your immune system, carrying a substance referred to as **lymph** around your body to transport critical immune cells from **lymphatic organs** such as the thymus and spleen into the bloodstream. If you have ever had a cut to the skin, or experienced an insect bite, you may see lymph coming from the wound – it is a clear liquid. The lymph is transported around your body via the movements of your muscles, rather than by an organ tasked with its movement (like your heart does for your blood). Your general daily movement allows the circulation of lymph throughout your system, but sometimes it can be aided by certain activities or bodily positions, which is why it is sometimes better to have a swollen joint or appendage elevated, to aid in 'lymphatic drainage'. Your lymph passes through the capillaries of your system and through the almost 600 nodes scattered around your body (Figure 2.3). Some of these nodes are clustered together in key areas, and some of them are solitary. Some are very large, and others very small. You can feel your **lymph nodes** swelling sometimes when you experience a peripheral inflammatory response as a result of a viral infection or similar. You can probably feel them in your throat, either just under your jaw (submandibular) or down the length of your throat on either side (cervical), and sometimes if your peripheral inflammatory response is strong, you may also notice pain or tenderness in your underarms (axillary), or even your groin (inguinal).

The lymphatic system is almost like an interchange of cells and molecules, allowing cellular waste (including some bacteria) to be 'cleaned' up from the body. Some of the organs that feed into it (for example, your bone marrow, spleen or thymus) have a direct line from the brain, and as far as we currently know that communication seems to be unidirectional, with these organs receiving input from the brain. These direct neural communication routes are mostly sympathetic, but there are some parasympathetic inputs as well. This input is there for a few reasons, but one of those reasons is to send instructions to the organ about increasing or reducing its activity, particularly with relevance to the type of immune cells that organ may create, help to develop, or otherwise house. The lymphatic system also gets the neurochemical route from the brain, with tissues of these organs, the tissue of the capillaries and nodes, and the immune cells themselves all carrying receptors for different types of neurotransmitters. These two routes of communication will be referred to a lot in this book, as they are used by

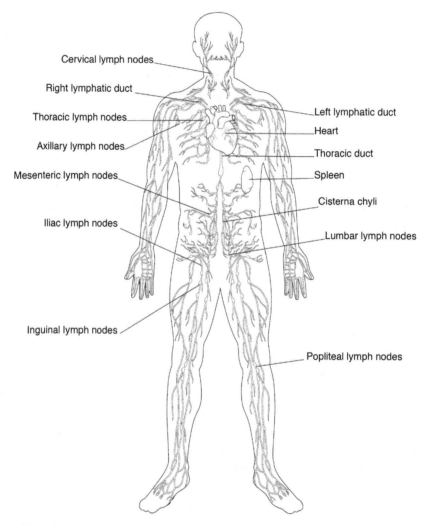

Figure 2.3   The lymphatic system.
Source: Boore et al. (2016), *Essentials of Anatomy and Physiology for Nursing Practice*, Sage

many of the processes we will discuss. Try to think about them as ethernet and wifi: a direct plugged-in physical route (neural route), and a diffuse, remote, signal broadcast route (chemical route: neurotransmitters, hormones etc.).

The general layout of the lymphatic system looks remarkably similar to that of the other two systems we have looked at so far, with far-reaching and extensive networks of vessels diffuse around the body. The key difference with the lymphatic system, however, is there is no central focal point as we have with the brain in the nervous system and the heart in the cardiovascular system. The lymphatic system almost looks like a template for the internal networks of all your systems, with nodes (and sometimes clusters of nodes) appearing at critical points around the body. These critical points might be close to vital organs like the liver, or at 'convenient' junction points where their purpose for serving as an interchange can be best served, such as at the junctions of your skeletal joints. As the lymphatic system provides good transport around the body, it can also be a system that provides a key *metastatic* delivery system for cancer. If a tumour can create circulating cancer cells, these can then be carried by the bloodstream and lymphatic system all around the body, resulting in *metastases* (sometimes referred to as 'mets'), providing multiple sites for tumours in the body. This is why mets are a key prognostic factor for cancer, as once it has spread to multiple sites in the body, it is far harder to treat.

Key Questions

- What aspects of our lives impact our lymphatic system?
  o Think about the health onion!
- What consequences do you think these impacts have for our health and wellbeing over time?
  o Are there other knock-on effects that result due to the impact on the lymphatic system?

The Skeletal System

We see skeletons all the time in museums, on Hallowe'en, Día de Muertos, or other similar pageantry, sometimes used as decoration in certain structures (for example in the Paris catacombs and the Ossuary chapels of Europe), and in movies and TV shows. We tend to think of our skeletons as passive structures that only spring into action when they need to repair themselves if they get broken, but this couldn't be further from the truth. Your skeleton is actually a system, and whilst it definitely does do remarkable things to repair itself when broken, it is also constantly changing, constantly working, and constantly supporting other systems and structures in our bodies. We have 206 bones in our skeletons, with two main 'sections': the **axial** (central core of the body: the head, spine, and bones of the torso) and **appendicular** (the appendages: the shoulders, arms, legs, and pelvis). Your skeleton is there to provide the shape of your body, allowing your internal organs to develop and function, to provide you with the ability to move, and to protect delicate internal structures. Healthy adult bones are very strong indeed, although their strength depends on the type of stress being exerted on them. However, in order for your bones to be strong, you need to be adequately nourished so

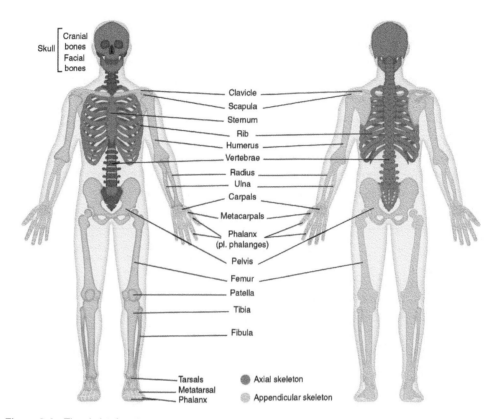

Figure 2.4 The skeletal system.

that your bones can develop and retain their strength and integrity. Your skeletal system is not just your bones though; you also have tissues like cartilage that serve to cushion and protect your joints as well. Your skeletal system is created and maintained using nutrients from your diet: zinc, calcium, potassium, and magnesium, as well as vitamins such as C, D, and K; so, having a diet that is rich in these is extremely important.

We sometimes think of our skeletons as being more or less passive, and maybe even lifeless once we have completed our physical development into adulthood, but this is far from the case. During childhood our bones are very busy indeed. They are growing and developing in all sorts of different ways as we mature. Their very structure changes over time also, allowing us to rapidly grow internally without stifling the growth of our most vital organs, such as our brains, but finally hardening and strengthening once they (and we) have reached adult size. As adults, though, our bones are still busy carrying out some very important functions, not just to maintain themselves, but also to support other key processes in our bodies. Our bones grow, maintain, and repair themselves through a fascinating process called **remodelling**, which requires processes local to the bone, but also processes initiated in other tissues in your body (particularly endocrine [hormonal] tissues like the thyroid). To repair your bone once it has broken, or even once it has experienced a micro fracture (some micro fractures happen as a consequence of growth, so they are not all significantly painful and traumatic), scaffolding is set up to provide a basic structure and some support whilst the intricate internal repair is being done. You have two main cell types that engage in the process of remodelling: **osteoclasts**, immune-like cells that resorb (re-absorb) damaged, old, or dysfunctional cells; and **osteoblasts**, that help to build new bone. Bone maintenance is therefore a bit like most other things in the body, some creation but also some destruction.

You have four main types of bones in your bodies: long bones, short bones, flat bones, and irregular bones. **Long bones** are any bones in your body that are longer than they are wide, so bones like your femur and humerus are good examples of these. Short bones are usually small cube-shaped bones that tend to be as wide as they are long, so the bones of your ankles and wrists are good examples of these. Flat bones are exactly as they sound, flat, and the bones of your cranium (skull) are examples of these. Irregular bones are pretty much any other type of bone that doesn't fit in any of the previous categories. Your **vertebrae** (the bones that make up your spinal column; singular: vertebra) fall into this category. All of these bone types have self-regulatory (and self-healing) properties that ensure the bones are in good condition to support their required functions, but long bones also have another important function to serve. Long bones are sometimes referred to as **trabecular** bones (and, also, cancellous bones), because they have matrix-like structures inside called *trabeculae* (singular: *trabecula*). These bones are therefore not completely dense, but have spongey and almost honeycombed internal morphology, and provide extra strength and integrity to the bone without the 'cost' of excessive weight. Your long bones also provide some other extremely important cells for your body: immune cells.

The larger **white blood cells** (WBCs) in your immune system are called **lymphocytes** (called *lymph*ocytes because they are the predominant cells found in lymph). You have three main classes of lymphocytes: **B-cells** (so called as they originate from your Bone marrow), **T-cells** (from your Thymus), and **Natural Killer cells** (more on these later). Your long bones create your B-cells along with many other of your blood cells as part of the **haematopoietic system**, which is a super-system made up of your lymphatic system, liver, and bones, and is tasked with creating your blood cells. Your bone marrow is deep inside your long bones, heavily vascularised (i.e., it has a lot of blood vessels running in, out, and around it), and is constantly working to create new cells (stem cells, in fact) that create your blood cells (both red and white). You make about two million **erythrocytes** (red blood cells) every second. About 1% of your body's

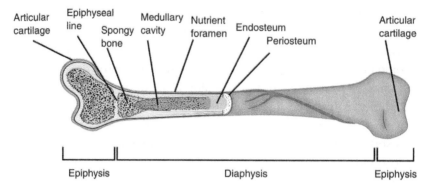

Figure 2.5 The anatomy of your long bones. Your marrow is in the medulla, which is where *haematopoiesis* happens.

Source: Boore et al. (2016), *Essentials of Anatomy and Physiology for Nursing Practice*, Sage

blood cells need to be replaced every single day regardless of whether you injure yourself, donate blood,[2] or menstruate. There are a variety of factors that can influence the ability of your bone marrow to create these stem cells, including cancers of the blood, ageing (as we age, our bone marrow can become fattier, taking up vital haematopoietic space), and nutritional status.

Your long bones, as well as having a rich blood supply, are also heavily innervated (i.e., there are also a lot of nerves running in and around them). This is why breaking a bone can hurt so much – there is a lot of neural tissue there to let you know if you have sustained an injury. That is not the only reason we have neural input to our bones, however, as we also know that the brain can talk directly to your bones to influence growth and the regulation of haematopoiesis. Yes, that's right, your brain talks to your bones. Not only this, but alongside this ethernet route, there is also evidence of a wifi route as well. Bone tissue itself has been shown to contain a wide variety of signalling molecules such as neurotransmitters and **neuropeptides**, AND there is evidence of receptors for neurotransmitters and hormones also being present on the cells of our bones. If you remember back to the earlier section about the sympathetic nervous system and our fight-or-flight response, you will notice I mentioned there about bone growth being inhibited. Hopefully now it will make more sense as to why shutting this process down might be so important in trying to prioritise our metabolic efforts. Growing, repairing, and maintaining bones, along with funding bone function, is metabolically very expensive.

---

2 I have donated 54 units of blood in my life and hope to continue doing so for a long time. Please do consider giving blood if you can, it is always needed and it is an easy way to give the gift of life.

Key Questions

- What aspects of our lives impact our skeletal system?
  - o   Try to think of something in all layers of the health onion.
- What consequences do you think these impacts have for our health and wellbeing over time?
  - o   What other systems might also be involved in these situations?
  - o   What might counteract them?

The Integumentary System

The last system we will discuss in detail in this chapter is the **integumentary system**. The integumentary system is made up of the skin, hair, nails, and our *exocrine* **glands**.[3] The skin is the largest sensory organ of our bodies, and it enables us to do some fascinating things. Like bones, our skin grows, repairs, and maintains itself. It keeps all our inside bits in, but also allows some of our inside bits out when they are needed as well. Sweating is a key function of the integumentary system, and without the ability to sweat, we would not be able to thermoregulate and would massively overheat whenever we exert ourselves or are in hot weather. About 10 pounds (4.5kg) of your adult bodyweight is made up of your skin, and like your bones it is constantly working. The skin and integumentary system also protects us from harmful things (like filtering UV radiation, pathogens, and toxins) by acting as a barrier between our delicate insides and the harsh surroundings. Not only this, but your skin also directly manufactures nutrients from its environment. Your skin creates vitamin D from exposure to the UV rays from sunlight and can do this from a very modest amount of sun exposure. Vitamin D is essential for a variety of processes in the body, and lack of sufficient UV exposure has been suggested to be associated with *Seasonal Affective Disorder* via its impact on vitamin D creation. Your skin is also an important information centre. It is covered in sensory receptors so that we know when we are hot or cold to initiate homeostatic behaviours to adjust. We also sense our environment through our skin – especially the skin on our hands. To understand the temperature of objects we touch (to know if we will be harmed by any extreme temperature), whether that object is still or has movement (and the speed of that movement), what its conformation is (solid/liquid/gas),

---

3 I have mentioned the endocrine system. That is the system or hormonal tissues (glands) throughout our body. *Endo* and *exo* are prefixes to denote where they dump their secretions – endocrine glands dump hormones into our bloodstreams (inside), and the exocrine glands secrete substances into the surface of the body: i.e., the skin (outside).

what its consistency and viscosity are, what gradient and texture it has, and whether touching it is painful, to name just a few. This is a tremendous amount of information to be able to receive, and the hardware required to perceive it is all packed in very tightly to provide as much information as possible.

The skin acts as an important barrier for our bodies in many different ways. It is obviously a literal barrier that prevents our internal bits and bobs from coming into contact with harmful things in our environment, but it also has immune properties that act as a first line of defence against invading pathogens and parasites. It also needs to let some things in, as we have seen with UV radiation, and can be an important and useful mechanism for the dosing of certain types of drugs as a result of its ability to absorb. Your skin also needs to let stuff out. Anyone who has worn rubber or nitrile gloves will know that your skin needs to breathe to function well. So, your skin needs to keep outside stuff out, let some outside stuff in, keep inside stuff in, and also let some inside stuff out. It also has to do all this whilst being the most likely contact point for damage. How many times have you cut, grazed, burned, or otherwise damaged the skin somewhere on your body? Once we do this, this is a literal pathway straight into our most vulnerable parts. Therefore, the skin, just as the gut does because we are always putting external stuff into it, needs to have a pretty sophisticated means of protecting our most vulnerable insides from invasion.

Your skin has several layers, and within those layers are immune cells ready and waiting for a problem to happen. When damage does occur, it is important for your skin to neutralise any invading threat, but also to block off the gap in the barrier that has just occurred in the short term to prepare the surrounding tissue for close immune surveillance, and to prepare for healing in the longer term. All of these actions are carried out by specific components of the immune system, and they mobilise into action very quickly indeed. Sometimes your skin has a special conformation that provides additional security, such as a mucous membrane. We have mucous membranes in many areas in our bodies, and these allow a more specific and concentrated immune surveillance area for invading pathogens. Essentially, we have mucous membranes around most of the places that provide a 'way in' for dangerous invaders: our mouths, noses, eyes, the gastro-intestinal tract, and our genitalia. These mucous membranes provide a variety of functions to allow the passage of molecules in and out, but also to host a variety of immune-related cells and chemicals to keep us that little bit safer in these high-exposure areas. Like our guts, too, our skin also plays host to bacteria and other micro-organisms that make up our microbiome. This external microbiome can also do all the same communications as that in our gut, and also assists in our mucosal barrier and immune barriers to invading pathogens. So we must be thankful to millions of tiny organisms that outnumber us and live on every part of our external selves for looking after us, and – of course – we need to look after them too. All of the factors mentioned previously that may harm the microbiome in the gut (such as poor diet, stress, and toxins) can harm the microbiome of the skin. This harm can upset the ability for your skin to maintain its barrier, and can cause infestations and infections within the skin itself.

Key Questions

- What aspects of our lives impact our integumentary system? Try to think of something in all layers of the health onion.
- Are there times in our lives when these impacts may be more or less important?

Using the information you have absorbed up until now, try thinking about other systems in the body, and what biological, psychological, and social factors may impact them.

- What might this do to our health over all?
- What other systems interact or overlap with those we have already looked at?
- Are the same 'players' appearing in terms of factors that will cause problems?
- What can we do about these?

Learning Outcomes Summary

- Understand some of the key systems in place in the human body and how they are regulated.

We have covered some of the key systems in the body, how they work, what can go wrong, and what they need in order to work well.

- Have an appreciation of the intersecting influences of human health on the systems level.

We have looked at several systems that overlap in terms of their physical infrastructure, their function, or their communication.

- Be able to explain some of the key psychological factors that have implications for health on the system and person levels.

We have considered a variety of psychological factors and how these can impact various systems in the body.

We have learned that stress, and the fight-or-flight response that it initiates, is a key vector for psychological-to-biological harm.

- Evaluate the influence of a variety of factors on individual health with a critical lens.

Through using the health onion, you will be able to work out which factors of our lives may have potentially harmful impacts on these systems.

Consider now how they may work together, but also how they can work through different mechanisms (e.g., through our behaviour when we are stressed, or through our nutritional status as a result of our life situations).

RESOURCES AND FURTHER READING

Arah, O. A. (2009). On the relationship between individual and population health. *Medicine, Health Care and Philosophy, 12*(3), 235–44.
This paper is a good one to read before you go on to the next chapter. It will help form a bridge between the things you have learned in this chapter and what you will learn from the next one.

Cryan, J. F., O'Riordan, K. J., Cowan, C. S., Sandhu, K. V., Bastiaanssen, T. F., Boehme, M., … & Dinan, T. G. (2019). The microbiota–gut–brain axis. *Physiological Reviews, 99*(4), 1877–2013.
This paper provides a detailed overview of the interplay between your microbiome and the gut–brain axis for those who would like to find out more.

McCorry, L. K. (2007). Physiology of the autonomic nervous system. *American Journal of Pharmaceutical Education, 71*(4), 78.
This review looks at the ANS in more detail. It is written for pharmacy students, and gives some good examples on how our bodily functions can be changed by agents that act on our ANS.

McLafferty, E., Hendry, C., & Farley, A. (2012). The integumentary system: anatomy, physiology and function of skin. *Nursing Standard (through 2013), 27*(3), 35.
This paper looks more closely at the skin and the integumentary system.

Ozturk, E. D., & Tan, C. O. (2018). Human cerebrovascular function in health and disease: Insights from integrative approaches. *Journal of Physiological Anthropology, 37*(1), 1–11.
This paper takes a closer look at cerebrovascular function. The focus in this chapter and in Chapter 10 is more on cardiovascular functioning, so reading this paper will give you more insight into the ways that our vascular system in our head and brain functions, and what can go wrong and why.

A subway map of human anatomy: https://www.openculture.com/2019/06/a-subway-map-of-human-anatomy.html

This is an excellent resource that shows all of the intricate and complex interconnections between the various systems in our bodies.

National Institute of Health anatomy and physiology: https://training.seer.cancer.gov/anatomy/

This is a useful guide on various different systems in the body that will reinforce and extend what you have learned in this chapter.

REFERENCES

Boziki, M. K., Kesidou, E., Theotokis, P., Mentis, A.-F. A., Karafoulidou, E., Melnikov, M., Sviridova, A., Rogovski, V., Boyko, A., & Grigoriadis, N. (2020). Microbiome in multiple sclerosis: Where are we, what we know and do not know. *Brain Sciences*, *10*(4), 234. https://www.mdpi.com/2076-3425/10/4/234

Caldeira, L. d. F., Borba, H. H., Tonin, F. S., Wiens, A., Fernandez-Llimos, F., & Pontarolo, R. (2020). Fecal microbiota transplantation in inflammatory bowel disease patients: A systematic review and meta-analysis. *PLOS ONE*, *15*(9), e0238910. https://doi.org/10.1371/journal.pone.0238910

Colman, R. J., & Rubin, D. T. (2014). Fecal microbiota transplantation as therapy for inflammatory bowel disease: A systematic review and meta-analysis. *Journal of Crohn's and Colitis*, *8*(12), 1569–81. https://doi.org/10.1016/j.crohns.2014.08.006

Drekonja, D., Reich, J., Gezahegn, S., Greer, N., Shaukat, A., MacDonald, R., Rutks, I., & Wilt, T. J. (2015). Fecal microbiota transplantation for *clostridium difficile* infection. *Annals of Internal Medicine*, *162*(9), 630–38. https://doi.org/10.7326/m14-2693%m25938992

Ghezzi, L., Cantoni, C., Pinget, G. V., Zhou, Y., & Piccio, L. (2021). Targeting the gut to treat multiple sclerosis. *The Journal of Clinical Investigation*, *131*(13), e143774. https://doi.org/10.1172/JCI143774

Proença, I. M., Allegretti, J. R., Bernardo, W. M., de Moura, D. T. H., Ponte Neto, A. M., Matsubayashi, C. O., Flor, M. M., Kotinda, A. P. S. T., & de Moura, E. G. H. (2020). Fecal microbiota transplantation improves metabolic syndrome parameters: Systematic review with meta-analysis based on randomized clinical trials. *Nutrition Research*, *83*, 1–14. https://doi.org/https://doi.org/10.1016/j.nutres.2020.06.018

Shogbesan, O., Poudel, D. R., Victor, S., Jehangir, A., Fadahunsi, O., Shogbesan, G., & Donato, A. (2018). A systematic review of the efficacy and safety of fecal microbiota transplant for *clostridium difficile* infection in immunocompromised patients. *Canadian Journal of Gastroenterology and Hepatology*, *2018*, 1394379. https://doi.org/10.1155/2018/1394379

Zhang, Z., Mocanu, V., Cai, C., Dang, J., Slater, L., Deehan, E. C., Walter, J., & Madsen, K. L. (2019). Impact of fecal microbiota transplantation on obesity and metabolic syndrome – a systematic review. *Nutrients*, *11*(10), 2291. https://www.mdpi.com/2072-6643/11/10/2291

3
THE POPULATION

INTRODUCTION

The aim of this chapter is to introduce you to looking at health on the population level. If you come from a psychology background, you're probably used to looking at people on an individual basis, and the previous two chapters will have felt more at home. If you come from a public health background, the previous chapters may have felt very strange, but this one should feel more at home. If you are from a medical or nursing background, you may be familiar with some of the principles in each of these biopsychosocial approach chapters (as well as this one), but hopefully the way you will have been looking at these issues will have been slightly different.

Learning Outcomes

- Understand some of the ways population health is measured and start thinking critically about how suitable these measurements are to understand health.
- Have an appreciation of the influence of intersecting identities on health outcomes.
- Be able to explain some of the ways in which social exclusion is manifested in health.
- Close the loop on understanding how health is made from cell to society.

WHAT DOES PSYCHOLOGY HAVE TO DO WITH POPULATION HEALTH?

We saw in Chapter 1 how psychological factors can influence our cells and how they work. We found that psychological, behavioural, and social factors all contribute to the functioning of our cells, and can all create lasting impacts for our health through their influence on our cells. We saw that before we even consider our larger organs or systems, the very things that create these infrastructures are vulnerable to influence from our external world, and that sometimes these influences can reverberate down through generations. Chapter 2 looked at the systems of the body and how they work and can be influenced by psychological and behavioural factors. We found that our various systems run on similar infrastructures and networks to operate, and that the nervous system is connected to everything, either physically or virtually. Because our nervous systems are connected to everything, this means that whatever happens in them (i.e., those psychological factors that can change the biological workings of the brain and nervous system) can happen anywhere else in the organs, tissues, fluids, and signalling pathways of our bodies. The intertwined networks that support these various systems are delicately balanced, and when one system is set out of kilter, this can have an impact on many others too. Moving forward, we are going to look at the consequence of these impacts writ slightly larger on the group scale. We have looked at cell changes, and system changes at the person level; now we will look at groups of people and how health can be associated with who you are as well as how you function, and the things that you experience, do, and feel.

As a person you are who you are, but you are also a member of many groups as well. Think about how many groups or communities you may belong to – I'm sure you will end up with a very long list. Whether you think about your age group, your ethnicity, your socio-economic position, your employment status, your gender, your sexuality, your diet, or your nationality – you will be able to think of some associations with health that relate to that group. Just as our bodies are made up of interconnected systems, we as people are made up of intersecting identities, and some of those identities come with particular health associations. These associations can be biological, psychological, or social – but also, very frequently, they can be a combination of all three.

When we think of groups – or populations – of people, there are many mechanisms by which belonging to those groups can influence our health. These can be physical or practical things, such as being someone who lives in a densely populated city, and therefore being exposed to high levels of pollution, being vulnerable to road traffic accidents, or not having sufficient green space around you. They can also be abstract and intangible influences, such as being someone from a group that is marginalised, experiencing stigma and discrimination, not having your medical needs properly addressed by your healthcare system, or by being left out of mainstream consideration for education. At every stage in our lives, and in almost everything we experience, we are more or less likely to be included in the big conversations that dictate our health across our life course depending on which groups we belong to. Some groups have advantage in social issues, some in biological, some in psychological, and some in all three. The ways that these influences affect us can happen on the cellular and system level, so it is important to remember what you have learned from the first two chapters. We will put the cell-to-society perspective into practice in later chapters to illustrate how all this works, but for now we will focus on the larger end of the scale, examining how groups are impacted as groups rather than clusters of individuals (or clusters of individuals' clusters of cells and systems), so for now things will be kept as simple as possible.

Key Questions

- What psychological factors determine health at the population level?
- What factors about humans as groups within a population are important to understand in health psychology?

MEASURING HEALTH AT THE POPULATION LEVEL

Before we can really consider what health looks like at the population level, we need to know how to measure it. We have discussed ways to measure health on the cellular level (looking at immune cells, hormones, and other **biomarkers**), and measurements on the person level (such as looking at blood pressure, incidence of heart attacks, or prescriptions for peptic ulcers), but when we get up to thousands, or even millions, of people, we need to think about measuring health in different ways. There are obviously ways we can look at some of these person-level metrics through public health data. We can use available data on hospitalisations, infection rates of disease (as we have seen with Covid-19), numbers of prescriptions written each year, or average mortality rate, but these only really tell us about what's going on. We can learn a great deal about a population from studying these metrics, but then what? We can identify that population A in country 1 has a lower mortality than population A in country 2, or population B in country 1, but when we are looking at populations and groups, we need to start looking deeper, to understand why. If you were a public health employee, would it be sufficient to you to say that women of Southeast Asian descent in your local area have shorter lifespans than a similar group in your neighbouring town or county? When we are considering public health, we are interested in understanding people's experience of health, not just a raw metric. This helps us to understand the *why* of group-level health, so that policies can be shaped to support the health of the population more effectively.

Looking at population health, there are a variety of metrics that help us to understand not just the health of particular groups, but also what that means and – critically – what needs to be done to improve health. Instead of just looking at mortality rate per year, or average life expectancy, we can look at metrics like healthy life expectancy (or the period of time people in a population live in good overall health), years in poor health (or even percentage of years spent in poor health), disability-free life expectancy, years with disability (or percentage of years spent with disability), health-related quality of life (HRQoL), and avoidable mortality rate (avoidable through timely and effective care, or public health interventions). A similar metric is Quality-Adjusted Life Years (QALY), a measure of remaining years in good health where one QALY is equal to one year of perfect health, which is often used to understand the efficacy of interventions. Another take on the QALY is the DALY, or the Disability[1] Adjusted Life Years measure, which measures the years of perfect health lost. Effectively, what all these metrics seek to capture is the consequence of things going wrong – whether that be the onset of a chronic condition or a change of health status because of injury. If we were simply to look at life expectancy of a population – which is helpful to a very basic degree – we can establish very high-level and basic understandings of health. If people in country

---

1 I should state here this is the formal phrasing given for this construct, and it is one that I find uncomfortable and outdated. 'Disability' is a very loaded term in this context, with the inference being that disability is suboptimal. For many with disabilities, they do not consider their standard of living to be suboptimal at all. For others, any suboptimal life standard might not be attributed to the disability *per se*, but rather due to the social conditions that the stigma and marginalisation that those with disabilities experience. What I believe this phrasing is getting at is that someone's health conditions are so severe that they are disabling and result in a reduced **quality of life** experience that would otherwise not be there without that health condition. I am hopeful this phrasing will be revised at some point in the near future to something more appropriate for the context.

A live on average to 84.6 years and people in country B live on average to 58.3 years, we know there are some key differences between those nations regarding the health of their inhabitants. This is a real example, by the way: as shown in data from the Organisation for Economic Co-operation and Development (OECD)[2] from 2019, the average life expectancy in Japan is 84.6 years, 26.3 years longer than that in Guinea-Bissau. But what does this tell us about this situation? Well first, it tells us that our world is hugely, and horrifically, unequal. Second, it tells us that our lives are very much dictated by a factor we have no control in – where we were born. But beyond this, what does it show? Actually, very little. It gives us a very large alert signal to indicate that something could – and perhaps should – be fixed, but we need to know more. We should also consider that to many people the quality of their life is just as important and meaningful as its duration. There is no easy answer to this at all, but the important thing to remember is subjectivity – we cannot place a ruler on someone's life experience and say that it is better or worse than someone else's without understanding their own interpretation. That's not to say that population health measures generally ask people their experience or their position on their own health – far from it; but what they do tend to do is take 'average' or commonly accepted understandings of what quality may mean in order to make sense of an aggregate level of experience. If you're thinking this all sounds very vague and imprecise, you would be right, but consider for a minute if we didn't look at health on the population level. If we just dealt with people on a person-level basis this may be fine for some, but for many we are missing the bigger picture of health inequalities between groups of people (or nations as we saw before) that we could put right if we tried. There is obviously no one-size-fits-all, but it is the best we can do without completely ignoring the bigger picture altogether.

Key Questions

- Generally speaking, what social groups can you think of that may have specific health-related issues?
- Do these groups have similar health outcomes across the country? Across the continent? Across the world?
- Do these groups have similar health outcomes across the life course? Are there particular 'pinch points' where some of these issues may be more (or less) relevant than others?

2 Do have a look at the excellent website www.ourworldindata.org where you can explore all manner of data from around the world.

THE SOCIAL GRADIENT OF HEALTH

When we look at health on the population level, and we can pull apart demographics to understand similarities and differences, we get to understand more about some of the social dynamics of health. These differences are termed **health inequalities**, as they are usually unfair, preventable, avoidable, or otherwise changeable systemic disparities in whichever metric of population health you may wish to choose (e.g., life expectancy, HRQoL, DALY, disease morbidity etc.). Examining these differences can be very powerful when we look within countries that exist under one overarching government whose directives shape all aspects of the social world of that nation (e.g., education, healthcare, housing, transport etc.). We will take a look at an example to illustrate this but remember that such examples exist all over the world, and with the exception of a handful of countries, health inequalities are prevalent almost everywhere you may choose to look.

The United Kingdom

I will use the example of the UK because this is the country I know best, seeing as this is where I live, but also because to me the level of health inequality in the UK should be a point of national shame, but it is not sufficiently high up on the socio-political agenda as yet. The UK is currently the fifth largest economy in the world (World Population Review, 2022), but it is also a country of staggering inequality. Despite its economic prowess, which for a very small nation is significant, there are still people in my country that require access to food and clothing banks because they do not have enough money to survive, and their number is increasing. We may rank our country by its gross domestic product (GDP) and come out feeling very pleased with ourselves, but our country in my opinion is only worth as much as its poorest citizens hold. Our unequal society is exemplified by the fact that the richest 10% in this country own over 43% of its wealth, with the bottom 50% holding just 9% (Office for National Statistics, 2022). The inequalities in the UK have been around for a long time, but there is evidence to suggest that instead of decreasing (which we would hope for in any society that commits itself to social progress), they are actually increasing.[3] Health inequality in the UK is so

---

3 There is a scholar in the UK named Prof Sir Michael Marmot who has dedicated his life to researching and highlighting this inequality and pushing tirelessly for change. If you put his name into a search engine you will find many publications (journal articles, government reports, and books) on the matter, and a wealth of powerfully shocking information about the state of a supposedly wealthy and advanced society.

bad now that for some men where they are born can mean they can expect to live 9.4 years less than another man in a more privileged area of the country, and for women that gap is around 7.4 years (The King's Fund, 2022). In the UK, those in lower socio-economic groups tend to have a much larger burden of disease too, with a much higher proportion of chronic illness, and higher severity of those illnesses the lower down the socio-economic stratifications you may be. Effectively, in the UK the more money you have, the longer you will live and the better quality your life will have with regard to your health. Unfortunately, these inequalities also exist along barriers between peoples within society not just on socio-economic position, but also on racialised identities. Racism and its direct and indirect influences on health will be a recurring theme throughout this book. The unpacking of how and why this happens will be the subject of this chapter and later chapters, but it is referred to as a social gradient to health, with causative factors being referred to as social determinants of health.

Social Determinants of Health

The **social gradient of health** is not just something bounded to the UK, it is observable in many – if not most – countries around the world to varying degrees. The gradient of life expectancy is not the only one that we can see, however, as there are gradients of many different types of health measure. In any system with a hierarchy of wealth or social status, we unfortunately see a corresponding impact on health. Work carried out looking at civil servants in the UK[4] has shown that there is a gradient of health within this system regarding standard and quality of health, regardless of the fact that, as a group, civil servants tend to be a relatively advantaged group in terms of their wealth and overall social position. Here, the gradient sits with employment grade, which somewhat depressingly suggests that even if we take away one gradient (country-level socioe-conomic position), another (organisation-level socio-economic position) emerges in its place to influence health.

Much of public health and epidemiology is centred on trying to identify the reasons for disparities within a population and has led to great advances in understanding how to prevent poor health outcomes. For example, we know from large-scale population-level analyses that heart disease is associated with (amongst other things) central adiposity (the fat carried around the abdomen), high levels of cholesterol, and having high blood pressure. Epidemiological studies have also looked at what behaviours underlie those factors in order to mount public health initiatives to support more healthy ways of living. After all, it wouldn't be very helpful if we just told people to have lower blood

---

4 The Whitehall Studies. There have been many papers published using these data, and some very fascinating findings.

pressure or cholesterol, would it? So, campaigns here can be spearheaded to promote a more balanced and heart-healthy diet, to discourage the consumption of saturated fats, and to advise moderate engagement with or overall reduction of behaviours such as alcohol use and tobacco consumption. These are causes of these particular issues, and by targeting those causes we will ensure our whole population stays healthy, right? Sadly, not so. For some, there is no amount of information, suggestion, or encouragement that can change some of these causes of heart disease, and that is because some of the factors that underlie whether we can make healthier choices are not that simple. The research into the social determinants of health instead allows us to identify the *causes of the causes*. Taking the prior example, if we were just to focus on poor diet as being a predictor of heart disease (due to its association with central adiposity, cholesterol, and high blood pressure) we would just recommend that people eat better, and we know that that doesn't work. Instead, and in order to inform more effective and accessible interventions and public health advice, we need to look behind that to understand what predicts poor diet. Poor diets can just happen by accident, but very frequently they are associated with multiple issues that are not simply personal choice and are not necessarily about the here-and-now. Poor diet can be associated with food affordability, food supply and accessibility, cultural behaviours associated with food, education around what a good diet is and how to facilitate it, and (as a very small aspect) personal preference. The social determinants of health here help us to make sense of why someone may have a poor diet – and if their diet is due to poverty, then what use is a very general health promotion campaign espousing the benefits of a well-balanced diet? Quite aside from whether people can afford good quality food, think about the other issues that poverty presents and how this relates to food. Poverty means you may not have access to your own form of transport, and therefore carrying bulky shopping a large distance may be very hard. The use of local convenience stores that have less choice, higher prices, and greater amounts of processed long-storage food may be your only viable option. Poverty also means that other aspects of your life beyond food are also financially strained – and that means stress. When was the last time you ate a healthy, well-balanced plate of freshly prepared food when you were stressed? Stress also (as we saw in the last chapter) completely derails many of our systems and means that even if we were able to eat healthily, we are more prone to having the high cholesterol, high blood pressure, and high central adiposity anyway. And that is just for starters.

Culture and Health

The issue of culture is also an interesting point to take into consideration when thinking about health on the population level. Culture is a very large and complicated thing to break down, and would take an entire book to explain properly, but it is an important point of consideration when we are thinking about people's behaviours. A lot of what we do is influenced by what we know, what is the norm for us, and people like us, and what we were brought up to be aligned to – and a lot of this is culture. I'm going to give you a very small crash course on some anthropology here to illustrate how important cultural aspects are in health, and it will only scratch the surface.

Culture is generally defined as a set of learned behaviours or beliefs that characterise a society or group of people – but remember we are all many different groups rolled into one person, so our personal culture will be quite different from the culture of any of the groups we belong to. We have culture at the international level (e.g., marriage, funerary rites) and national level (e.g., Sundays are an official holiday in Chile), and also subcultures within and across these other cultural frameworks (e.g., those associated with religion or other ethical/moral practices). For those from a psychology background, have a think about social identity theory (Tajfel & Turner). There is a lot there with regard to our group membership and the behaviours and attitudes those groups (and, therefore, we) ascribe to. Culture itself can also be a lot more subtle and can exist on several levels within an individual. We can look at culture as existing on three levels: macro, meso, and micro. Macro is the largest – this might be the culture of your nation, your ethnicity, your gender, or some other large higher-order cultural framework. You exist within that large macro culture, but also have a meso level of culture too – this could be your social class, your racialised identity, your sexuality, your age group (or generation), or your religion (this could also be a macro-level group, depending on how centralised that group is to your identity). Finally, whilst fitting into those macro and meso levels, you also have micro-level cultures that influence your behaviour. Micro-level cultures can be almost anything that incorporates a set of attitudes and behaviours along with it, such as being a vegetarian, being strongly pro-environmental, being a recovering addict, or being a yoga practitioner. Cultures are effectively systems of shared meanings and attitudes, which are likely to influence a whole host of behaviours (both positive and negative). Culture is so important to understanding health that there is an entire field associated with it: medical anthropology. Whilst it is an entire field in itself, a good interdisciplinary scholar or practitioner will find various aspects of the learnings generated by this field both fascinating and incredibly useful.

Biological Pathways in a Social Context

As we have seen in the last two chapters, biological pathways underpin all our health processes, but somewhere along the line our social experiences get under our skin to influence these processes. To make sense of this, we can consider psychosocial and material conditions of living. As an example, infant mortality in Denmark in 1900 was around 125/1000 live births – today it is around 3/1000. The conditions surrounding infant mortality back then are easy to guess: poor sanitation, poor quality/ absent medical care, dirty water, poor nutrition, and so forth. These were all things we could consider to be material conditions, in that they were due to a lack of scientific knowledge and/or technological advancements. However, infant mortality today still varies hugely between countries. In 2020, the infant mortality rate for the world was 27.4/1000 live births (The World Bank, 2022), but the variation around this figure (much like the figures we previously looked at for life expectancy) vary hugely. The lowest figure is around 2/1000, which is recorded mostly in European countries such as Iceland, Belarus, and Estonia, as well as some Asian countries like Japan and Singapore. At the other end of the spectrum there are records of 70–80/1000 (almost four times the world average) in countries such as Sierra Leone, Lesotho, Somalia, and Nigeria. Infant mortality, like many other higher-level health metrics, can also vary hugely within countries, across either regions or specific subpopulations of peoples. The reasons behind this may still be poor sanitation, poor quality/absent medical care, dirty water, poor nutrition etc., but because the necessary advancements have been made to understand and compensate for these, they are now what we could consider to be psychosocial conditions. Whether that is due to governments being unable or choosing not to spend money on health infrastructure (for whatever reason), down to the collective (in)efforts of humanity, or through the exploitation of individuals and groups can be debated, but it still stands that as we have the knowledge and technology to ensure that children are given a fighting chance to survive their birth, the fact that so many inequalities remain can no longer be considered strictly material. Psychosocial conditions of living concern pretty much everything – and can be causes of material conditions too, if the material conditions exist but are not available to some for whatever reason. If we take the example of the United States, black men in deprived areas of the US have a 20-year shorter life expectancy than their white counterparts. This is ascribed to a variety of factors, including an increased prevalence of HIV in the black community, increased level of violent crime, and increased prevalence of cardiovascular disease. Underneath each of these factors exist biological processes and mechanisms; but black people in the US are not 'wired' towards these health conditions, rather it is the psychosocial conditions in which they live that make these conditions far more likely. As you read more of this book and engage in its activities, you will come to realise that that last sentence starts to become less and less clear. It is absolutely the case that black people in the US are not 'wired' towards these health conditions on the surface of things, but if their psychosocial lives are such that they are funnelled down a path towards these health issues by the cultural institutions they are subjected to, then unless we change those contexts, it will be a situation that repeats itself generation after generation.

Key Questions

Before going on to the next section, have a think to yourself about a health condition that is a problem in your country or community, and have a go at considering what material factors and what psychosocial factors drive these particular health conditions.

- How many of these are shared by other sections of the community?
- How many of the material factors are likely to be addressed in your lifetime?
- How many of the psychosocial factors could be addressed with the political and social will?
- What can and does need to change in order to address these issues?

SOCIAL EXCLUSION

Everything that we have discussed so far in this chapter has hopefully led you to the conclusion that societies can simply be unfair. Sometimes this unfairness is directed at certain groups of people, sometimes the unfairness spreads across vast groups of people, but either way this all contributes to the concept of social exclusion. Social exclusion refers not just to the hardships experienced in economic poverty, but also to the psychosocial hardships of marginalisation and disenfranchisement. Exclusion, like many other psychosocial issues, exists on a continuum, and is often multi-dimensional. Social exclusion can be considered at the institutional level (so whether the policies of the government of your country consider or act in the best interests of people like you), but these very often filter down to the individual level as well (being manifested in things like stigmatisation and marginalisation). To think about it another way, if we are socially *included*, we are much more likely to enjoy access to quality education, healthcare, political consideration, civil protection, social networks, social support, and employment opportunities. Social inclusion/exclusion also affects us at every stage of our lives too. Before going on to the next section, have a go at the activity in the box. Think about what groups you may belong to (this could be based on any way you might wish to group yourself), and think about how well represented the needs and views of your group are in your community and your country.

Key Questions

- Do you feel like the health concerns of your particular social group (however you may wish to define yourself) are understood, prioritised, or sufficiently catered for by your local government officials? Or your central government?
  - o What do you think the impact is if government (local, federal, or national) does not include the concerns of your particular group(s) in their policies?
  - o What sorts of policies have an impact on the health of people in your group(s)?

Processes of Social Exclusion

When we think about the ways we can be socially excluded, we can split this up into three specific pathways. First, we have economic processes. This is where the social exclusion you may experience may be driven by your local or national unemployment rate, the overall job security relevant in your sector or profession, or even through larger sweeping financial factors such as austerity. Second, we have demographic processes. This is where social exclusion can occur through the way population trends change over time, such as the increase in single households, the ageing population, or the distribution of immigration and emigration. Finally, we have spatial processes, which are where there are direct barriers to inclusion. This might be through social mechanisms such as a lack of community integration, the lack of affordable housing creating pockets of people grouped by their socio-economic banding, or gentrification that drives out certain communities by pricing them out of the housing market, or even a lack of diverse local employment. We will have a look at some clear examples of social exclusion soon, but just think to yourself now – are you a member of a group for whom your elected officials speak for or to? Or are you a member of one (or several) groups that may not be on 'the political agenda'? Go to the next box and have a think about these issues and where you fit in your socio-political landscape.

Key Questions

- What groups are socially excluded from health and welfare considerations in your country?
- Do intersecting identities (that is where someone may belong to several socio-demographic groups) make this issue better or worse?
- What levels of the way that health is made and defined are experienced by those who are excluded?

One of the biggest problems with social exclusion is that it **self-perpetuates**. If some-one like you isn't high up on the agenda of the government in your country, things will likely only continue to get worse. Part of this complicated process is the fact that marginalisation filters down and is internalised by individuals and groups. We learn from the policies our governments deliver, and from their behaviour and conduct as individuals, whether 'people like us' are who our government looks after. We know by the faces of the people in our panel of elected government officials whether 'people like us' are even represented by that group of people tasked with making our policies. So does everyone else. Policy is a very socially powerful tool – it not only has the power to directly help and support (or not, as the case may be), but it also serves as a social and cultural narrative to the rest of the country about who is or isn't worthy of support and consideration. We are obviously all agents of our own choices when it comes to how we conduct ourselves with others, but policymakers and political rhetoric very frequently set the tone. This is very much the case in cultures that have a high level of political populism, which we are seeing more and more of in our modern world. We learn through observing who our governments do and do not prioritise, or who they legislate for and against, that there are preferred groups. This message gets internalised, and if we happen to live in a very unequal society, we can hardly help but build an internal social hierarchy where we position ourselves and others. Not only this, but if we feel 'left out' of political decision making, this may also make us less likely to vote, which – in turn – means that the issues and needs of 'people like us' have less of a chance to be voiced. If we don't vote, we have no voice, and that also makes us feel disempowered, disenfranchised, and marginalised. Of course, it can be argued that your electoral institutions may render your vote meaningless anyway (as they can do in many countries that do not have systems such as proportional representation), which is another powerful means of disenfranchisement. By default, any sitting government will have got where they are through the electoral system they succeeded in, so they are in no way incentivised to change it. Unfairness breeds unfairness.

PUTTING KNOWLEDGE INTO PRACTICE: SOCIAL EXCLUSION OF THOSE OF ETHNIC MINORITY STATUS

Regardless of what *type* of minority group you may belong to (this could be associated with your nationality, the colour of your skin, your religious practices, your sexuality, your gender identity), just being a minority in any society is sufficient to constitute social exclusion. You don't even necessarily need to be a minority as such – social exclusion can occur to certain groups even in the case of reasonable balance, as we see in nations where males and females are afforded different social and political liberties. However, for now we will focus on situations where individuals are in minority status. Both migrants and other minority groups experience significant social exclusion in policy and in social participation across the world. A study led by Ikram and colleagues (2016) set out to understand how ethnic minority status might be associated with all-cause mortality (literally death from any cause) by examining demographic public health data from six western European nations. They found that ethnic minority status of those that moved into the country was associated with different patterns of mortality compared to those born in the country. They found that most migrant populations had higher mortality due to infectious diseases and homicide, but lower rates of mortality due to cancer and suicide. Moreover, they found that migrants from some regions did better than those who were locally born, and some worse. For example, women from countries in the Sub-Saharan African region had higher risk ratios than women locally born, but women from East Asian countries had lower risk ratios. For men, those from Latin American countries had lower risk ratios than locally born men, but those from Eastern Europe had higher. What might explain this?

Key Questions

- If we are in a group that is socially marginalised, what do you think this means for our biology (and that of our future generations)?
- Think about your nation during the Covid-19 pandemic – were there groups in your country that were more vulnerable to getting Covid, or suffering serious illness if they did get Covid?
- What factors do you think underlie this enhanced vulnerability?

RACISM AND HEALTH

Racism is an important underlying component of many social determinants of health, in terms of its overt impact on us if we experience it, but also in the subtle mechanics of how racism functions through the various layers of our society. The same is true for other types of discrimination, and if we happen to be a member of several groups that are discriminated against in our society, the impact this has will last a lifetime (and potentially beyond).[5] Racism is such a well-established factor in health that there have

---

5 For a beautiful example and celebration of what it means to live with intersecting identities, take a look at the website of The Triple Cripples: https://thetriplecripples.uk/about-us

been several large-scale systematic reviews and meta-analyses on the work that has been carried out. One of these published in 2015 from Paradies and colleagues outlines how both physical and mental health are impacted by racism, even after controlling for a vast number of other factors. Racism affects the health and wellbeing of children and young people also, both directly and vicariously. A study using population-level data found that children born to mothers who experienced interpersonal racism experienced deficits in socioemotional development and some cognitive abilities (Kelly et al., 2013). A massive global review of 121 studies found that racism was a significant determinant of mental and physical health in children and young people, with detriment to markers of health in children as they grew, and at birth (Priest et al., 2013). When we consider the impact of racism, whether we have experienced it or not, we can understand that the impact of being discriminated against will cause significant psychological stress and distress, but racism exists beyond the interpersonal dynamics we can more readily see. Racism can be inherent in our societies. If our society is institutionally racist, then anyone who is not of the national majority group will be structurally marginalised in almost every way you can think of, from access to healthcare, to access and support with quality education, to just being able to operate as a free member of society. This also holds if that group is no longer the majority but has previously held (and therefore maintained) the majority privilege through institutional racism. We will consider more about how specific elements of policy filter down to affect our health in Chapter 9, where you will be able to gather a deeper understanding of how institutional racism (or any other type of institutional exclusion or marginalisation) can impact people in very subtle but extremely profound ways across their life course. Overall, racism is associated with higher levels of perceived stress and lower levels of social capital (Heim et al., 2011). Social capital is an important aspect when considering any level of social exclusion – it is the sense that who you are as a person has social currency, that you are well thought of, included, and valued.

Key Questions

Taking what you know now, from information from this chapter and the last two, reflect on the statistic highlighted earlier in this chapter about black men from deprived areas in the United States.

- What reasons can you think of that may be behind this statistic?
- Think about the layers of the health onion.
- Think about it from cell to society.

CLOSING THE LOOP: SOCIAL EPIGENETICS

In the social gradient to health, there is no one factor that is responsible for the gradient (in terms of its steepness or magnitude). We are all intersections of identities, and each of those identities will sit somewhere on that social gradient. The pathways behind the social gradient can be material (e.g., poverty), biological (e.g., adiposity), behavioural (e.g., diet), and psychosocial (e.g., stress) (Arendt & Lauridsen, 2008; Blane, 2006). Cast your mind back to Chapter 1, where we learned about epigenetic changes. We know that nutrition during pregnancy is hugely associated with epigenetic changes and birth outcomes (Sullivan et al., 2011) – and we have learned in this chapter that nutrition is impacted by a variety of different sociodemographic factors – from poverty to policy to marginalisation. Parenting style and psycho-environmental conditions create epigenetic changes that impact health (Champagne, 2008), and if we look at this from the society level, we know that education, social policy, marginalisation, and poverty all contribute to those as well. Trying to bring this all together, a study examining epigenetic changes and socio-economic status in the UK examined a cohort from Glasgow in Scotland (McGuinness et al., 2012). They found that epigenetic changes were associated with severe deprivation and being in manual work. They also found that years in education were associated with the degree and number of epigenetic changes that occurred. When looking at the person-level correlates, they found these epigenetic changes were associated with cardiovascular diseases and a variety of inflammatory markers even when controlling for other health-modulating factors like diet and socio-economic position.

The significance of **social epigenetics** also extends to the impact of intergenerational trauma. There has been a vast amount of research that has sought to make sense of how social exclusion can echo through the generations via epigenetics. Research looking at First Nations peoples in Canada (e.g., Bombay et al., 2009) and Australia (e.g., Menzies, 2009) has uncovered a huge role for the health and wellbeing outcomes in the continued passing on of trauma via genetics and psychosocial transference. A whole area of research has sprung up to synthesise these multiple levels of health influence: DOHaD – Developmental Origins of Health and Disease (Dubois & Guaspare, 2020). This work is the very essence of cell-to-society and back again.

SUMMARY – FROM CELL TO SOCIETY AND BACK AGAIN

In this chapter, we have started to look at what population health is and how it is measured. We have found that our social groups have a lot to do with the way that our health is made – from psychosocial factors to more physical, material points. These population-level factors also creep back into our bodies, impacting us right back to the cellular level. Stress is a huge factor in our physical functioning on the population level and can be experienced from almost everywhere in our lives, from our individual experiences to the structural context in which we live.

To combine the learning of these first three chapters, we have seen that environmental factors can create cellular-level changes that then have an impact on the function of those cells, and how they contribute to our overall physical functioning. At the person level, our systems are extremely interconnected and require a great deal of balance to operate well. Cellular-level factors impact system-level functioning. At the population level, our social systems are highly interconnected, and our social groups can dictate almost every level of our ability to remain healthy – from being protected by public health policy to experiencing environmental stressors. Social exclusion can trigger epigenetic changes that then impact ourselves and our future generations, making some groups born into cellular disadvantage.

Learning Outcomes Summary

- Understand some of the ways population health is measured and start thinking critically about how suitable these measurements are to understand health.

We have examined how population health can be quantified, and what measures may be used.

- Have an appreciation of the influence of intersecting identities on health outcomes.

We have taken a critical view of how social groups and identities may or may not be supported through our social and political systems, and how this impacts health.

- Be able to explain some of the ways in which social exclusion is manifested in health.

We have looked at the pathways of social exclusion, and have discussed how certain factors such as racism and minority status are associated with health.

- Close the loop on understanding how health is made from cell to society.

We have examined how these population-level factors have been associated with epigenetic outcomes, meaning that population-level health has a direct influence on both cellular- and person-level health.

FURTHER READING

Barry, A. M., & Yuill, C. (2011). *Understanding the sociology of health: An introduction*. Sage. This book takes a sociological perspective on health. The topics covered here are similar to others you may find in psychology-oriented books, but there is a stronger focus on social dynamics and political contexts that is particularly helpful.

Dubois, M., & Guaspare, C. (2020). From cellular memory to the memory of trauma: Social epigenetics and its public circulation. *Social Science Information*, 59(1), 144–83. An excellent primer for social epigenetics.

Marmot, M., & Wilkinson, R. (eds.). (2005). *Social determinants of health*. Oxford University Press.
This is a great book that will provide you with some interesting perspectives on public health and the social determinants of health. The chapters within this book are written by some brilliant authors in the field whose work you can also look up to learn more about the issues raised here.

Pool, R., & Geissler, W. (2005). *Medical anthropology*. McGraw-Hill Education.
As with the text on medical sociology, this book will provide you with the anthropological perspective – giving you a closer look at the impact of culture on health, health behaviours, and the systems that influence our wellbeing.

Sniehotta, F. F., Araújo-Soares, V., Brown, J., Kelly, M. P., Michie, S., & West, R. (2017). Complex systems and individual-level approaches to population health: a false dichotomy? *The Lancet Public Health*, 2(9), e396–e397.
This is a paper written by some top names in health psychology. It gives a very philosophical and integrated overview of how the cell-to-society perspective can and should work.

REFERENCES

Arendt, J. N., & Lauridsen, J. (2008). Do risk factors explain more of the social gradient in self-reported health when adjusting for baseline health? *European Journal of Public Health*, 18(2), 131–7. https://doi.org/10.1093/eurpub/ckm096

Blane, D. (2006). The life course perspective, the social gradient, and health. In M. Marmot, & R. Wilkinson (eds.), *Social Determinants of Health* (pp. 54–77). Oxford University Press.

Bombay, A., Matheson, K., & Anisman, H. (2009). Intergenerational trauma: Convergence of multiple processes among First Nations peoples in Canada. *International Journal of Indigenous Health*, 5(3), 6–47.

Champagne, F. A. (2008). Epigenetic mechanisms and the transgenerational effects of maternal care. *Frontiers in Neuroendocrinology*, 29(3), 386–97. https://doi.org/https://doi.org/10.1016/j.yfrne.2008.03.003

Dubois, M., & Guaspare, C. (2020). From cellular memory to the memory of trauma: Social epigenetics and its public circulation. *Social Science Information*, 59(1), 144–83. https://doi.org/10.1177/0539018419897600

Heim, D., Hunter, S. C., & Jones, R. (2011). Perceived discrimination, identification, social capital, and well-being: Relationships with physical health and psychological distress in a U.K. minority ethnic community sample. *Journal of Cross-Cultural Psychology*, 42(7), 1145–64. https://doi.org/10.1177/0022022110383310

Ikram, U. Z., Mackenbach, J. P., Harding, S., Rey, G., Bhopal, R. S., Regidor, E., ... Kunst, A. E. (2016). All-cause and cause-specific mortality of different migrant populations in Europe. *European Journal of Epidemiology, 31*(7), 655–65. https://doi.org/10.1007/s10654-015-0083-9

Kelly, Y., Becares, L., & Nazroo, J. (2013). Associations between maternal experiences of racism and early child health and development: Findings from the UK Millennium Cohort Study. *Journal of Epidemiology and Community Health, 67*(1), 35–41. https://doi.org/10.1136/jech-2011-200814

McGuinness, D., McGlynn, L. M., Johnson, P. C. D., MacIntyre, A., Batty, G. D., Burns, H., ... Shiels, P. G. (2012). Socio-economic status is associated with epigenetic differences in the pSoBid cohort. *International Journal of Epidemiology, 41*(1), 151–60. https://doi.org/10.1093/ije/dyr215

Menzies, P. (2009). Homeless Aboriginal men: Effects of intergenerational trauma. *Finding home: Policy options for addressing homelessness in Canada* (pp. 1–25). Toronto: Cities Centre, University of Toronto.

Office for National Statistics. (2022). *Household total wealth in Great Britain: April 2018 to March 2020.* Retrieved 30 Sep 2022 from https://www.ons.gov.uk/peoplepopulationandcommunity/personalandhouseholdfinances/incomeandwealth/bulletins/totalwealthingreatbritain/april2018tomarch2020

Paradies, Y., Ben, J., Denson, N., Elias, A., Priest, N., Pieterse, A., ... Gee, G. (2015). Racism as a determinant of health: A systematic review and meta-analysis. *PLOS ONE, 10*(9), e0138511. https://doi.org/10.1371/journal.pone.0138511

Priest, N., Paradies, Y., Trenerry, B., Truong, M., Karlsen, S., & Kelly, Y. (2013). A systematic review of studies examining the relationship between reported racism and health and wellbeing for children and young people. *Social Science & Medicine, 95,* 115–27. https://doi.org/https://doi.org/10.1016/j.socscimed.2012.11.031

Sullivan, E. L., Smith, M. S., & Grove, K. L. (2011). Perinatal exposure to high-fat diet programs energy balance, metabolism and behavior in adulthood. *Neuroendocrinology, 93*(1), 1–8. https://doi.org/10.1159/000322038

Tajfel, H. & Turner, J. C. (eds.), (2010) *Social Identity and Intergroup Relations* (reissue edition). Cambridge University Press.

The King's Fund. (2022). *What are health inequalities?* Retrieved 30 Sep 2022 from www.kingsfund.org.uk/publications/what-are-health-inequalities#life

The World Bank. (2022). *Mortality rate, infant (per 1,000 live births).* Retrieved 30 Sep 2022 from https://data.worldbank.org/indicator/SP.DYN.IMRT.IN

World Population Review. (2022). *GDP Ranked by Country 2022.* Retrieved 30 Sep 2022 from https://worldpopulationreview.com/countries/countries-by-gdp

4
THE CELL-TO-SOCIETY OF THE LIFE COURSE

INTRODUCTION

The aim of this chapter[1] is to cover the cell-to-society factors of health from fertilised egg to death in very old age, and introduce you to how biopsychosocial factors influence development and health. Within the earlier sections (embryo, baby, child) the prime focus is on the coverage of the development of the brain, how and when things may go very well or very poorly, and how these have correlates with health. The teen section will cover the biological developmental factors of health, and how changes in brain development influence behavioural changes, and ultimately health. The young adult section will discuss the influence of work on health, as well as other life events that are both influencers of and influenced by health issues (such as fertility and parenthood). The final two sections will discuss key factors of ageing that are relevant to biopsychosocial gradients of health such as menopause and immunosenescence.

---

1 This chapter was developed with the excellent advice and support of Dr Samantha Dockray, a remarkable academic whose expertise and support have been extremely valuable both in the development of this book, and in my own development as an academic. Thank you, Samantha.

Learning Outcomes

- Understand how major influences on health differ across the life course.
- Have an appreciation of critical points where health outcomes can be impacted by biological, psychological, and social influences across the life course.
- Appreciate the ways that social and environmental influences on health may change over time, and how others may remain providing lifelong influence.

EARLY LIFE

When it comes to understanding how health is made and impacted during early life, it is important to remember that this is probably the only part of any human's life on which their own personal conduct has very little impact – or, rather, that seeing as their own personal conduct is so very limited due to infancy, this is one aspect of health influence that we can more or less rule out at this stage. In the very early beginnings of life, the developing cells that eventually turn into a baby are most influenced by their direct environment. In this case, that is the uterine environment, which is largely dictated by the health, environment, and experiences of the pregnant person.[2] Once born, the baby is still very limited in their ability to survive independently, so influences on their health and their brain development are now the result of their lived environment, the influences of those people that are in their life, and the choices that are made on the behalf of the baby by their caregiver(s).

You should have picked up by now that the brain has a great deal to do with how our bodies and health function. So much of our health relies on the way that our brains receive, interpret, and react to our environments. In this way, some of the best ways we can make sense of health influences in very early life come from understanding how our brains are built, and what factors may influence that development either to advantage or disadvantage.

---

2 The term 'parent' is very socially loaded. There are many people that carry a foetus to full term who may not identify with being the parent of the child after birth. 'Pregnant person' is used in this chapter to denote the person that gestates and carries the foetus to full term and birth, but remember that someone who does this may not ultimately be the parent, guardian, or caregiver of that child after birth.

The Embryo and the Foetus

Building a brain relies on five distinct stages of neural cellular development. A fertilised egg (**blastocyst**) is considered an embryo once the beginnings of the amniotic sac start to develop, and is called an **embryo** until week 11 of gestation, at which point it is then referred to as a **foetus**. In the embryonic stage, templates for future structures such as the central nervous system and vital organs are created. During the foetal stage, these templates are 'filled' with iterative phases of cellular production, growth, and maturation to create functioning organs, and networks within the body.

First, neurons are created. This is referred to as **proliferation** or sometimes **neurogenesis**. This happens in a huge flurry of activity in the early weeks of gestation. It is currently accepted that this starts at about week 10 post conception, and decreases in speed at about week 18, but neurogenesis continues even after birth. In fact, we create neurons throughout our lifetime, so this process never really stops, but it is at its most productive whilst we are building the brain. Once we have started to create the neurons we need, we then need to start building the three-dimensional architecture of the brain, and this is done through the process of **migration** (see Figure 4.1). Migration happens very quickly after neurons start to be created, and continues well into the later term of gestation. It is facilitated by the radial positioning of supporting cells within the brain (referred to as **glia**), which the neurons travel across to reach distal areas of the future brain structure. Once in place, these very basic neurons are then developed to create neuronal specialisation in a process called **differentiation**. This is what makes a motor neuron different from a sensory neuron, and what will ensure the fundamental underlying networks of communication that give our brains the skills they have. This process creates the neuron's physical characteristics (its **morphology**) as well initiating the final stages of neuronal maturation. Within this last stage, there are two other critical processes: **myelination** and **synaptogenesis**. Myelination refers to laying down of *myelin* (essentially fatty coatings) of the axons of the neuron. The axons of a neuron send electrical impulses from the head of the neuron (the **soma**, or cell body – where the nucleus and cellular machinery are present) to the ends where they can communicate with other neurons. These axons can be incredibly short, but also can be very long too, and they create the networks across the brain (and throughout our nervous systems as well). Myelin is created by glia, and serves two functions: to facilitate electrical conductivity (to send the 'message' along the axon), and to protect it. As it is made of fats and proteins, it makes sense to initiate myelination after neurons have migrated to their final location to save weighing them down. The final part is synaptogenesis, which is where the connections between neurons are created. A 'junction' between one neuron

Left: Immature neurons migrate from the inner layer, where they were "born," to their destination between there and the outer layer. Right: A close-up of one of the neurons climbing a radial glial cell scaffold.

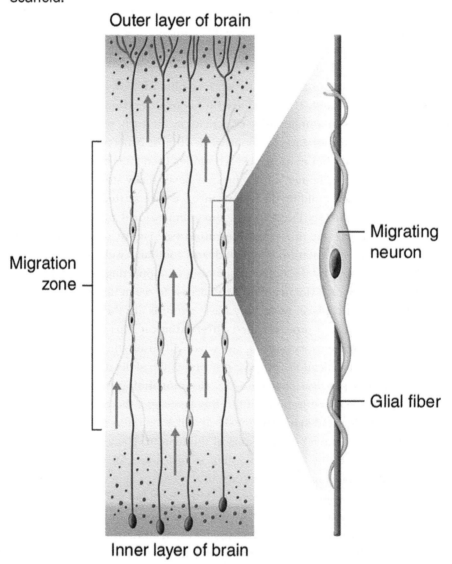

Figure 4.1   The process of neuronal migration. The neuron uses radial processes of glia to pull itself along to further out areas of the brain and central nervous system tissues.

Source: Garrett & Hough (2018), *Brain and Behavior: An Introduction to Behavioral Neuroscience*, Sage

and another is referred to as a synapse (see Figure 4.2). Here, the electrical impulse that is sent along the axon of a sending cell is converted into a chemical message by eliciting the release of neurotransmitters. These neurotransmitters are then 'received' by the next neuron to tell the next neuron what it should do. The phase of synaptogenesis is the initiation of the multiple connections between neurons across the brain. There is

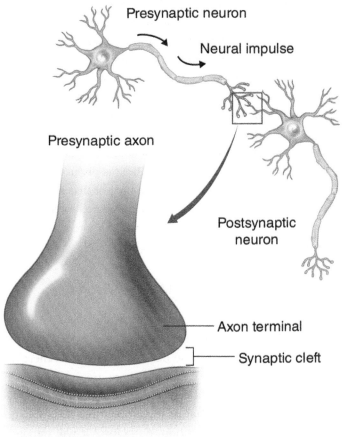

Notice the separation between the presynaptic axon terminal and the postsynaptic neuron.

Presynaptic neuron

Neural impulse

Presynaptic axon

Postsynaptic neuron

Axon terminal

Synaptic cleft

Postsynaptic neuron

Figure 4.2 Communication between neurons. The axon is wrapped in myelin, and the communication between neurons is facilitated electro-chemically. The synapse is the junction between neurons – you have billions of these in your nervous system.

Source: Garrett & Hough (2018), *Brain and Behavior: An Introduction to Behavioral Neuroscience*, Sage

a focus on quantity over quality at this stage, with a huge number of new connections being made in these very early stages of development. These latter stages of neuronal maturation tend to start at about 27 weeks' gestation and continue to beyond birth.

As the brain and central nervous system (and other structures such as vital organs) are being built through these processes, their functions will be enabled as soon as there is sufficient infrastructure and connection there to be able to support them. The need to connect systems, structures, and networks within the central nervous system drives the mass proliferation of synaptic connections (synaptogenesis), which occurs rapidly and intensely to support the incredibly diverse and complex functions that the future human will have. Brain development starts with the basics, and becomes more sophisticated as time progresses, in iterative stages of proliferation, migration, and maturation, in spurts and surges of inconsistent pace. The brain is developed from the inside out and from back to front, and this is because our most basic and fundamental life-sustaining functions are in the very deepest (and evolutionarily oldest) parts of our brains. It is quite a logical format really; there is very little need to be able to understand the complexities of hypothetical thought if you are not able to make the muscles in your ribs and diaphragm move to support your breathing. So, our brains start simple. This is important to note because the impact of external influences that can alter typical brain development, for example the damage resulting from being exposed to certain medications or alcohol (as discussed later), will depend on what parts of the brain are being developed at the time of that exposure. The earlier that damage may occur to a gestating embryo or foetus, the more fundamental the damage can be, as it affects the brain functions central to life as well as potentially damaging other vital organs that may be under development at the time.

Where Things May Go Wrong

The embryo/foetus cannot sustain life independently of the pregnant person. However, there are a variety of different factors that influence the way the embryo and foetus develop for better or worse. Some of these may be genetic, and there is very little that can be done to control or change those factors. There are, however, many factors that influence *in utero* development that can be changed or otherwise prevented, supported, or carefully managed. These types of factors tend to fall into three categories: exposure to disease, exposure to toxins, and nutrition. As before, it will depend at what point during gestation these incidents that induce damage or trauma (sometimes referred to as *insults*) occur as to what the resultant damage will be for the embryo or foetus.

A clear demonstration of the way that exposure to disease can impact the development of gestating foetuses unfortunately came from the outbreak of **Zika virus** of The Americas in 2015–16. Primarily transmitted through mosquito bites, the virus induces

Zika Fever in adults, a cold- or flu-like illness that is not generally fatal. The Zika virus is able to cross the placenta to a gestating foetus, and as a result we saw thousands of babies being born with *Congenital Zika Syndrome*, often characterised by *Microcephaly* (or being born with a very much smaller than typical head). Microcephaly is caused by a fundamental lack of sufficient brain development, which results in the cranium (upper portion of the skull that houses the brain) being significantly smaller, due to not having sufficient cerebral structure growing below to help form it. Microcephaly in and of itself results from an underdevelopment of brain structures, and is associated with a wide range of functional deficits, ranging from motor difficulties to intellectual disabilities to longer-term issues such as seizures. Congenital Zika Syndrome is also characterised by an atypically thin cerebral cortex, subcortical (deep brain) calcifications, atrophy to certain structures within the brain, overall asymmetry in the brain, and *hydrocephalus* (an over-accumulation of cerebrospinal fluid in the brain). Depending on when during gestation the Zika infection occurs, there can also be a complete absence of brain areas, and the development of profound brain conditions such as Cerebral Palsy in those born with Congenital Zika Syndrome. The damages that occur to the developing brain as a result of Zika exposure are irreparable, and we are still trying to understand the longer-term prognosis for those who were born during this time.

Foetal Alcohol Spectrum Disorder (FASD), previously referred to as Foetal Alcohol Syndrome (FAS), illustrates the potential damage of toxin exposure. Alcohol, like the Zika virus, can also be transmitted to the developing foetus through the pregnant person's bloodstream and past the placental barrier. Alcohol is a highly toxic substance that adults are able to successfully filter from their blood via their liver, meaning that a very large dose is required to fatally or critically damage an adult. A foetus' liver is one of the last organs to fully develop, primarily because other structures can be prioritised for development due to the protection provided by the placental barrier in preventing the passing of a whole variety of harmful microbes and substances from the pregnant person's bloodstream. Therefore, for a foetus, alcohol may remain far longer in the circulation, and also may be of much higher concentration, and so much more likely to cause damage. This is why there is such inconsistent and changeable advice on how much alcohol a pregnant person may be able to drink without potentially harming the foetus they are carrying. The condition of FASD is usually associated with chronic or prolonged consumption of alcohol throughout pregnancy, and impacts the foetus in very specific ways. Alcohol effectively interrupts or disturbs the development of networks in the brain, meaning there are a variety of functional, structural, and neurological impairments that may result. Like Zika, the timing of alcohol exposure during gestational development will determine what damage may occur. FASD is associated with microcephaly in some cases (as with Congenital Zika Syndrome), but also with a wide variety of other impacts on neurological, developmental, and cognitive function. There may be social and emotional issues as a result of FASD as certain areas of the brain responsible for emotion regulation may become damaged by *in utero* alcohol exposure, resulting in some children having difficulty in regulating their emotions, and in relating socially to those around them as they grow older. Various functional impairments may occur as well, with some children with FASD having issues with movement and balance, or with sensory processing such as vision and hearing. Cognitively, children with FASD may have impaired intellectual development, experience difficulty concentrating, or struggle to acquire knowledge or retrieve learned information. As a result of cognitive and emotional impacts, their behaviour may also be impacted, with some showing hyperactivity and issues with impulse control. Not only can the brain incur damage during development, but other organs in the body may as well, which can mean that children are born with defects or vulnerabilities to their heart, liver, kidneys, or even joints and muscles. It is also a condition of spectrum, meaning that there is a sliding scale with which the damage may occur, and therefore many children are affected to a lesser extent that may be less easy to detect. This means that there are likely many more children who have FASD-type damage that may not be diagnosed and reported. These issues resultant from foetal alcohol exposure continue to adulthood, and whilst the ability for the brain to compensate for some of these deficits may be seen post birth, some of them may remain for the life course.

In the case of nutrition, we know that a well-rounded diet full of the nutrients that support our physiological functioning is needed at any age, but during gestation nutrition requires much finer tuning, and can have immediate and significant effects the development of the embryo/foetus. One condition that we know is associated with nutrient intake is *Spina Bifida*, a condition characterised by the incomplete formation of the membrane layers around the spinal cord in the early stages of pregnancy, usually present in the lower portion of the spine. Whilst there are genetic factors associated with the likelihood of developing Spina Bifida, we also know that it is much more likely to occur when the pregnant person does not consume enough folate (sometimes referred to as Folic Acid, it is essentially vitamin B9) before and during early pregnancy. As a result, a baby with Spina Bifida may experience a vast range of functional issues, such as impaired bladder or bowel control, impaired lower limb function, and sometimes brain issues such as hydrocephalus. Having sufficient levels of folate before and during the early stages of pregnancy is recommended to prevent the majority of potential cases of Spina Bifida. Nutrient impact on developing foetuses is not just about getting enough vitamins, sometimes it is also about having just the right amount. In the case of retinol (vitamin A), if the pregnant person does not consume enough of it, the baby might be born blind, but if they consume too much of it, this can result in other birth defects such as malformations of the central nervous and cardiovascular systems. This is one of the many reasons that there are very specific multivitamin supplements designed for those who are planning to become or who are pregnant.

Key Questions

Have a think now about the various influences on *in utero* development. Reflect on all the processes that you have learned from the previous three chapters when considering this. Whilst the developing foetus has no control over these aspects, how much control do you think the pregnant person has?

- Consider the various layers of the health onion and where some of these influences may be more or less common.
- What social or societal situations and contexts can be changed to help reduce the potential for these health influences?

The Baby and the Child[3]

Once born, there are very many more influences on the development of a baby. They are able to interact with the world around them, they will often encounter many people, and their social and emotional development begins alongside their continuing physiological development. After birth, the greatest amount of brain development happens through the neuron maturation phases – synaptogenesis and myelination. At birth, a human brain is about 400g, about a third of its future adult weight, meaning a relatively good chunk of brain growth has already occurred at this very early stage. Whilst some of the senses begin to develop *in utero*, it is after birth that they begin to come fully online. Vision is very poor to begin with, but develops significantly in the first six months after birth. Hearing is also rather rudimentary at birth, but at this early stage the baby will have a preference for its pregnant parent's language. The cerebral cortex begins to myelinate to facilitate much of this 'switching on' of sensory functions, followed by motor areas thereafter. Myelination increases rapidly up to two years old, but actually continues up to 30 years of age as your brain continues to develop. Growth and development of the brain at this stage tends to be due to the increasing size of neurons and the growing number of glia (supporting cells in the brain) and their deposition of myelin onto neuronal axons, and this (like all infant human growth) tends to happen in spurts.

---

3 Ruby, you were about 10 months old when I wrote this (because I was massively behind on schedule, you should have been no more than six months old really). At this point your favourite things were grabbing my hair and kicking me, which I hope won't still be the case by the time you eventually read this. I'm sure you will be just as adorable though.

One of the key aspects of this stage of brain development is the preferential enhancement of well-used motor circuits. In these very early stages of life (from pre-birth up to a few years after birth) there is an explosion of network connections being made across the central nervous system (through the expansion of neuronal dendrites and synaptogenesis). This is very much a quantity over quality arrangement. Effectively, the growing organism (and this goes for other vertebrates too, not just infant humans) tends to wire almost everything up, creating over 50% more connections than we will ever really need. Over time as these circuits are used more and more, those that are used more frequently are preferentially supported, and those that are used less may be subject to a process called **pruning**. Think of it a bit like when you might study a new topic – you will head off to the internet to find as many papers as you possibly can on the topic you are interested in (quantity over quality). Over time, and as you start to mould and shape what aspects of your topic you are interested in, there will be some resources that are very important (and used all the time), some that are quite important (used sometimes, but not critical), and some that no longer serve the purpose you need. At this stage, you may well end up deleting those resources you no longer need in order to concentrate on those that you do. This is exactly the principle of neuronal network establishment and refinement. We connect everything up we possibly can, just in case we need it, and then through the process of understanding which routes and pathways are most used, we prune away those connections that are not used enough. I know this seems a bit of a shame – if we could retain all of those connections, how smart we would be! Well, yes and no. We may well have a superbly connected brain, but those connections would never be developed sufficiently to allow fast and efficient use of those pathways. We would end up with a neuronal map of thoroughly connected but very slow and sluggish pathways. Instead, our brains strike a beautiful balance of multiple well-served connections. So, at some point we switch to quality over quantity. The process of pruning is facilitated by a cellular mechanism called **apoptosis** (also referred to as 'programmed cell death'). Apoptosis is a very normal, healthy cellular process. In the case of neural pruning, it occurs in our nervous systems, but apoptosis actually occurs everywhere in your body. As an adult, you lose about 50–70 billion cells each and every day due to apoptosis; for a child this number is about 20–30 billion across the whole body. Apoptosis is needed to ensure that your cells are functioning at their best. Our cells (like us) age, and as we all may know, when you age your function may well decrease. As a result, apoptosis helps to ensure that at any one given time our cells are working in tip top condition, clearing out those that are getting a bit old and tired. During the pruning stage, it is not because your neurons have got old and tired of course, it is triggered by them not being used. Apoptosis in neurons occurs by the cell secreting a signalling chemical on its membrane. This chemical attracts brain-based immune cells called *microglia* (the cleaners of the brain) to munch them up and clear them away. Those neurons that start to initiate the process of apoptosis during pruning are most likely to be those that have made non-useful or incorrect connections (for example, your visual centre does not need to be connected to the neurons that move your toes). Once they have been cleared away, the space left over can then be grown into by those neurons and connections that are being used – allowing them to grow strong and fast. An interesting example of how neuronal pruning can be observed in children comes from work looking at the ability of infants to discriminate between phonemes, the very distinct hard sounds in any given language (for example, the sound of 't' that makes the words 'cat', 'cab', and 'cap' sound different). You may have come across the work of Werker and Tees (1984) if you have studied any aspects of developmental or cognitive psychology. Their work was pivotal in developing the understanding how speech perception is organised and refined in the developing brain. They found that infants around six to eight months old could distinguish between some of the characteristic phonemes in various distinct languages (this was indicated by conditioning a response to turn the head on hearing a novel sound), but after a year those infants were far less able to distinguish between phonemes of languages that they were not used to hearing (i.e., not any of the languages spoken in their family home). This is also partly the reason that if you are learning a language that is very different from your own, you may not be able to physically create the sounds used in that language. Think of the language Xhosa spoken in South Africa. This language includes very distinct clicking sounds not present in many other languages across the world. If you don't learn how to create (and – critically – practice creating) that sound in early life, then chances are you will never be able to truly create it as an adult if you are learning. So, neuronal connections and the functions and processes they support are a tale of survival of the fittest. Use it or lose it!

The Importance of Social-Emotional Development

As in the previous section, the infant brain is also extremely vulnerable to impact from malnutrition, toxins, and pathogens that can be encountered. Many illnesses that would be manageable in adults can prove to be catastrophic for the developing baby's brain. Things like hypothyroidism (the insufficient functioning of the thyroid), the experience of fevers, and having low blood sugar can all cause illness in adults, but are capable of causing irreparable damage to the developing brain in early life, so care must still be taken after birth to keep the baby safe from harmful situations. Not only this, but the development of the brain is now highly dependent not just on being kept safe and adequately nourished, it is also responsive to the social and psychological experiences of living too. A stimulating environment for a child can make the difference between a 25% greater ability to learn or 25% less in an environment with little stimulation. In studies that have examined the neurological consequences for children who have unfortunately been subject to abuse, we now know that such abuse can seriously (and, in some cases, irreparably) inhibit the development of the brain. So as we saw in previous chapters, where our environments influence the way that our genes, our cells, and our internal systems work, much of the way our brain develops and functions is also influenced by our environment. This is a term referred to as 'neuroconstructionism', and is another aspect of how our lives and health are never entirely predetermined by any biological factors. A word of warning: some of the following may not make for easy reading as it contains references to abuse and neglect.

Where Things May Go Wrong

One of the most important social mechanisms for supporting brain development is through the process of *serve and return*. Serve and return is about the reciprocal gestures babies make with their immediate caregivers and other regularly appearing humans (such as siblings, aunts, uncles, grandparents, friends etc.). These gestures are usually eye contact and facial expressions in very early life, but move on (as the baby's capabilities develop) to touch, sound, and movement too. Many of us when faced with a cute smiling baby will find it impossible to do anything but smile back (and possibly make some cute burbling noises as well to try and make that smile bigger), but for some babies their facial expressions and initiations of reciprocal emotional displays will not be returned. This can happen for a variety of reasons, both involuntary and deliberate. In the case of post-natal depression or following traumatic births, parents may find it very hard to respond with outward displays of positive emotions whilst their internal state is in so much pain. For this reason, and for the sake of the mental health of the parent who is suffering, there should be a lot of support given to the adult in such cases, as these can often be made worse by the parent's guilt about being unable to meet the emotional needs of their child. There are also situations where there may be deliberate neglect and abuse, where the baby's initiations of reciprocal emotional display are deliberately not met, or are otherwise countered with negative emotional displays instead. Unreliable, inappropriate, or absent reciprocal behaviours can disrupt the development of the brain through both a lack of positive stimulation and the induction of stress or distress.

For cases of neglect, we can consider that neglect can be both emotional and cognitive, and there are often underlying mitigating factors in these cases (for example, parental depression), and it is a minority occurrence of cases of overt and deliberate neglect. Emotional and cognitive neglect can result from limited exposure to language (and attempts at conversation), to touch and emotional communication, or social interaction altogether. We know that this type of neglect results in structural differences in those children and adults who have those experiences in childhood compared to children who receive typical levels and varieties of emotional and cognitive stimulation. Studies have shown that those people who have experienced neglect are more likely to have a lack of brain growth beyond what has been seen through poor nutrition, and neuronal depletion beyond that which normally occurs through pruning. Some of the most powerful evidence we have of the neurodevelopmental effects of neglect comes from studies that have followed the progress of children from Romanian orphanages in the Bucharest Early Intervention Project (2022). This project was initially a joint collaboration between researchers at Tulane University, University of Maryland, and Boston Children's Hospital to follow children from these institutions to understand the impact of their early deprivation, and (in some cases) whether this could be remedied by being adopted into high-quality foster care. This project has been quite controversial for a number of reasons, but has shown us a great deal about the potential damage that can be done through the environmental and social under-nourishment of children. Amongst the wealth of publications that have come out from research in this project, it has been found that there are areas of stunted white matter (i.e., axons, the connections between neurons) volume in several areas of the brain relating to emotion and behaviour (limbic system), cognitive functioning (frontostriatal circuit), sensory processing (medial lemniscus), and structures essential for interconnectivity (such as the corpus callosum, corona radiata, and retrolenticular internal capsule) (Bick et al., 2015). Over time, those children who were able to go into high-quality foster care showed some normalisation of these deficits. The timing of the exposure to neglect and intervention is critical here, however. As with other examples of brain development influences, when this happened (and what is being developed at that time) will be very much related to the potential outcomes. Similarly, when the intervention occurred will also have an impact on the potential outcomes as well. Some of these children are still being followed today, and we are still trying to understand the consequences for their mental and physical health as a result of being institutionalised, and which impacts – if any – may normalise over time when the children are provided with a loving and stimulating environment.

Alongside the evident consequences to brain development that appear to be associated with a lack of supportive, caring environments and relationships, there are also the potentially toxic effects of stress and distress that have a bearing on the developing brain, and consequently life course correlates of mental and physical health. Stress in adulthood is more or less everywhere. If we don't experience enough of it, we are in some ways certain to seek it out ourselves in one way or another. However, in childhood, the experience of stress should be less frequent and ubiquitous, but it can, in some cases, prove damaging to the brain long term. This is referred to as *toxic stress*, and is usually stress is either extensive and/or prolonged, and may also occur as a result of the absence of adequate support from loved ones. Much like the insults to brain development that can happen *in utero*, the timing of toxic stress experience during child development will impact what longer term outcomes may result. In the case of abuse, children can overdevelop areas of their brains relating to fear, anxiety, and impulsive behaviours, along with underdevelopment of areas associated with love, happiness, and longer-term planning.

This is, therefore, a bit of a double whammy of damage, with areas that reinforce negative emotions and behaviours being prioritised, and areas that support positive emotions and behaviours being under-prioritised. If you consider this in relation to key stages of neural pruning, this could potentially have very long-lasting implications indeed. Not only this, but chronic exposure to stress in childhood (and this stress can be environmental, interpersonal, or the type of multifaceted stress associated with childhood poverty) can also alter the hormonal stress response such that it will be initiated at lower levels of psychological stress, potentially harming all of the other systems that this hormonal axis interacts with as well (more on this in Chapter 5). Neural circuits that deal with stress are highly adaptable (*plastic*) during childhood, and they can adapt very quickly to 'expect' stress, and this is more likely to occur when a child experiences persistent or repeated stress. Similarly, hormonal systems that support the stress response and other physiological functions associated with it (as we have discovered, almost all other systems) can also become chronically dysregulated through over-exposure to toxic stress. High exposure to toxic stress in childhood can impact the person across all domains of their life, including behaviour (anger, impulsivity), cognition (learning, memory), psychological function (depression, anxiety), neurological processes (delayed or altered development), and physiological processes (hormonal dysregulation), and these impacts can be experienced across the entire life course. Some of these changes are neurobiological in nature (with areas of the brain being over-/under-developed in response to the psychosocial environment), and some are through epigenetic changes. Recent evidence has shown that DNA methylation from childhood trauma is associated with a huge array of health and wellbeing outcomes up to 17 years later (van den Oord et al., 2022). Toxic stress in childhood is so reliably associated with health problems in adulthood such as cardiovascular disease, diabetes, substance abuse and dependence disorders, and anxiety and depression, that many studies that seek to understand the aetiology of these conditions need to take into account what is referred to as **ACEs** (**A**dverse **C**hildhood **E**xperiences).

Where Things Can Go Better than Expected

Ever since there have been parents, there have been concerted efforts to understand how babies can be given an extra boost to their development, to give them the best possible start in life. Whilst there have been techniques developed to facilitate neurological and cognitive development to help accelerate brain development, such as the practice of hothousing, where children are given intensive and extensive study of certain topics or activities to enhance learning and cognitive capacity, these are not consistently well supported in the available research. Other methods of attempting to increase cognitive development come from environmental enrichment, in the form of brightly coloured toys or exposure to music, but the evidence here is also somewhat weak and very frequently mixed. However, newer brain imaging technologies available in recent years have allowed us the opportunity to really see how and whether such interventions can enhance biological brain development. There is a whole host of developmental techniques to ensure optimum experiences and care for every child to have healthy, positive development, but as examples I will focus on two that are particularly well-researched and supported: the benefits of learning to play music, and learning other (or several other) languages.

Studies that examine the brains of musically trained adults have shown that they tend to have much more highly connected brains than those who do not play a musical instrument. Unsurprisingly enough, areas that show higher development tend to be associated with sound, with some musically trained adults having up to 30% larger temporal cortices (Schneider et al., 2002). This is not just an advantage for super-hearing, however, as this area of the brain is responsible for a variety of other processes as well, including memory. In a study seeking to understand the potential benefits of musical training on cortical activity in children, Habibi and colleagues (2016) decided to track the progress of children who had been provided with specialised musical training called *El Sistema*. In order to understand whether it was actually music, or whether it was just some sort of enriching extra-curricular activity that may provide benefits, they took three groups of equally matched children (matched in socio-economic status and age). One third received the musical training, another received some sports training, and the other group just experienced their normal day-to-day activities. Prior to the intervention, there were no differences in cognitive task scores or EEG activity between each of the groups. After two years of these activities, the researchers tested the children's auditory discrimination using *event-related potentials* (ERPs: electrical impulses recorded on the scalp that indicate neuronal activity in response to cognitive processes). Children in the music group performed better at auditory discrimination tasks that were associated with determining different tones. As would be expected with growing children, all groups showed greater reactivity to different tones, but the ERPs of the musically trained children were more similar to older, more developed children providing some evidence that musical training accelerates the maturation of auditory processing. Importantly, this study also included sports-related training, and this is important because we also know that physical activity has been shown to be as relevant to cognitive development in children, as it is to their physical development (Khan & Hillman, 2014). When children learn to play music, their brains begin to hear and process sounds that they couldn't otherwise hear. They also learn and refine their physical dexterity (which can also be enhanced through physical activity). This auditory aspect helps them develop 'neurophysiological distinction' between certain sounds that can aid literacy. Children with one to five years of musical training were able to remember 20% more vocabulary words read to them off a list than children without such training. Advanced growth in areas associated with motor and auditory skills have been shown in comparison to children participating in singing/percussion classes (Hyde et al., 2009). Just three years of musical training in childhood produces measurable differences in brain response to sound (Skoe & Kraus, 2012). Providing musical training to children can be very expensive, however, so it is definitely worthwhile noting that there are also comparable cognitive benefits to engaging in physical activity throughout child development that have been evidenced in both neuropsychological tests and brain imaging studies (Khan & Hillman, 2014).

Multilingualism is another gift for the brain development of children, if not also for the future benefits that being able to communicate with many more people, and to develop a deeper understanding of many more cultures, that speaking other languages provides. There are many cultures where learning languages is cemented into compulsory education; however, some individuals start learning more than one language from birth if they are in a multilingual household. Learning more than one language from birth was initially thought to be a bad thing for children's brain development. It was thought that acquiring, retaining, and using more than one language would be cognitively too complex, and would lead to children not developing sufficiently in any of the languages that were being attempted. However, recent studies have shown that the brains of multilingual children are more highly connected, and process information much quicker than those who are monolingual. Multiple language acquisition from birth has the strongest effect on the brain; however, secondary language acquisition later in life also enhances brain connectivity and efficiency (Mohades et al., 2012). It is never too late to get the cognitive, social, and experiential benefits of learning another language.

Key Questions

We have seen through out this section how the social and psychological environment of the child can impact the way its brain develops, and the consequences this can have for health in the future. Whilst the baby has no control over these aspects, how much control do you think the parent, guardian, or other caregiver has? As before, think back to the first three chapters of this book and what you have learned from them, and consider some of the aspects you may have covered in the previous key questions activity in this chapter.

- Consider the various layers of the health onion and where some of these influences may be more or less common.
- What social or societal situations and contexts can be changed to help reduce the potential for these health influences?

The Teen and the Young Adult

Much could be written to make sense of the various twists and turns of this period, and how this affects health across the life course. The following will be quite brief. It will be focused on typically developing cisgender children, but will also likely be relatable to those with different identities and developments. I have included some recommended reading at the end of this chapter that will help to start you on a track to learning more about development in other identities and experiences.

At this stage in development, where the young person becomes more individualised and independent, the impact of their personal choices and preferences starts to become just as important in shaping their health as the more long-standing influences of the social-emotional environment directed by their caregivers. It is perhaps the time in someone's life where the bio, psycho, and social are closest interlinked, with clear and strong multidirectional relationships between those three health influences. What happens to the person at this stage can also shape not just their physical and mental health across the life course, but also their social status and 'fit' within the world, setting the lifelong tone for their position in society, and their chances and opportunities for inclusion, exclusion, and equity.

One of the largest hallmarks of this stage of development is the onset of **puberty**, and all the changes that brings both physically and psychologically. There are increases in circulating levels of gonadal hormones such as **testosterone, oestrogen**, and **progesterone**, and these increases initiate physiological changes that will facilitate development of the reproductive system. The increase and fluctuation of these hormones causes a variety of cellular-and systems-level changes in the developing adolescent that contributes to their overall health and wellbeing. Some of these changes are necessary to facilitate the future capability of the person to create new life, and some are side-effects in those processes. As we saw in previous chapters (particularly Chapter 2), all our internal systems are intimately interlinked. You simply cannot play around with one system without there being a subsequent impact on others, and that is precisely what puberty is. Puberty starts when there is a healthy and sufficient level of communication within your **hypothalamic-pituitary-gonadal axis**. The communication between the pituitary and hypothalamus (which also communicate for other endocrine functions such as the stress response) links to the gonads also (the ovaries or the testes). It is a delicate and intricate cascade of hormones that communicate between these structures, allowing the onset of sexual maturation (overviews here: DiVall & Radovick, 2009; Lewis & Lee, 2009). There are many hormones involved in these processes aside from the big-hitter sex hormones listed above, and they all have multiple functions and can create multiple consequential effects on other systems in the body. If we take just the three big steroid hormones and look at the non-pubertal/non-sexual impacts they can have, this may give you some clue as to the remarkable and quite rapid physiological changes that happen during this stage of life. Oestrogen, testosterone, and progesterone are implicated in the maintenance of every system in your body. They are involved in the regulation of the sleep/wake cycle, in bone development/maintenance, the maintenance of blood sugar levels, circulation and blood flow, muscle mass and tone, cognitive functions, collagen production (which supports healthy joints, but also the overall functioning of your skin), and communicate with your immune system cells (Morales-Montor et al., 2011; Shah, 2018). It is no wonder that this period of life (and other periods of life where these hormones change, such as menopause) is so often represented as dramatic, but most young people experience these psychological, emotional, and physiological changes without too much disruption or discontent, although it can be a period of enhanced vulnerability for some young people.

Not only do young people need to adapt to these biological changes, but their health and wellbeing can also be affected by the subjective reactions to those changes, both personally and interpersonally as these changes are accompanied by an enhanced sensitivity to social experience. There are the psychological reactions to the changing body that can and will shape their mental health, their health choices, and ultimately their overall health. This stage can be influenced strongly by culture. Earlier maturing girls, whilst initially reporting more body satisfaction, can be more vulnerable to emotional and behavioural problems (e.g., depression, eating disorders, engaging in risky behaviours, and early sexual behaviour) (Wiesner & Ittel, 2002). This is partly due to earlier maturing girls socialising with older peers where they are drawn into riskier behaviours through peer influence without necessarily having the emotional maturity to counterbalance actions with consequences long term. The impact of earlier puberty on boys has been less consistently described, but recent work has suggested that it is associated with similar negative outcomes, and that these relationships for both boys and girls are due to the discrepancy between physiological and social development (Mendle & Ferrero, 2012). Early puberty and its effects on a variety of outcomes (from health to occupational and educational domains) has been contested over the years. There are theories that early puberty may alter cognitive and social developmental trajectories, or that it may simply amplify pre-existing adverse conditions, or that these outcomes may depend on the social-environmental context that the developing person is in. A wealth of aging literature has been relatively negative in the prospects of those who develop early, with suggestions that this impacts educational attainment and future employment prospects (initiating all of the other social and cultural impacts that these factors have on health), but a recent review suggests that this may only be the case when the environment context in some way exacerbates the potential adverse social and interpersonal aspects of early maturation (from peers, parents, and teachers) (Laube & Fuhrmann, 2020).

The consequences of early or late maturation may not last into adulthood, but could have repercussions that have lifespan implications if they impact interpersonal relationships, the ability to engage with education, or the motivation or confidence of the person.

During the teen years, the brain is still developing, but most of this development is focused on 'higher' brain areas that are located at the very front and/or very outermost regions of the brain. This is a period of time characterised by more pruning in these higher areas, with this refinement continuing until the age of 25.[4] Interestingly, and somewhat obviously to anyone who may have spent time with a teen, there can be a mismatch between what hormones are making the brain interested in, and what brain development is making the person capable of handling, both emotionally and cognitively. The influx of pubertal hormones creates emotional arousal of far higher intensity and far lower set-point, and all the while the areas of the brain responsible for impulse control, for careful, forward planning, and for reward/risk monitoring are very far from being fully developed. We have two main growth 'spurts' of the brain during adolescence. One during ages 13–15 where the cortex becomes thicker, and neuronal communication becomes more efficient as pathways strengthen and consolidate (through pruning). There is an accompanying rapid development in motor and spatial areas of the brain also. This period is characterised by a massive amount of glucose metabolism in the brain – the largest amount in the whole lifetime. The second spurt occurs at about 17 continuing to early adulthood. Here, the frontal lobes of the cortex develop, providing enhancements to problem solving, logic, and planning. Our judgement is probably the very last thing to finalise in terms of our neural development between 20 and 25 (Gogtay et al., 2004).

Sensation seeking is at a peak during adolescence, and can lead to reckless behaviour in some cases, which has direct implications for health. Risky behaviours are lauded by peers, and are therefore sought after more; they also distance the individual from parental or societal control, so they form an important part of the developing identity of the adolescent as an autonomous and distinct individual. This drive to autonomy is compensated for later by the developing areas of the pre-frontal cortex that govern judgement and problem solving. Teens are more likely to make risky choices than adults, and this is illustrated by a broad literature showing comparatively high rates of unprotected sex, accidents, and drug abuse amongst others. At this stage, teenagers may know the risk, but emotional and social factors may overcome the perception of likelihood or severity of that risk (Crone & van der Molen, 2004; Slovic, 1998; Steinberg, 2007). Not only this, but risk taking can be enhanced by societal perceptions and expectations.

---

4 We are legally capable and socially expected to be doing a great deal before this age. It is interesting to think that both legal and social expectations on individuals have not adjusted in line with our enhanced understanding of how long it takes brains to develop these critical judgment and impulse inhibition capabilities.

Media portrayals of teens as risk takers are likely to be attended to more by those that are higher in sensation seeking (Greene et al., 2002), making exposure to these common narratives potentially more harmful for those already pre-disposed to risky behaviour. Risky behaviours also often compound, with research finding that risky behaviours such as risky driving being far more likely in those that already engage in other risky behaviours such as early onset tobacco, alcohol, or marijuana use (Shope & Bingham, 2008). It is important to note, however, that common cultural narratives and media depictions of puberty and teen-aged years as being turbulent and altogether unpleasant for everyone involved are not generally characteristic of what happens. It is perhaps because of some of these narratives that some teens experience more distress during this developmental phase than they would otherwise have experienced if there were no expectations placed on them.

Key Questions

Consider the various factors that we have discussed that impact the health and development of adolescents. During this time, the influences on an adolescent are driven by their caregivers, but also by themselves. We often see key health issues arising in teens that can have lifelong consequences. Once again, also consider what you have learned in previous chapters and reflect on what you considered in the previous key questions activities in this chapter. To what extent do you think the teen/their parent or guardian has control over these factors? To what extent do you think society has a responsibility for creating or preventing these circumstances?

- Consider the various layers of the health onion and where some of these influences may be more or less common.
- What social or societal situations and contexts can be changed to help reduce the potential for these health influences?

Older Adulthood and the Oldest Old

Once we have cleared our period of adolescence, we then enter two rapidly passing decades of semi-stability (biologically speaking) before physiological changes set in once more. Adult life is bursting with opportunities for stress to seep into the body and impact health, and depending on where you fit in your particular society, the various factors that we see on the health onion will play a part in dictating your health and welfare. This time is usually characterised by working, which constitutes a significant source of stress for most people, but also a significant source of purpose and motivation. As well as being stressful (and potentially rewarding), our work can also be a meaningful mediator of health, with many pathways to poor or good health from the type of work you do, the context in which you work, and the support that is provided through your work for your health and wellbeing. The engagement in risky or hazardous work will have direct impacts on health if the person becomes injured or incapacitated at work, and depending on the extent of these injuries may have lifelong consequences for mental and physical health. Even work that is not necessarily risky, but requires a lot of manual activity, can be harmful to health over time, resulting in musculoskeletal injuries and damage. Those whose work requires rotating hours can have their health harmed through lack of proper sleep and the dysregulation of their sleep/wake cycles, which is associated with a variety of health outcomes such as diabetes, cardiovascular disease, and gastrointestinal disorders, as well as putting them at increased risk for workplace accidents when they are poorly rested (Costa, 2010). Work can be beneficial to health too, however. If we earn enough money to support a good lifestyle, and to keep us free from debt stress, this is a useful buffer to some of the stresses and strains that can cause us harm. If our employer has a suitable workplace health and wellbeing support package for their employees this may also have direct benefits in the form of financial support to seek specialised and general medical help when needed, and high-quality, rapid-access care. Equally, our employment may well allow the accrual of a supportive pension to support our health and wellbeing beyond the end of our working years. Of course, our work may also have none of these perks, which not only means we do not experience the benefits they can provide, but our health can also be impacted by the added stress that can be experienced through the daily and profound worry of debt stress, the inability to source healthcare, and the apprehension of managing on a small state pension in the future.

Some people may also choose to have a family, which similarly has its stresses and joys. The bearing and birth of children, and subsequent breastfeeding, can impact the person's chances of gynaecological and breast cancers in the future (Anderson et al., 2014). Similarly, the use of hormonal contraception has an impact on these types of cancer outcomes (White, 2018). Some people may have their family choices limited by financial constraints; others may have their financial choices limited by family constraints. Having children costs a significant amount of money, and that is if you are fortunate enough to have healthy children. Bringing up a child with extra needs, from either physical or developmental disability, can be extraordinarily expensive, adding to the additional strain experienced by just being a parent. Needing to care for another person, whether that is a child with additional needs or even a parent (which many in adulthood do), can also be a source of chronic stress. At the time of writing, around

6000 people a day in the UK take on a caring role (Carers UK, 2022) for a child, a parent, or another relative, and the overwhelming majority of the unpaid care burden falls on women. Caring in itself can be a richly rewarding and wonderful thing to do. Regardless of who it is for, the opportunity to support someone you love can be profoundly beneficial to both the person caring and the care recipient. Caregiving can also be extremely stressful, however. It can be so reliably stressful that it has served as a model for chronic stress in a huge volume of research over the last few decades. We will look at this more in Chapter 7, but it is an important aspect of family life to consider in understanding how health in adulthood can be impacted, particularly for those most frequently affected, and those most frequently affected by other societal inequalities that impact their health: women (I have included some important and highly recommended reading on this at the end of the chapter). Socially, caring for another may reduce opportunities for socialising with support networks as time is taken up with caring. There may also be increased pressures from work if employers or colleagues are not supportive in accommodating the need to provide care for another within that working role. This may also lead to financial strain, particularly if the person's job is not secure, or if extra costs are incurred as a result of caring (for example extra transport costs, unpaid leave, or if the care recipient needs financial support with groceries or other expenses). Psychologically, the changed dynamic between the carer and the care recipient may cause stress and worry. It may remind the carer of the care recipient's (and, indeed, their own) mortality. Depending on the needs of the care recipient, there also may be interpersonal issues that take their toll. If the care recipient is a child with a developmental disorder, or an adult with a cognitive impairment, challenging behaviour, emotional outbursts, and confusion can all create uncomfortable and distressing interpersonal scenarios. Simply seeing someone you love in a situation where they are so vulnerable, or witnessing a change in their capacity over time, can be a very distressing thing to have a front-row seat to. The changing dynamic between carer and care recipient, particularly when the care recipient is a parent or other older loved one, can be difficult for both to experience. Biologically, a whole host of things can occur in the prolonged stress of being a carer, and this will be the main focus of the discussion of this issue in Chapter 7.

Adulthood and older adulthood also include biological changes as we age. Everyone encounters hormonal changes as they age. For people with functioning ovaries and a uterus, there is a very specific and inevitable hormonal event – essentially a process – that occurs, whereas for those with functioning testes, ageing tends to happen steadily over time. The process I'm referring to here is the **menopause**. The fact that women have a very abrupt (biologically speaking) and ultimate change to their fertility status, whereas men do not, has been a question that has stumped scientists for a very long time.[5] There are a variety of theories as to why this might be the case, with very little consensus of opinion.

Regardless of the evolutionary reasons for this, the menopause constitutes a significant change of direction for health in the people that experience it. It is characterised by another large hormonal balance change, with a gradual waning of oestrogen starting from the mid-30s, and reduced fertility over time. Menopause as a medical phase is considered to have finished once menstruation has ceased for 12 consecutive months with no other medical mitigating factors, and this occurs at an average age of 51. However, endocrinologically, menopause continues to up to five years after this point with continued hormonal changes that have an impact on other bodily systems and functions. Menstrual cycles require highly regulated communication between the structures in the hypothalamic-pituitary-gonadal axis, and are reasonably well established one to three years after initiation of menstrual periods (also referred to as **menarche**) in adolescence. Menopause usually begins around four years before menstrual periods (menses) cease, and is characterised by increasing irregularity of menses, the intermittent stopping and re-starting of menses, and then eventually the ceasing of menses altogether. Along with this, the cyclical variability of the various hormones that support menstruation also de-regulate. With oestrogens and progesterone having monthly peaks, over time these peaks become more erratic and irregular, may be less high, and eventually even out so that these hormones are produced and circulated at a relatively constant rate. If you cast your mind back to the prior section where we looked at all the other physical functions and processes that are influenced by sex hormones, you can probably also imagine the various other physiological issues that may come along with fluctuating and then gradually decreasing levels of these hormones. Oestrogen is very important in a variety of physiological functions, including the maintenance of bone integrity and health, and in the general functioning of the immune system. It is because of this that we may often see people develop conditions like osteoporosis (a condition characterised by loss of bone density) and a variety of auto immune diseases post menopause.

Ageing is an inevitable part of life. However, we are living in a world with an increasing ageing population with a focus on the needs of the young, so many countries and cultures across the world experience highly stressed and unwell ageing groups. It is estimated that by 2050, there will be more older people than younger people in the world for the first time. In terms of population health, this already has important implications

5 I will refer to 'women' here for ease, but there are non-binary individuals and trans men who do not undergo hysterectomies or hormonal therapies and will experience menopause as well.

due to the general decline in functioning that happens in the ageing process, but can also have a descending impact on other generations that may need to support the care of these ageing people. In response to this, the United Nations has launched the Madrid International Plan of Action on Ageing (MPIAA), which seeks to tackle three key challenges: older persons and development; advancing health and wellbeing; and ensuring enabling and supportive environments (there will be more of this in Chapter 7). As with everything in the body, the immune system ages. This process is called **immunosenescence**. As the thymus ages, this changes the T-cell production and their function over time. This is partly due to the age-related degeneration of the thymus (**thymic involution**), but also due to *replicative senescence* caused by the **Hayflick limit** (the limit to the number of cell divisions a cell can undergo). Thymic involution is associated with the passing of time, but replicative senescence is less bound to time, and more associated with the amount of exposure we have had to pathogens (which might also be considered to be a function of time) (Castle, 2000). There is a change in the balance of pro-inflammatory and anti-inflammatory immune patterns over time (Pawelec et al., 2002), which can lead to difficulty in mounting effective responses to infections, as well as the increased likelihood of chronic illness. There will be more on this in Chapter 5. **Endocrinosenescence** refers to the ageing of the endocrine system. Not only do older people tend to have higher levels of anxiety and psychological stress, but we also see elevated **glucocorticoid** levels. These elevated stress hormone levels may play a part in thymic involution and general decline in white blood cells seen in older age, as we can see similar changes after younger people have been treated with glucocorticoids (Collaziol et al., 2004). Sex hormones also decline with age, and may also play a part in immunosenescence since oestrogen and testosterone can regulate some pro-inflammatory processes (Ershler & Keller, 2000). Cognitive decline also occurs in older age, accompanied sometimes by neurocognitive disorders associated with old age such as Alzheimer's Disease and various types of dementia. Some cognitive decline has been associated with sedentary behaviours (Wheeler et al., 2017), meaning that exercise – as helpful as it is in childhood development – can continue to be supportive of good health for brain and body across the life course.

Alongside the general processes of biological ageing that impact health, there are also specific psychosocial stressors associated with being at an older age that impact health. Generally speaking, mental health is more vulnerable in older age, with the likelihood of anxiety, depression, and **loneliness** increasing as we age (Singh & Misra, 2009). Add onto that the decreased mobility, increased likelihood of bereavement, decreased financial independence, loss of social role in retirement, and cognitive decline – there is a lot to consider in terms of how the social and psychological environment may influence health outcomes at this stage of life. In many countries and cultures across the world, the oldest of our society tend to be less protected and less well-served than other demographics. In some countries, there are few or no laws that protect elders from abuse, and in very rural or poor areas, the problems that many adults encounter in regard to having easily accessible healthcare can be very much more complicated for those who are less mobile and autonomous. Loneliness, neglect, and psychosocial stress can all impact neurocognitive decline in older age (Boss et al., 2015). Neurocognitive decline is also associated with physical frailty in old age (Fabrício et al., 2020), meaning that the good functioning of the brain is as important for physical health in old age as it is for early development.

Key Questions

Consider the various factors that we have discussed that impact the health and development of adults and the oldest old. During this time, the influences on the health of adults vary depending on their autonomy, which can change over time. The influence of having others to care for (either a growing family, or through a change of health status for a loved one) can have profound impacts on the various layers of influence on our health. As before, reflect on what you have learned from previous chapters, and on the things you have considered in the previous key questions activities. To what extent do you think society has a responsibility for creating or preventing these circumstances?

- Consider the various layers of the health onion and where some of these influences may be more or less common.
- What social or societal situations and contexts can be changed to help reduce the potential for these health influences?

Learning Outcomes Summary

- Understand how major influences on health differ across the life course.

We have looked at key stages across the life course to discuss some of the relevant health influences that occur at these critical points. We have seen how control over these influences changes from being located with others, to the self, then sometimes back to others.

- Have an appreciation of critical points where health outcomes can be impacted by biological, psychological, and social influences across the life course.

We have discussed the various biological, psychological, and social influences on health at differing times during the life course. The activities provided throughout the chapter will help to guide you in considering other aspects that may influence health at this time. Try to think beyond your own country or cultural context, considering factors mentioned in previous chapters, to deepen your appreciation here.

- Appreciate the ways that social and environmental influences on health may change over time, and how others may remain providing lifelong influence.

We have seen how people may have increased or decreased levels of control over the influences in their health and wellbeing across the life course, and where some responsibility has been shared. The activities in the chapter will help you to consider where society may play a key role in creating some of these health influences, and what may need to change to make health more equitable for all, across the ages of life.

FURTHER READING

Berken, J. A., Gracco, V. L., & Klein, D. (2017). Early bilingualism, language attainment, and brain development. *Neuropsychologia, 98*, 220–7.
An interesting article summarising some key research in the field of multilingualism and brain development.

De Bellis, M. D. (2005). The psychobiology of neglect. *Child Maltreatment, 10*(2), 150–72.
A specific article addressing psychobiological aspects of neglect.

Dorn, L. D., Hostinar, C. E., Susman, E. J., & Pervanidou, P. (2019). Conceptualizing puberty as a window of opportunity for impacting health and well-being across the life span. *Journal of Research on Adolescence, 29*(1), 155–76.
A fantastic paper that rallies against the very common doom-and-gloom approach towards puberty. The paper provides some examples of how puberty can function as a junction between earlier life experiences (and the help or harm they may incur) and later life consequences.

Geist, C., Greenberg, K. B., Luikenaar, R. A., & Mihalopoulos, N. L. (2021). Pediatric research and health care for transgender and gender diverse adolescents and young adults: Improving (biopsychosocial) health outcomes. *Academic Pediatrics, 21*(1), 32–42.
A good overview of where the literature is (or, rather, isn't) with regard to the key questions for the biopsychosocial health and wellbeing outcomes for trans and nonbinary adolescents and young people.

Glaser, D. (2000). Child abuse and neglect and the brain – a review. *The Journal of Child Psychology and Psychiatry and Allied Disciplines, 41*(1), 97–116.
A review on relevant research in neglect and brain development.

Hall, J. E. (2015). Endocrinology of the menopause. *Endocrinology and Metabolism Clinics, 44*(3), 485–96.
Useful article going into more detail on the hormonal changes that precede and develop menopause.

Larkin, M. (2013). *Health and well-being across the life course*. Sage.
An excellent text that covers this chapter in far greater detail.

Nokoff, N. J., Scarbro, S. L., Moreau, K. L., Zeitler, P., Nadeau, K. J., Juarez-Colunga, E., & Kelsey, M. M. (2020). Body composition and markers of cardiometabolic health in transgender youth compared with cisgender youth. *The Journal of Clinical Endocrinology & Metabolism, 105*(3), e704–e714.
A paper comparing insulin resistance and body composition between cis- and transgender adolescents.

Perez, C. C. (2019). *Invisible women: Data bias in a world designed for men*. Abrams.
An important book that I recommend all to read. This book (and the one next in this list) provides a shocking overview of how male norms do a disservice to women in every way. The impacts on health and welfare are particularly complex and multifaceted. A must read for all.

Saini, A. (2017). *Inferior: How science got women wrong – and the new research that's rewriting the story*. Fourth Estate.
A wonderful book that will introduce you to all the many ways that women have been wronged by science over history. There are some interesting points that relate to development and psychobiology in the latter chapters.

Sisk, C. L., & Romeo, R. D. (2019). *Coming of age: The neurobiology and psychobiology of puberty and adolescence*. Oxford University Press.
A whole book dedicated to the inter-twining of neurobiological and psychobiological changes during adolescence.

Suppakitjanusant, P., Ji, Y., Stevenson, M. O., Chantrapanichkul, P., Sineath, R. C., Goodman, M., … & Tangpricha, V. (2020). Effects of gender affirming hormone therapy on body mass index in transgender individuals: A longitudinal cohort study. *Journal of Clinical & Translational Endocrinology, 21*, 100230.
A study looking at the impact of gender-affirming hormone therapy on body-mass index over time.

VIDEOS

TED Ed has wonderful videos that describe some of the elements introduced in this chapter in greater detail. My favourites are:

Dr Anita Collins: How playing an instrument benefits your brain: www.ted.com/talks/ anita_collins_how_playing_an_instrument_benefits_your_brain?language=en

Dr Mia Nacamulli: The benefits of a bilingual brain: www.ted.com/talks/ mia_nacamulli_the_benefits_of_a_bilingual_brain?language=en

REFERENCES

Anderson, K. N., Schwab, R. B., & Martinez, M. E. (2014). Reproductive risk factors and breast cancer subtypes: A review of the literature. *Breast Cancer Research and Treatment*, *144*(1), 1–10. https://doi.org/10.1007/s10549-014-2852-7

Bick, J., Zhu, T., Stamoulis, C., Fox, N. A., Zeanah, C., & Nelson, C. A. (2015). Effect of early institutionalization and foster care on long-term white matter development: A randomized clinical trial. *JAMA Pediatrics*, *169*(3), 211–19. https://doi.org/10.1001/jamapediatrics.2014.3212

Boss, L., Kang, D.-H., & Branson, S. (2015). Loneliness and cognitive function in the older adult: A systematic review. *International Psychogeriatrics*, *27*(4), 541–53. https://doi.org/10.1017/S1041610214002749

Bucharest Early Intervention Project. (2022). *Bucharest Early Intervention Project.* Retrieved 5 Oct 2022 from www.bucharestearlyinterventionproject.org/

Carers UK. (2022). *Facts and figures.* Retrieved 5 Oct 2022 from www.carersuk.org/news-and-campaigns/press-releases/facts-and-figures

Castle, S. C. (2000). Clinical relevance of age-related immune dysfunction. *Clinical Infectious Diseases*, *31*(2), 578–85. https://doi.org/10.1086/313947

Collaziol, D., Luz, C., Dornelles, F., da Cruz, I. M., & Bauer, M. E. (2004). Psychoneurodendocrine correlates of lymphocyte subsets during healthy ageing. *Mechanisms of Ageing and Development*, *125*(3), 219–27. https://doi.org/https://doi.org/10.1016/j.mad.2003.10.009

Costa, G. (2010). Shift work and health: Current problems and preventive actions. *Safety and Health at Work*, 1(2), 112–123. https://doi.org/https://doi.org/10.5491/SHAW.2010.1.2.112

Crone, E. A., & van der Molen, M. W. (2004). Developmental changes in real life decision making: Performance on a gambling task previously shown to depend on the ventromedial prefrontal cortex. *Developmental Neuropsychology*, *25*(3), 251–79. https://doi.org/10.1207/s15326942dn2503_2

DiVall, S. A., & Radovick, S. (2009). Endocrinology of female puberty. *Current Opinion in Endocrinology, Diabetes and Obesity*, *16*(1), 1–4. https://doi.org/10.1097/MED.0b013e3283207937

Ershler, W. B., & Keller, E. T. (2000). Age-associated increased Interleukin-6 gene expression, late-life diseases, and frailty. *Annual Review of Medicine*, *51*(1), 245–70. https://doi.org/10.1146/annurev.med.51.1.245

Fabrício, D. d. M., Chagas, M. H. N., & Diniz, B. S. (2020). Frailty and cognitive decline. *Translational Research*, *221*, 58–64. https://doi.org/https://doi.org/10.1016/j.trsl.2020.01.002

Gogtay, N., Giedd, J. N., Lusk, L., Hayashi, K. M., Greenstein, D., Vaituzis, A. C., … Thompson, P. M. (2004). Dynamic mapping of human cortical development during childhood through early adulthood. *Proceedings of the National Academy of Sciences*, *101*(21), 8174–9. https://doi.org/doi:10.1073/pnas.0402680101

Greene, K., Krcmar, M., Rubin, D. L., Walters, L. H., & Hale, J. L. (2002). Elaboration in processing adolescent health messages: The impact of egocentrism and sensation seeking on message processing. *Journal of Communication*, *52*(4), 812–31. https://doi.org/10.1111/j.1460-2466.2002.tb02575.x

Habibi, A., Cahn, B. R., Damasio, A., & Damasio, H. (2016). Neural correlates of accelerated auditory processing in children engaged in music training. *Developmental Cognitive Neuroscience*, *21*, 1–14. https://doi.org/https://doi.org/10.1016/j.dcn.2016.04.003

Hyde, K. L., Lerch, J., Norton, A., Forgeard, M., Winner, E., Evans, A. C., & Schlaug, G. (2009). Musical training shapes structural brain development. *The Journal of Neuroscience*, *29*(10), 3019–25. https://doi.org/10.1523/jneurosci.5118-08.2009

Khan, N. A., & Hillman, C. H. (2014). The relation of childhood physical activity and aerobic fitness to brain function and cognition: A review. *Pediatric Exercise Science*, *26*(2), 138–46. https://doi.org/10.1123/pes.2013-0125

Laube, C., & Fuhrmann, D. (2020). Is early good or bad? Early puberty onset and its consequences for learning. *Current Opinion in Behavioral Sciences*, *36*, 150–56. https://doi.org/https://doi.org/10.1016/j.cobeha.2020.10.005

Lewis, K., & Lee, P. A. (2009). Endocrinology of male puberty. *Current Opinion in Endocrinology, Diabetes and Obesity*, *16*(1), 5–9. https://doi.org/10.1097/MED.0b013e32832029be

Mendle, J., & Ferrero, J. (2012). Detrimental psychological outcomes associated with pubertal timing in adolescent boys. *Developmental Review*, *32*(1), 49–66. https://doi.org/https://doi.org/10.1016/j.dr.2011.11.001

Mohades, S. G., Struys, E., Van Schuerbeek, P., Mondt, K., Van De Craen, P., & Luypaert, R. (2012). DTI reveals structural differences in white matter tracts between bilingual and monolingual children. *Brain Research*, *1435*, 72–80. https://doi.org/https://doi.org/10.1016/j.brainres.2011.12.005

Morales-Montor, J., Togno-Pierce, C., & Munoz-Cruz, S. (2011). Non-reproductive effects of sex steroids: Their immunoregulatory role. *Current Topics in Medicinal Chemistry*, *11*(13), 1714–27. https://doi.org/http://dx.doi.org/10.2174/156802611796117630

Pawelec, G., Barnett, Y., Forsey, R., Frasca, D., Globerson, A., McLeod, J., … Solana, R. (2002). T cells and aging, January 2002 update. *FBL (Frontiers in Bioscience-Landmark)*, *7*(4), 1056–83. https://doi.org/10.2741/a831

Schneider, P., Scherg, M., Dosch, H. G., Specht, H. J., Gutschalk, A., & Rupp, A. (2002). Morphology of Heschl's gyrus reflects enhanced activation in the auditory cortex of musicians. *Nature Neuroscience*, *5*(7), 688–94. https://doi.org/10.1038/nn871

Shah, S. I. A. (2018). Systemic non-reproductive effects of sex steroids in adult males and females. *Human Physiology, 44*(1), 83–7. https://doi.org/10.1134/S0362119718010188

Shope, J. T., & Bingham, C. R. (2008). Teen driving: Motor-vehicle crashes and factors that contribute. *American Journal of Preventive Medicine, 35*(3, Supplement), S261–S271. https://doi.org/https://doi.org/10.1016/j.amepre.2008.06.022

Singh, A., & Misra, N. (2009). Loneliness, depression and sociability in old age. *Industrial Psychiatry Journal, 18*(1), 51–5. https://doi.org/10.4103/0972-6748.57861

Skoe, E., & Kraus, N. (2012). A little goes a long way: How the adult brain is shaped by musical training in childhood. *The Journal of Neuroscience, 32*(34), 11507–10. https://doi.org/10.1523/jneurosci.1949-12.2012

Slovic, P. (1998). The risk game. *Reliability Engineering & System Safety, 59*(1), 73–7. https://doi.org/https://doi.org/10.1016/S0951-8320(97)00121-X

Steinberg, L. (2007). Risk taking in adolescence: New perspectives from brain and behavioral science. *Current Directions in Psychological Science, 16*(2), 55–9. https://doi.org/10.1111/j.1467-8721.2007.00475.x

van den Oord, C. L. J. D., Copeland, W. E., Zhao, M., Xie, L. Y., Aberg, K. A., & van den Oord, E. J. C. G. (2022). DNA methylation signatures of childhood trauma predict psychiatric disorders and other adverse outcomes 17 years after exposure. *Molecular Psychiatry, 27*, 3367–73. https://doi.org/10.1038/s41380-022-01597-5

Werker, J. F., & Tees, R. C. (1984). Phonemic and phonetic factors in adult cross-language speech perception. *The Journal of the Acoustical Society of America, 75*(6), 1866–78.

Wheeler, M. J., Dempsey, P. C., Grace, M. S., Ellis, K. A., Gardiner, P. A., Green, D. J., & Dunstan, D. W. (2017). Sedentary behavior as a risk factor for cognitive decline? A focus on the influence of glycemic control in brain health. *Alzheimer's & Dementia: Translational Research & Clinical Interventions, 3*(3), 291–300. https://doi.org/https://doi.org/10.1016/j.trci.2017.04.001

White, N. D. (2018). Hormonal contraception and breast cancer risk. *American Journal of Lifestyle Medicine, 12*(3), 224–6. https://doi.org/10.1177/1559827618754833

Wiesner, M., & Ittel, A. (2002). Relations of pubertal timing and depressive symptoms to substance use in early adolescence. *The Journal of Early Adolescence, 22*(1), 5–23. https://doi.org/10.1177/0272431602022001001

5

PSYCHOBIOLOGY: A PRIMER FOR PNI, PNE, AND PNEI

INTRODUCTION

The aim of this chapter is to offer a crash course on integrating knowledge from psychology, neuroscience, and immunology/endocrinology. The material covered in previous chapters (particularly Chapters 1 and 2) will be advanced to provide you with an overview of these fascinating fields of interdisciplinary research – the field of research I call my home. You will be given an introduction to bidirectional brain–body communication, and how this is modulated by psychological, social, and behavioural factors. You will be walked through some of the basics of the ways our immune systems and hormone systems work, and critically which aspects are vulnerable to psychosocial influence. We will also take a look at one of the applied fields of research that uses this information to deepen our understanding of one of the world's biggest health issues.

> ## Learning Outcomes
>
> - Understand what psychology has to do with the immune system and endocrine system.
> - Have an appreciation for the interplay between the immune and endocrine systems.
> - Understand how psychological factors can be the result of immune/endocrine dysfunction.
> - Understand how psychological factors can influence cancer.

As a small warning before we start, there are a lot of complicated terms and a whole ton of synonyms or parallel terms in this chapter, but please don't be put off. Nobody expects you to remember all the complicated terms and names, and nobody expects you to have a sophisticated understanding of how all these systems and processes interlink. The point of this chapter is to provide a crash course on two very, VERY complicated systems. It will hopefully serve to be a point of reference for you, and will give you some confidence to start reading some journal articles in these areas so that you might get as excited about this huge field of research as I get. The best take-home from this chapter will be to understand that no processes happen in exclusion – and that health is created/changed by a diverse set of processes and systems that interlink.

WHAT IS PSYCHOBIOLOGY?

Psychobiology is an interdisciplinary field that takes learning from a variety of other disciplines and scientific traditions. In the UK, there is a Psychobiology section of the British Psychological Society, so it is a well-established field that has a growing interest. It is essentially (as the name would suggest) the intersection between psychology and biology, and takes influence and learning from neuroscience, medicine, and behavioural sciences, as well as potentially incorporating broader cognate fields such as medical anthropology and medical sociology. My particular corner of psychobiology is the cell-to-society perspective that has been discussed throughout this book so far. Psychobiology can incorporate cellular-level fields (such as those in focus in this chapter), but it can also be systems-level considerations as well, such as the field of **psychophysiology**, which looks at (amongst other things) the way psychological factors influence cardiovascular functioning. Two large fields within the broader discipline of psychobiology are **psychoneuroimmunology** (PNI) and **psychoneuroendocrinology** (PNE). PNI is all about understanding how psychological factors (including social influences and behaviour) can change the physical workings of our central nervous system, and how this then has an impact on our immune system. PNE is about understanding how psychological factors (including social influences and behaviour) can change the physical workings of our central nervous system, and how this then has an impact on our endocrine system. Of course, these factors don't actually tend to work in exclusion of each other (as you will see throughout), so we can bring these disciplines together to form **psychoneuroendocrinoimmunology** (PNEI), which is a natural and logical integration of these fields, and covers a lot of work in the broad field of psychobiology. If you are from a psychology background, it is critically important to have a good grasp of the fundamental aspects of biology and medicine that support learning in this field if you want to make sense of how health is made from cell to society. I did this myself, being advised by my supervisor during my PhD that in order to understand PNI, you must understand the 'I' as well as any of the other parts. This was tremendously good advice, and I wrote a whole chapter of my thesis on the natural history and pathophysiology of **Human Immunodeficiency Virus (HIV) and Acquired Immune Deficiency Syndrome (AIDS)**, providing me with an excellent foundation on which to build an entire career of research. The point of this chapter is to try to give you some of that foundation as well, so that you will be able to make sure that each of your 'P's, 'N's, and 'I's (or 'E's) are equally shored up with knowledge.

The learning that is garnered through psychobiology can be applied in research (both academic and clinical), but can also be directly applied to specific medical-oriented fields of practice. Psycho-oncology (how psychobiology is associated with cancer) will be discussed later in this chapter, but there are many other fields of applied work as well, including psycho-dermatology (psychobiology and skin diseases/disorders), psycho-cardiology (psychobiology and cardiac health), and psycho-rheumatology (psychobiology and musculoskeletal disorders/diseases). Each of these areas is fascinating, and there are career pathways associated with them in various types of working environments: academia, clinical practice, and clinical research. Whilst psychobiology looks at individual-level (and cellular-level) information, we can still learn a lot about social groups and populations in terms of their psychobiological profiles. Population-level datasets have started to include the collection of biomarkers (e.g., cortisol, blood lipids, inflammatory factors etc.) in their datasets to build a better picture of systems-level functioning in large groups (population level) of people. Looking at this type of cellular functioning across generations can also help us to understand epigenetic changes.

Warning

Sadly, like any exciting/interesting/technical-word-heavy discipline, the various aspects of psychobiology (particularly psychoneuroimmunology and psychoneuroendocrinology) are often associated with bad science. A quick look at YouTube reveals videos from people on 'beating inflammation', 'anti-inflammatory foods', and 'clean living' to improve your gut health. Aside from these being outrageously misinformed, they are potentially quite harmful because they take ideas from *real* science, but don't do any of the work required to substantiate their claims. Unfortunately, good science will always be used by bad people for money or to fuel their self-importance. However, as I said at the beginning of this book, a lot of that is about how we as researchers fail to communicate effectively. Our research is often hidden behind academic journal paywalls (where only the title and abstract are viewable), and even if it isn't, it is often written so obscurely that everyday people find it impenetrable. If we communicate our work in plain language when we can, the people that use it to sell their pills and potions will have less to stand on. I would argue we have a responsibility to do this - not just to deter those seeking to capitalise from obscure-sounding concepts and ideas, but because a great deal of science is in some way or other publicly funded, and it should be available (and *accessible*) to the public.

BRAIN-BODY COMMUNICATION

We took a look at some of the important hardware involved in the cross-talk between the brain and the body in Chapter 2. Almost everything is connected to the brain in some sort of physical or chemical communication network. The brain and the body have to talk to each other all the time for you to be able to do the things that you can do with your body. Talking, walking, running, playing a musical instrument, playing football, swimming, dancing – they all require rapid and intricate communication between the brain and the body. Our senses rely on this cross-talk too, allowing us to see, smell, hear, feel, taste, and balance. But what if I told you that not only does something like your immune system receive information from your brain, but it also talks back? The first time I found this out it absolutely blew my mind.

One of the ways our brains and immune systems talk that you will probably all have noticed at least once in your lifetime is the brain-to-body direction. Think of a time – any time – when you have been really stressed. Maybe it was during a period of exams, or when you had a serious disruption to a relationship. It could be a house move, a job change, or being tasked with a high-stakes project. Did you become ill at some stage either during or after this point? Most of us at one time (or, more likely, very many times) will experience something stressful followed by a heavy cold or other type of circulating infection. This is not because being stressed gives us a cold, but it does make us more likely to pick up a circulating infectious disease, and – if we do pick something up – we are more likely to have heavier symptoms for a longer period of time. This is an example of how your brain talks to your immune system. We discovered in Chapter 2 how our fight-or-flight system prepares us for action in the case of danger. This is powered by the **hypothalamic-pituitary-adrenal (HPA) axis** – you encounter something stressful, and this initiates a cascade of hormones to put you into the fight-or-flight state, and this sympathetic activity has an impact on our immune systems too. Our immune systems are very sensitive to stress hormones (glucocorticoids), partly because some of the functions our immune systems regulate are not critical at that fighting or running away event. It is one of those occasions where 'non-essential' systems and functions are deprioritised in favour of those that are essential in that critical moment.[1] So, during one of those examples of peak stress, your body will be very frequently lurching into this pattern of acute stress – sometimes it may become chronic stress too – and all the while when this happens, your immune system is being instructed to stand down (more on this in Chapter 6). This means you are much more likely to pick up that cough, cold, or stomach bug that might be circulating, and if you do you may also suffer worse from it. It may also mean that if you were already successfully fighting off an infection, all of a sudden your immune system is not fighting so hard anymore and you may end up getting a full-blown illness from it. It could also manifest in taking a prolonged time to heal from an injury – and many studies have looked at wound healing time as an outcome in psychobiological research. All of this is evidence that you can directly observe of your brain talking to your immune system.

Your brain talks to your immune system in several ways. As we briefly considered in Chapter 2, there are hard-wired routes but chemical routes too. The organs in your body that are associated with the creation, maintenance, or instruction of your immune system have direct lines of communication from your brain, usually in sympathetic networks. Your thymus, bone marrow, and spleen all have built-in nerve routes from your brain. Your lymph nodes may have sympathetic fibre input to them as well. Beyond

---

1 There are some aspects of immunity that are heightened in acute stress, such as the ability to clot our blood, or the immune functions that serve to protect against trauma-related immune compromise. This makes sense because at the time of fighting or running away we may be more likely to become injured, so we will need to stop bleeding out (by clotting) and also make sure that pathogens are prevented from entering the body at the site of trauma.

this, many of your immune-associated tissues will also receive information chemically from your brain as they are receptive to various types of neurotransmitters, brain-based hormones, and other neuropeptides. Not only this, but the cells of your immune system have these receptors too. There is not one cell in your immune system that does not carry receptors for at least one type of brain-originating signalling chemical. So, your brain can talk to your immune system in a variety of different ways, with the potential to modulate a large spectrum of functions and processes. This also means that anything that changes the way your brain is currently working (such as stress) has the potential to affect many of your immune processes as well.

As for the other way around, you have probably been able to see examples of this as well, but may not have realised it at the time. Have you ever felt 'a bit off' or 'a bit run down' or similar just a few days before becoming ill? That period of time where you don't have any symptoms of whatever illness you are obviously brewing, but you *just don't quite feel right?* It is only when a few days later you start showing the symptoms of the illness you have picked up (sneezing, coughing, etc.) that you put this all together and realise that the reason you have been feeling this way is because you were coming down with an illness. Before reading any more, have a quick go at the activity – this will help with several points later in this chapter.

Key Questions

If you have ever felt 'run down', 'slightly off', 'a bit peaky', or any other similar phrases for this period of time before you start showing symptoms of an infection - what are the consequences of this?

- What did you do (or not do)?
- How did you feel?
- Are there any clinical conditions that seem a bit similar to these patterns of feelings and behaviour?

This period of feeling run down, and the consequent impact this has on our behaviour, is a prime example of our immune system talking to our brain. When our immune cells encounter a pathogen (a virus, bacterium, or parasite) in our bloodstream, they do their best to clear it away, but they also send out a distress signal. Just as our neurons talk to each other through signalling molecules (neurotransmitters, neuropeptides, etc.), our immune cells talk to each other with signalling molecules too (called **cytokines**). These molecules serve several purposes, but one of those is an early-warning signal system that covers the entire body. If you have watched a film or read a book about historic societies (that far predate the communication tools like telephones and the internet), you may be familiar with signal fires. This is where there may be a lookout on the coast somewhere, and when the lookout spots an enemy ship approaching, they light a signal fire. There are many signal fire attendants miles apart stretching from key areas like the coastline right up to the final point where the message is needed (usually a castle, chieftain's longhouse, fort, or other place of central power), with signal fires being spotted and then lit sequentially until the distress signal is received at the final destination, usually within minutes. This facilitated fast communication of a simple message ('warning – enemy incoming') to where it was needed over a vast amount of space, which provided critical extra response time that would have been lost with a single messenger. Your cytokines are doing something a bit like this. Some immune cells can produce cytokines, and they will do this once they have encountered and neutralised the threat of a pathogen (so they light the first fire), or if they receive a signal from another immune cell to indicate they have encountered something (lighting subsequent fires in the chain). These cytokines then travel around the bloodstream effectively warning other immune cells of the incoming attack, which then send off their own cytokines to amplify this message, and soon the message will also get picked up by the brain (the castle or longhouse in this metaphor). We are only beginning to understand the fascinating complexities of these processes, but it is through this mechanism that we think that **inflammation** (which is an immune process – more on this soon) can play a key role in a variety of neurological and psychological disorders. The purpose of all this signalling is to initiate that pattern of behaviour that I hope you have identified through the activity – and this is called **sickness behaviour**.

Sickness behaviour is a sort of suite of behaviours and responses that are designed to keep us safe whilst we are under attack from within. We become tired and lethargic – this makes us want to rest (so our immune system can use our body's energy to fight the infection) and probably makes it less likely that we will go out (making it less likely we will come under further attack from other pathogens). We may feel more hungry or thirsty, which will be helpful if we are fighting a pathogen that will require energy to neutralise, or that we can otherwise flush out via our kidneys. Conversely, we may feel less hungry too, which will help in the case of us being infected with a pathogen that may have come into our bodies through ingestion (such as those bugs that give us food poisoning), thereby preventing us from potentially consuming more of them. We may feel a little down, or a little less sociable. This means that we minimise our chances of picking up more viruses or bacteria from other people, and that we rest and look after ourselves. These seemingly very simple behaviours with very sophisticated mechanisms for preserving ourselves come from these unbelievably tiny molecules. The activity also asked you to consider what clinical conditions might seem similar to this pattern of behaviour – being lethargic and slow, eating a lot more or a lot less, feeling a bit grumpy or low, and not wanting to be around others or do exciting things – hopefully you would have suggested depression. Depression is remarkably like sickness behaviour in many ways, and that is one reason why we think that there may be an inflammatory aspect of the onset or maintenance of depression. Cytokines are sometimes prescribed to patients in some cases of cancer or complex viral infection, and these patients often end up showing marked symptoms of depression as a result (Capuron & Dantzer, 2003). The relationship between depression and inflammation is not at all straightforward, but it is clear that this is one of those prime examples of the interconnectedness of our systems, and how conditions that we once thought were associated with just one system (in this case, the brain) also have very complex interactions with other systems and networks (Dantzer, 2012). Similarly, the immune and endocrine systems also have very complex interconnections and – in some cases – shared communication infrastructures. **Corticotropin-releasing hormone** (CRH) is classically thought of as being released from the brain during stress to signal down to the adrenals; however, CRH can also be created by **leukocytes** (white blood cells) in response to trauma and acts as a messenger to (partially) initiate the pain response (Blalock & Smith, 2007). This is a very good example of how the endocrine and immune systems can talk to each other without needing to involve the brain, so the cross-talk between the brain and each of these systems (and between the systems themselves) is complex and multifaceted.

HOW THE IMMUNE SYSTEM WORKS

Now we have looked at some examples of how the communication between the brain and the immune system happens, you will hopefully be beginning to understand and fit into place all of those exercises you have done in this book up until now. You will be able to appreciate that more or less anything that happens in the brain can have an impact elsewhere in the body. Now we will look at the way the immune system works in more detail so that you can get a feel for the ways that psychological and social factors can impact us on the cellular and system levels.

The immune system is more of a mechanism than a specific structure in itself, although it does rely on some specific infrastructures within the body in order to work. As we saw in Chapter 2, the lymphatic system is the network within the body that supports many of the immune system's functions, and the circulatory system does as well, as that is where our immune cells patrol to defend us from attack. Your immune system is responsible for some extremely important processes, both regulatory (i.e., keeping things running correctly) and adaptive (i.e., responding to change or challenge):

- Protection – the immune system is involved in searching for and destroying invading pathogens.
- Maintenance – it helps to clean up waste products, dead cells, and general junk in the body.
- Defence – it also tells your brain you are under attack, and allows your brain to initiate sickness behaviour patterns to allow you to convalesce in safety.

There are many different subdivisions of the immune system, which can be classified according to types of cells, types of functions of cells, or even patterns of response. We can look at the immune system as originating with two main 'arms': the innate and adaptive.[2] **Innate immunity** refers to the cells we are born with that have general bug-killing capacities with no real specificity. These types of cells are white blood cells like T-cells (also referred to as T-lymphocytes) that originate in the thymus, and B-cells (B-lymphocytes) that originate in the bone marrow. There are also other types of cells like Natural Killer cells, **monocytes**, **macrophages**, **basophils**, **neutrophils**, and eosinophils. They serve a lot of functions, but are general all-rounders that destroy pathogens (through a process called **phagocytosis**) when they encounter them, and also support some of the immune signalling in the early detection mechanisms that were mentioned in the previous section. The other cluster of immune cells and their functions is referred to as adaptive immunity. As the name suggests, this part of the immune system has the ability to 'learn' about the pathogens we encounter and to build our immunity to diseases over time. The cells of our immune systems develop before we are born, so we are able to have some sort of basic immune response from birth. We also receive some antibodies from our pregnant parent *in utero*, particularly if they receive a vaccination during gestation. Antibodies can also be passed on through breast milk, providing some boosts to early immunity. During gestation, the immune system learns about what is 'self' and what is 'not self' – anything that is not self is then a potential invader. After birth, your immune system retains this un-specialised general purpose (i.e., innate) immunity, but also then learns to attack pathogens as they are encountered (i.e., acquired/adaptive immunity). Some of our 'innate' cells can also learn

---

2 They can also be referred to as 'cellular' and 'humoural' (also 'humoral'). Cellular refers to your innate (cell-based) immunity, and humoural/humoral refers to your adaptive immunity. The latter is named after substances in your bodily fluid (lymph, blood), which were previously called 'humours'.

(particularly **memory T-cells**), and we will likely discover far more cells and signalling molecules that have multiple functions and purposes. I have provided some reading on memory T-cells at the end of this chapter for any of you that have not found this section confusing enough!

One of the best ways of understanding how the immune system works is to think of it like an army – there are ranks and roles that are involved in doing some quite different actions, but together they are there to defend you, maintain your defences, and win the war against invaders. Some soldiers are general all-rounders (like infantry) who are there just to get anything that moves and looks slightly suspicious. Some are highly specialised intelligence officers that work on known information to seek out and target specific invaders. General infantry cells are there to keep the attack at bay, and the specialised soldiers are in the background waiting in case the line is breached. Communication within the various lines of the immune system is necessary to mount a coordinated attack. You have a huge number of cells that support your immune system, and many different types of cells too. Some cells may be highly specialised, some may be good all-rounders, but they all work together to protect and maintain the body. An important aspect of your immune system is that it has memory – both in terms of its cells and as a system. Your immune system cells learn about pathogens and produces specific antibodies to combat them, and it is through that process that we are able to inoculate people against diseases, by effectively priming the immune system to recognise a certain pathogen so that it can destroy it if it ever happens to invade the body. Your immune system itself learns about how pathogenically risky your life is over time and will deploy circulating immune cells accordingly. The fundamental way that your immune system does all this is by your innate immune cells knowing what is, and what is not, you. Your white blood cells do not have a complex library of different types of cells to refer new information against, they simply use cell-surface molecules to detect what belongs to you and what does not. Our white blood cells patrol our blood vessels all the time, and if a cell is recognised as non-self then a chemical cascade occurs to trigger a response (such as the release of cytokines). Ideally, what our immune systems should understand to be non-self should be pathogens (viruses, bacteria, fungi, parasites) or toxins (both toxins we get from outside, but also toxins created internally as part of regular cellular processes and food digestion etc.), allergens, and a handful of virtually anything else foreign that we introduce to our bodies, like medications and molecules from food. The determination of self to non-self is complicated, and is part of what goes wrong in auto-immune disorders (where our immune system fails to recognise our own cells as 'self', and then consequently attacks our own cells or tissues). Many of your immune cells can recognise patterns of molecules expressed on the surface of cells, and if these are determined to be non-self, then attack is initiated. That very simple process is basically how your immune system keeps you alive, although exactly how this development of recognising self and non-self is mastered within the immune system is still a matter of debate today.

Th1/Th2 Immunity

There are other ways of classifying the immune system and its function that go beyond the simplistic born/not born with it distinction of innate/adaptive. Whilst that is a useful way of understanding which cells are all-purpose and which are specialised, our immune systems tend to behave in ways that incorporate the mobilisation and suppression of cells or molecules in either arm in order to respond to attack or to carry out regular maintenance. In fact, the way our immune systems work in response to any given reaction or regulatory function is incredibly sophisticated, and it is said there may be as many patterns of the immune system working as there are cells in the immune system itself. Work in animals in the 1980s discovered that there were proliferative patterns of immune system function that originate with certain classes of T-cells –T-helper (Th) cells in this case, and this has since been well-established in humans also. T-helper cells are thought to be almost the architects of immune responses (perhaps the colonels to extend the metaphor further), capable of mobilising the cells of all other classes within the immune system, including initiating the secretion of antibodies from B cells. This is obviously very important for understanding how our health functions at this level, as if there are any psychological, social, behavioural, or environmental influences that change either the number or function of these T-cells, then this can have a very significant impact on the immune system as a whole. Whilst research in this area is rapidly evolving as we are able to learn more and more about the immune system, it is thought there are two regulatory 'profiles' of immune system operation. These profiles are important particularly in psychobiology as they have helped us to understand the consequences of certain psychosocial conditions, where a switch from one profile to another can explain many of the health consequences we observe in those cases. These profiles are referred to as **Th1** (T-helper 1) and **Th2**, and they exist in a relative balance, much like the divisions of the autonomic nervous system (the sympathetic and the parasympathetic). We have different cells and signalling molecules that are associated with each of these profiles, and each profile largely serves to support distinct cellular mechanisms and overall immune functions. These two profiles are characterised by two distinct patterns of cytokine signalling. Every immune cell is capable of synthesising and secreting molecules that serve to signal other cells, and these send a message (much like neurons and their neurotransmitters) to act or to stand down (in immune system parlance: upregulate and downregulate). Cytokines are proteins or **peptides** (complex molecular chains of amino acids) that work as a communication network in the immune system. We have a lot of different types of cytokines (and similar molecules called chemokines, which help to signal to white blood cells), including **interleukins** (often noted as IL-), **interferons** (noted as IFN-), and other 'factors' like **tumour necrosis factor** (TNF), transforming growth factor (TGF), and several types of **colony-stimulating factors** (CSF). The Th1 profile of immunity is by and large pro-inflammatory, and is responsible for the seek-and-destroy elements of immunity that target pathogens and toxins, but also function in autoimmunity. These processes involve more of the innate (cell-mediated) immunity classes of cells, the infantry of your immune system. The Th2 profile relies on a complex combination of (intelligence officers) antibodies (adaptive/humoural immunity), but uses some innate cells also (such as **eosinophils**), and can present a more anti-inflammatory action. Just as we see with the autonomic nervous system, where there is a balance of sympathetic and parasympathetic – the sympathetic constituting autonomic arousal, and the parasympathetic de-escalating that arousal – the effect of Th1 (aggressive and largely pro-inflammatory) is balanced out by Th2 (targeted and anti-inflammatory). Unlike the autonomic nervous system, however, in an immune response we should be using both of these profiles, not one over the other. A preferential swing either way could lead to problems in executing any of the core regulatory or effector functions of the immune system. We are still trying to work out what all of this means, and – in doing so – we are also discovering other profiles of immunity that are led by types of T-cells, such as T-regulatory cells and Th17 cells (T-helpers that rely on IL-17 to initiate their cascade) amongst others.

The balance between Th1 and Th2 is regulated to an extent by our endocrine systems, and can be influenced by stress – with acute stress shifting to Th1 and chronic stress to Th2. The balance between Th1 and Th2 has been demonstrated to be affected by depression (Myint et al., 2005), so this is a good example of how nothing that goes on in our brains simply stays there. We talk about stress and its impact on immunity a lot, and this is easy to demonstrate because of the well-established ways in which stress impacts the endocrine system, but depression (whilst having impacts on our hormones) is more subtle in the ways it may descend to the rest of our bodies. However, it is still nonetheless important in immunity. The balance between Th1 and Th2 is known to impact a variety of different health conditions, meaning stress and depression have a direct mechanistic impact on conditions such as atopic dermatitis (Grewe et al., 1998), various cancers (e.g., Hou et al., 2013; Reiche et al., 2004), atherosclerosis (Gu et al., 2012), and chronic pain (Kaufmann et al., 2007), to name just a handful. You could spend a lifetime trying to make sense of all of this (many have!), but for now try to keep the Th1/Th2 balance in mind, as this will come up again when we look at examples of how health is impacted at this cellular and system level.

HOW THE ENDOCRINE SYSTEM WORKS

Much like the immune system, the endocrine system has no channels/routes that belong specifically to it, but is a collection of glands throughout the body and uses the infrastructure of other systems. **Glands** talk to each other via hormones, which are usually dumped into the blood for broad circulation to be picked up by tissues and cells as needed. Your HPA axis is an example of an endocrine loop that we have already considered several times in this book. The endocrine system (Figure 5.1) is the communication network between a variety of systems and structures around the whole body, rather than just at local points. Hormones are released into the bloodstream to circulate around the body, they then interact with receptors on target cells and tissues. What makes hormones hormones is that they are produced in endocrine tissues (glands), but they can function over large distances or even very short distances as neurotransmitters as well.

We can classify hormones into two main groups depending on how they are made. We have **steroid hormones**, which are made from cholesterol, and are created as and when required. Their onset tends to be quite slow, but their effects last longer. These types of hormones can interact directly with cellular DNA to alter how the cells work. Examples of steroid hormones are sex hormones like testosterone and oestrogens, and stress hormones like cortisol. We also have **peptide hormones** that are made

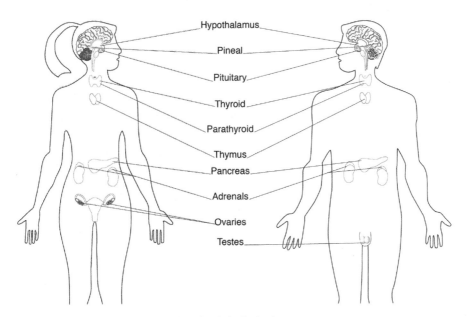

Figure 5.1 The major endocrine endocrine glands in the body

Source: Boore et al. (2016), *Essentials of Anatomy and Physiology for Nursing Practice*, Sage

from complex amino acid chains and are stored until signals have been received to release them. These hormones often have quite fast effects, but do not last long. They interact with receptors on the cell surface that can cause cellular changes to alter DNA transcription rather than interacting with DNA itself. Examples of peptide hormones are those that provide homeostatic processes like vasopressin (antidiuretic hormone), and melatonin. As well as performing internal functions, our hormones can and do have a direct impact on our behaviour. One of the easiest examples of how hormones impact behaviour is to consider a behaviour central to life, like maintaining water balance (osmolarity). Vasopressin is made in the hypothalamus and then stored in the pituitary. When the brain establishes lower than optimal levels of water in the blood, the pituitary releases vasopressin. This then changes the permeability of some of the hardware in the kidneys, allowing water to be reabsorbed into the body, and decreases the frequency of urination. However, vasopressin also does some interesting things in the brain. It appears to be related to social behaviour as well as in the neurocognitive processes that are involved in interpreting social signals from others (Heinrichs et al., 2009). In Chapter 4, there was a lot of talk of sex hormones and how these are related to different developmental stages but also are related to a variety of regulatory functions in other ways that influence our health. All our hormones have multiple purposes – some of which we have not yet discovered or otherwise have not fully understood – and all add up to ensuring the careful balance of our internal systems.

The Thyroid Gland

To illustrate the importance of hormones and the endocrine system in both health and psychology a little bit further, I will use the example of the **thyroid** gland. Your thyroid secretes a variety of hormones that are responsible for your metabolism, but it can malfunction in 1–5% of the population (Vanderpump, 2011). There are two ways in which your thyroid may malfunction (but several different conditions lead to this malfunctioning): you may have an overactive thyroid (*hyperthyroidism*) or an underactive thyroid (*hypothyroidism*). Both malfunctions have very distinct pathopsychology (i.e., psychological processes as a result of disease/disorder) as well as pathophysiology (i.e., physiological processes as a result of disease/disorder). Table 5.1 outlines some of the different psychological and physiological impacts of these two patterns of dysfunctional thyroid behaviour. Do you notice anything interesting here?

Table 5.1 An overview of some key characteristics of conditions associated with hypothyroidism and hyperthyroidism

Hypothyroidism (underactive)		Hyperthyroidism (overactive)	
Physical	*Psychological*	*Physical*	*Psychological*
Weight gain	Depression	Weight loss	Anxiety
Lethargy	Flat affect	Hyperactivity	Mood swings
Sensitivity to cold	Slow thoughts	Sensitivity to heat	Irritability
Hypersomnia	Tiredness	Insomnia	Tiredness
Muscle aches, weakness, and cramps		Palpitations	

The keen-eyed of you will have noticed that many of the physical and psychological characteristics of hypothyroidism are the reverse in the case of hyperthyroidism. You will also have noticed that there are almost as many psychological characteristics of these conditions as there are physical characteristics. This will hopefully underline to you just how important something that isn't in your brain can be to those things that we classically assume to be almost entirely under our brain's control (like our moods, our attention, and our ability to think). The thyroid gland is primarily responsible for **metabolism**. Most people consider metabolism to just be about how quickly you digest your food, but that is just one aspect. Your whole body clock is wound up in your metabolic processes. You can probably quite easily see from the examples of hypo/hyperthyroidism that they are almost completely opposite patterns of symptoms, and some of these are to do with digestion (such as being over-/underweight), some are about your sleep/wake cycle, such as being unable to stay awake (hypersomnia) and unable to fall or stay asleep (insomnia), but others are far more subtle. Think about the last time you were kept awake all night – how did that make you feel and behave? It is not simply that being tired makes us cranky (although it most definitely does), it affects our concentration, our stress threshold, our emotional responses to situations, our appetite, and many other functions and behaviours. This is because all these internal systems and processes are interlinked, and whilst we know a great deal about these interlinking complexities, we still don't properly understand it all yet. There are also immune links with thyroid hormones, which may provide an inflammatory mechanism between thyroid dysfunction, physical ill health, and mental health symptoms. If you cast your mind back to thinking about sickness behaviour, whilst a lot of those patterns were similar to depression, they could equally be similar to hypothyroidism. Hypothyroidism can easily be missed when a person speaks to their doctor for exactly this reason.

Glucocorticoids

It just would not be possible to get past a section on endocrinology without mentioning some of the hormones that are the most well-studied in the field of psychoneuroendocrinology. They also serve to complete the loop between PNI and PNE, and show how we really need to be considering the integration of the two (PNEI) to make sense of the multiple influences that biopsychosocial factors can have on cellular and system-level health. Glucocorticoids are the hormones that support our stress system, the HPA axis (see Figure 5.2). One key aspect of fight or flight is the suppression of the inflammatory aspects of the immune system, which is why (cortico)steroids (e.g., cortisone, dexamethasone, prednisolone) are prescribed for inflammatory diseases and conditions like asthma and hayfever and auto immune diseases like rheumatoid arthritis and lupus. Glucocorticoids are released by the **adrenal glands** in response to hormonal cascade from the hypothalamus (corticotropin-releasing hormone: CRH) and pituitary (adrenocorticotropin-releasing hormone: ACTH). Various neurotransmitters can modulate the release of CRH (and therefore other glucocorticoids). Acetylcholine, **noradrenaline**, and serotonin can all increase CRH release. GABA (γ-aminobutyric acid), nitrous oxide, and Substance P can decrease it. Not only this, but CRH release is also sensitive to other hormones, with it being particularly sensitive to oestrogens that can enhance its release.

There are several ways in which glucocorticoids can influence the immune system. We have already seen that cortisol is one part of the HPA axis outflow that has a direct impact on immune function in order to downplay immune activity whilst we are fighting or running away, but other hormones in the stress response have immunoregulatory

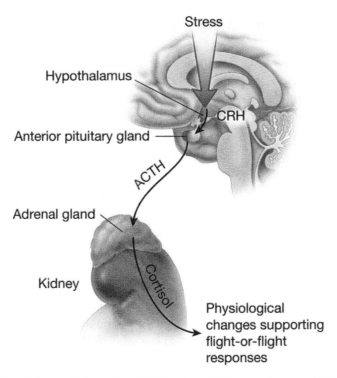

Stress

Hypothalamus

CRH

Anterior pituitary gland

ACTH

Adrenal gland

Kidney

Cortisol

Physiological changes supporting flight-or-flight responses

Figure 5.2   The hypothalamic-pituitary-adrenal (HPA) axis and its hormonal communication
Source: Amanda Tomasikiewicz/Body Scientific Intl. in Gaskin (2021), *Behavioural Neuroscience*, Sage

or immunomodulatory properties also. ACTH decreases antibody production (another reason that we get sick when we're stressed); it can also impact our in-built ability to kill cancers, and alter our cytokine messaging (McEwen et al., 1997). In animals, CRH has been detected in a variety of lymphoid tissues (the thymus, gastro-intestinal tract etc.), and it can promote the release of pro-inflammatory cytokines (Baigent, 2001). Glucocorticoids tend to have a mainly inhibitory effect on many parameters of immune function, including the patterns of immune defence that we have, such as Th1 to Th2 (Elenkov, 2004). Glucocorticoid impacts on the immune system are not unidirectional or unifunctional – they interact in a variety of ways. Glucocorticoids can also be influenced by activities within the immune system as well. CRH can be increased in response to pro-inflammatory cytokine action, and when all is functioning healthily this serves as a circuit breaker to down-regulate inflammation (Turnbull & Rivier, 1999). This may well be one of the mechanisms that also underlies the fact that we may get a bit cranky and irritable when we are unwell. We will put this knowledge into practice a little more in Chapters 6 and 7 where we are looking at the impacts of stress at both the individual and population levels.

CANCER[3] AND PSYCHO-ONCOLOGY

To put some of this knowledge into action, we will consider the case of cancer and its applied psychobiological area, psycho-oncology. **Cancer** is not one thing – there are a huge number of different types of cancers, even down to the variation in types of cancers that affect the same tissue or organ. There are more than 200 different types of cancer that have been identified at this stage, but they are all characterised by the rapid and uncontrolled growth of cells. It is estimated that one in two people in the world will develop cancer at some point or other in their lives, so it is one of the leading health concerns globally. The treatment of cancer can be very complicated, and usually involves some invasive and aggressive medical care, which can be variable depending on where you live in the world and what access you have to healthcare (and what access your healthcare systems have to types of therapies). Some cancers can be in some way predictable (if we have others in our family who have had cancer, for example) and others seem to come out of nowhere. Cancer is still a leading cause of death globally, and treatment (and whether that treatment will be effective) will be dependent on the stage at which it is detected. There are a huge number of biopsychosocial aspects that we understand to be related to the detection of and prognosis in cancer, but there are also biopsychosocial aspects in the **aetiology** (i.e., the causes) of cancer. That will be the prime focus of the rest of this chapter.

What Is Cancer and How Does It Develop?

Cancer is a condition that is referred to as being *neoplastic* (i.e., the novel initiation of cell plasticity). Neoplasms are the development of tumours (as a result of rapid cell growth) and may be non-invasive or invasive. Cancer is characterised by rapid and uncontrolled multiplication of cells in any tissue in the body. Cancer can occur in organs (such as the pancreas or lungs), structural tissues (such as the bones), endocrine tissues (such as the ovaries or adrenal glands), and even in the blood (these tend not to be in tumour form, but cancer cells may fill up the blood over time and invade the bone marrow, where tumours can form). Cancers can be categorised into five main groups: lymphomas (within the lymphatic system), leukaemias (within the blood and bone marrow), carcinomas (within epithelial cells lining the skin or organs), sarcomas (within the

---

3 This section was developed with the excellent advice and support of Dr Daniel Stones, an incredibly clever cell biologist who specialises in cancer.

bones and soft tissues), and brain tumours (within the central nervous system). Over time, and with the help of the excellent networks we have in our bodies in the form of our vascular and lymphatic systems, cancers may travel to other sites in the body to form **metastases**. This happens in usually a very advanced stage of cancer, and makes cancer very hard to treat and much more likely to be fatal.

Tumour growth generally starts because there is some sort of error made in the replication of normal healthy cells. What triggers this error can vary, but we know that there are (epi)genetic causes, where we may carry a gene that makes control of tumour growth more difficult, as well as the experience of oxidative stress (as briefly discussed in Chapter 1). Tumourigenesis (i.e., the development of a tumour) can also be associated with exposure to certain chemicals or DNA-damaging environmental influences like radiation (including the ultraviolet radiation from the sun, which we know can lead to *melanoma* – skin cancer). Tumours develop as a result of accidents or errors over time as our cells divide and multiply naturally (mutations), and this needs to happen multiple times before a tumour will manifest. There can be two mechanisms for this. Either a mutation will fail to suppress abnormal cell proliferation (an error in tumour suppressor genes), or a mutation may occur that accelerates dysfunctional cell division (an error creating what is referred to as an *oncogene*). You may have noticed that I mentioned a specific immune cell type earlier called tumour necrosis factor (TNF), and that is because your immune system is to an extent primed to watch out for errors in irregular or erratic cell proliferation. In your lifetime you may have hundreds, if not thousands, of cellular events that *could* lead to cancer, but these can be kept in check by several mechanisms in the immune system. Cancer occurs when all these fail-safes are exhausted.

The Evolution and 'Hallmarks' of Cancer

There are several distinct stages that cancer goes through that can be related to its ability to be treated and the prognosis of the patient. You may have heard of people referring to 'Stage One' or 'Stage Four' before, and that is because it is clinically useful to gauge the life stage of the condition to understand what treatment may be available. There are actually two main ways of categorising the stage of cancer, and these are associated with the size and magnitude of the original tumour site (if present), and whether it has metastasised, or may be likely to metastasise. If we focus on the primary tumour itself to begin with, there are a few stages that a tumour goes through as it develops (Figure 5.3). First, it will simply be mutated cells, and then over time these mutated cells will replicate and grow in number. This overgrowth of cells is referred to

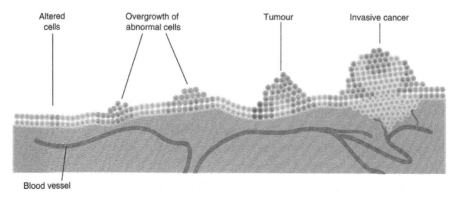

Figure 5.3   The development of cancer

Source: Cook et al. (2019), *Essentials of Pathophysiology for Nursing Practice*, Sage

as *hyperplasia* (*hyper* meaning too high, *plasia* referring to plasticity), and at this stage, despite there being a cluster of too many of them, they will most likely look normal under a microscope. The second part of this overgrowth is *dysplasia*, where the cells will look abnormal if examined. The growing cluster of cells is categorised as a tumour (or cancer *in situ*); this is where the cells have changed to being cancerous but are still located to one distinct location. Finally, we reach the stage of invasive cancer. Here, the tumour may have developed its own blood supply (*angiogenesis*) in order that it can grow more efficiently. Once a tumour has been connected to the vascular system, this also means that it may be able to spread as cells break away from the tumour and may travel via the vascular or lymphatic systems. For the staging systems associated with cancer, Stage 1 and some of Stage 2 cancers are usually in the pre-invasive phases (although some cancers can still be classed as Stage 2 if they have invaded local lymph nodes). Treatment of Stage 1 and Stage 2 cancers usually can be done effectively via surgery and through other types of treatment such as radiotherapy and chemotherapy. Stage 3 cancer is where the tumour is quite large, may have invaded local tissues, and has been found in lymph nodes around the body. Stage 4 cancer is where it has spread to and established itself in another bodily structure such as an organ – this is sometimes referred to as *metastatic* cancer.

This all understandably sounds terrifying. When put together with all the other things discussed in this book so far, and the multiplicities of doom and gloom that we can be subject to through biopsychosocial influences on our health, you would be forgiven for thinking that cancer is inevitable in all of us and at any time, but this is not the case. In order to develop right through to cancer, cells must be able to satisfy 10 (originally 6) distinct cellular mechanisms – referred to as the hallmarks of cancer (Hanahan & Weinberg, 2000, 2011).

The hallmarks of cancer (Hanahan & Weinberg, 2000, 2011)

1 Growth signal autonomy - *cells can divide through a self-directed mechanism without the need for the external signals that usually initiate mitosis.*

2 Insensitivity to growth inhibitory signals - *cells remain resistant to any external molecular signals to suppress growth.*

3 Evasion of apoptosis - *the ability to suppress the initiation of apoptosis, a mechanism that is inbuilt to cells and is usually triggered when DNA damage occurs.*

4 Limitless replicative potential - *the ability to surpass the Hayflick limit, governed by the shortening of telomeres.*

5 Sustained angiogenesis - *angiogenesis in normal, healthy functioning is usually regulated by a variety of signalling molecules that inhibit and stimulate this process. Cancer cells must be able to create their blood supply autonomously from that.*

6 Tissue invasion and metastasis - *beyond normal growth development, human cells tend to remain where they are. Cancer cells must develop the ability to invade surrounding tissues and to travel through the body to create secondary sites.*

7 Deregulating cellular energetics - *as cancer cells grow and replicate very quickly, they must be able to accelerate their metabolism beyond normal bounds to create enough energy and absorb sufficient nutrients to function.*

8 Avoiding immune detection - *our immune systems have in-built mechanisms to seek out and destroy abnormally replicating cells. The developing cancer must be able to evade this in order to continue growing and establishing.*

9 Genome instability and mutation - *cancers are typified by severe chromosomal abnormalities. There must be a sufficient number of mutations developed in the developing tumour in order to support the many qualities of the other hallmarks.*

10 Tumour-promoting inflammation - *tumours use our in-built immune mechanisms of inflammation to support their growth. The identification of immune cells within tumours was previously thought to be due to attempts by the immune system to control them, but cancer actually needs immune cells to create a suitable environment for the tumour to grow.*

Perhaps one of the most complex of these hallmarks is the ability for cancer to go unnoticed or unchallenged by the immune system. This is in itself an evolutionary process that the developing tumour undergoes, and it is suggested now that cancerous cells become cancer perhaps not in spite of immune intervention, but because of it. This can be the case with mutating viruses as well. A virus will become neutralised by the immune system, but viruses are very prone to mutations and if it can replicate fast enough (particularly before we can develop enough antibodies to combat it), it can also start to mutate to adapt to its oppressive environment. Those cells (either virus or cancer) that survive detection from our infantry-like immune cells will proliferate more in a very Darwinian process of survival of the fittest. Cancer similarly goes through phases of first being eliminated by the immune system, then managing to proliferate beyond the ability of the immune system to control it (establishing an equilibrium between cellular growth and destruction), and eventually developing mutations that allow it to evade immune detection altogether. This is referred to as the Three E's (elimination, equilibrium, evasion).

The Role of Psychobiology in Cancer and Psycho-Oncology

Psycho-oncology considers the combined biopsychosocial factors associated with the development and growth of cancers, and the psychological consequences of living with cancer (Holland, 2002). It is a much-needed area of health psychology given the rising numbers of cancer diagnoses, the lack of sufficient new treatments to compensate for this rise, and the corresponding growth of ineffective alternative/natural therapies. These techniques can range from guided imagery techniques (like imagining cells munching up tumours) to the consumption of shark cartilage, and now, worryingly, the use of fasting as it supposedly 'kickstarts' the immune system. Some may be completely harmless (aside from making therapeutic promises that it cannot deliver), but some can be very harmful indeed. Another indicator for the need for psychobiological approaches to cancer is that the variation in prognosis between individuals who are diagnosed with the same type and stage of cancer goes beyond simply being associated with biological factors – as does the variation in developing cancer (along with its timing and severity) in those who are deemed biologically at risk. There must be more going on than purely biological influence. As is arguably the case with all disease and disorder, the underlying causes are manifold. Not only this, but the complicated and delicate processes of living with cancer require arguably a lot more than purely medical care, meaning evidence-based interdisciplinary perspectives are very much needed.

We focused a bit before on the ability for cancer to evade detection by the immune system, and what biological factors underpin this. To illustrate where taking a psychobiological approach to cancer (i.e., psycho-oncology) can really help, we can look at what psychosocial factors may be associated with this as well. The *immune-surveillance hypothesis* outlines that cancer cells might arise really quite frequently, but are usually able to be targeted and destroyed by the immune system. If the immune system is suppressed (as happens during stress), the surveillance element is weakened, potentially allowing tumours to develop (Ostrand-Rosenberg, 2008). This may be associated with immunoediting, a process responsible for sculpting tumours as they develop (Dunn et al., 2002). There has been a wealth of research to support the thesis that psychosocial factors such as stress may play a key role in the weakening of immune surveillance that consequently provides a more favourable environment for cancer to develop (Forlenza & Baum, 2000). The debate about the contribution of stress to cancer pathogenesis and development has been a hot topic for some time. Activation of the sympathetic nervous system is associated with tumour growth, providing a direct link for neuroendocrine involvement (Cole et al., 2015). Inflammatory factors that are often modulated by stress are an important part of cancer cell growth (Mantovani et al., 2008). These inflammatory processes are thought to be associated with 15–20% of deaths from cancer, particularly breast cancer (Touvier et al., 2013). Stressful experiences often accelerate cancer progression and increase the likelihood of cancer-related mortality (Hamer et al., 2009). Stress is also known to limit DNA repair, which may impact the onset and progression of cancer (Kiecolt-Glaser et al., 2002). All of this is not to say that stress causes cancer – it is simply not that straightforward. However, stress is clearly a key contributor to cancer development that will likely add risk alongside other predisposing factors in the pathogenesis and pathophysiology of cancer.

Cancer also involves a fair number of genetic adaptations and changes. We know that some people have a genetic susceptibility towards certain types of cancer, but even then, there are variations in whether those people will go on to develop cancer or not. This is another one of those occasions where genetic predisposition requires an environmental trigger. For example, BRCA1 and BRCA2 are tumour suppressor genes, and mutations in these significantly increase the risk of breast/ovarian cancers (Zhong et al., 2015). However, some people with gene mutations associated with BRCA1 and BRCA2 do not end up getting cancer. It seems other environmental and behavioural factors are associated with the progression of cancer in these instances, including oral contraceptive or HRT use, smoking, alcohol consumption, postmenopausal weight-gain, and low levels of physical activity (Song et al., 2011). Even some associations have been made in terms of peoples' occupations (Palli et al., 2004). Behaviour is complex factor that has had strong links made to the likelihood of developing certain types of cancer. Obesity has been linked to many types of cancer (breast, bowel, uterine, oesophageal, gastric, pancreatic, renal, gallbladder) in about 5% of cases (Cancer Research UK, 2022). Our fat can speak to our immune and endocrine systems, so much so that fat is now thought of as being part of both systems, and this communication may be one of the common mechanisms by which obesity and being overweight can contribute to a variety of health outcomes including cancer (Huh et al., 2014; Trayhurn, 2005; Vieira-Potter, 2014). Exercise is known to be beneficial in prolonging life (and quality of life) in those with cancer (Eyigor & Kanyilmaz, 2014) – and its impact on reducing/managing the biological stress response may be important in preventing the impact of stress on cancer development.

So, the influences on our health that come from each part of the biopsychosocial paradigm are not only important indicators in themselves, they also very frequently relate to each other – mitigating or increasing the propensity of developing disease.

Key Questions

Thinking about the links you've found already between psychobiology and cancer, consider the approach of one of the psychobiology applied areas. Have a go at researching some of the immune and endocrine links to a type of illness. Once you have found some of these links, see if you can answer some of these questions in relation to the illness you are interested in:

- What in our psychological, social, and environmental worlds may drive some of these links?
- Can some of these links be more profound in certain populations of people?

Think back to the health onion, but try to link all of these to specific immune or endocrine changes to test your knowledge and expand your awareness of different mechanisms that drive disease pathways.

You may want to find one of your own, but you could start with some of those listed at the beginning of this section, such as psychocardiology or psychodermatology.

Learning Outcomes Summary

- Understand what psychology has to do with the immune system and endocrine system.

We have looked at how the brain and the body talk to each other and have seen some examples of how psychological factors can influence the immune system and vice versa. We have also looked at some examples of endocrine system dysfunction and how these impact psychological factors.

- Have an appreciation for the interplay between the immune and endocrine systems.

By looking at the ways in which both systems work, we have found common influences that affect both systems. We have also looked at particular situations where the immune and endocrine systems may speak to each other.

- Understand how psychological factors can be the result of immune/endocrine dysfunction.

We have used some examples of how psychological factors can be the result of immune system functioning (in the case of sickness behaviour) and the endocrine system (looking at thyroid dysfunction). The activities in this chapter will help you to expand your knowledge in this area further.

- Understand how psychological factors can influence cancer.

We have looked at the field of psycho-oncology as a case study for the way in which psychobiology can be applied to specific types of health concern. We have looked at the ways in which cancer develops and have then applied biopsychosocial factors that relate to the different ways in which cancer may develop.

FURTHER READING

Ader, R. (2000). On the development of psychoneuroimmunology. *European Journal of Pharmacology, 405*(1–3), 167–76.
A paper summarising the origins and development of the field of PNI, written by one of the 'founding fathers' of the field, Robert Ader. Contains some animal-based research.

Besedovsky, H. O., & Del Rey, A. (2007). Physiology of psychoneuroimmunology: A personal view. *Brain, Behavior, and Immunity, 21*(1), 34–44.
A great paper summarising over 30 years of work in the field of psychobiology. Contains some animal-based research.

Dinan, T. G., & Cryan, J. F. (2017). Microbes, immunity, and behavior: Psychoneuroimmunology meets the microbiome. *Neuropsychopharmacology, 42*(1), 178–92.
A paper introducing the integration between psychoneuroimmunology and the gut–brain axis.

Farber, D. L., Yudanin, N. A., & Restifo, N. P. (2014). Human memory T cells: Generation, compartmentalization and homeostasis. *Nature Reviews Immunology, 14*(1), 24–35.
For those of you wishing to enhance your immunology knowledge, this article gives a great overview of what we know about memory T-cells so far.

Lutgendorf, S. K., & Costanzo, E. S. (2003). Psychoneuroimmunology and health psychology: An integrative model. *Brain, Behavior, and Immunity, 17*(4), 225–32.
A good review paper summarising how PNI and health psychology are mutually driven and mutually beneficial.

Nicholson, L. B. (2016). The immune system. *Essays in Biochemistry*, *60*(3), 275–301.
A very detailed overview of what we know (or knew in 2016!) about the immune system.

Sapolsky, R. M. (2004). *Why zebras don't get ulcers: The acclaimed guide to stress, stress-related diseases, and coping*. Holt Paperbacks.
Robert Sapolsky is a wonderful writer, and whilst I would recommend that you read all his books, this is the one that really describes the core aspects of stress and psychobiology very well.

Turnbull, A. V., & Rivier, C. L. (1999). Regulation of the hypothalamic-pituitary-adrenal axis by cytokines: Actions and mechanisms of action. *Physiological Reviews*, *79*(1), 1–71.
An excellent overview of research demonstrating immune and endocrine cross-talk.

REFERENCES

Baigent, S. M. (2001). Peripheral corticotropin-releasing hormone and urocortin in the control of the immune response. *Peptides*, *22*(5), 809–20. https://doi.org/https://doi.org/10.1016/S0196-9781(01)00395-3

Blalock, J. E., & Smith, E. M. (2007). Conceptual development of the immune system as a sixth sense. *Brain, Behavior, and Immunity*, *21*(1), 23–33. https://doi.org/https://doi.org/10.1016/j.bbi.2006.09.004

Cancer Research UK. (2022). *Obesity, weight and cancer*. Retrieved 30 Sep 2022 from www.cancerresearchuk.org/about-cancer/causes-of-cancer/obesity-weight-and-cancer

Capuron, L., & Dantzer, R. (2003). Cytokines and depression: The need for a new paradigm. *Brain, Behavior, and Immunity*, *17*(1, Supplement), 119–24. https://doi.org/https://doi.org/10.1016/S0889-1591(02)00078-8

Cole, S. W., Nagaraja, A. S., Lutgendorf, S. K., Green, P. A., & Sood, A. K. (2015). Sympathetic nervous system regulation of the tumour microenvironment. *Nature Reviews Cancer*, *15*(9), 563–72. https://doi.org/10.1038/nrc3978

Dantzer, R. (2012). Depression and inflammation: An intricate relationship. *Biological Psychiatry*, *71*(1), 4–5. https://doi.org/10.1016/j.biopsych.2011.10.025

Dunn, G. P., Bruce, A. T., Ikeda, H., Old, L. J., & Schreiber, R. D. (2002). Cancer immunoediting: From immunosurveillance to tumor escape. *Nature Immunology*, *3*(11), 991–8. https://doi.org/10.1038/ni1102-991

Elenkov, I. J. (2004). Glucocorticoids and the Th1/Th2 Balance. *Annals of the New York Academy of Sciences*, *1024*(1), 138–46. https://doi.org/https://doi.org/10.1196/annals.1321.010

Eyigor, S., & Kanyilmaz, S. (2014). Exercise in patients coping with breast cancer: An overview. *World Journal of Clinical Oncology*, *5*(3), 406–11. https://doi.org/10.5306/wjco.v5.i3.406

Forlenza, M. J., & Baum, A. (2000). Psychosocial influences on cancer progression: Alternative cellular and molecular mechanisms. *Current Opinion in Psychiatry*, *13*(6), 639–45.

Grewe, M., Bruijnzeel-Koomen, C. A. F. M., Schöpf, E., Thepen, T., Langeveld-Wildschut, A. G., Ruzicka, T., & Krutmann, J. (1998). A role for Th1 and Th2 cells in the immunopathogenesis of atopic dermatitis. *Immunology Today, 19*(8), 359–61. https://doi.org/https://doi.org/10.1016/S0167-5699(98)01285-7

Gu, H.-f., Tang, C.-k., & Yang, Y.-z. (2012). Psychological stress, immune response, and atherosclerosis. *Atherosclerosis, 223*(1), 69–77. https://doi.org/https://doi.org/10.1016/j.atherosclerosis.2012.01.021

Hamer, M., Chida, Y., & Molloy, G. J. (2009). Psychological distress and cancer mortality. *Journal of Psychosomatic Research, 66*(3), 255–8. https://doi.org/https://doi.org/10.1016/j.jpsychores.2008.11.002

Hanahan, D., & Weinberg, R. A. (2000). The hallmarks of cancer. *Cell, 100*(1), 57–70. https://doi.org/10.1016/S0092-8674(00)81683-9

Hanahan, D., & Weinberg, Robert A. (2011). Hallmarks of cancer: The next generation. *Cell, 144*(5), 646–74. https://doi.org/10.1016/j.cell.2011.02.013

Heinrichs, M., von Dawans, B., & Domes, G. (2009). Oxytocin, vasopressin, and human social behavior. *Frontiers in Neuroendocrinology, 30*(4), 548–57. https://doi.org/https://doi.org/10.1016/j.yfrne.2009.05.005

Holland, J. C. (2002). History of psycho-oncology: Overcoming attitudinal and conceptual barriers. *Psychosomatic Medicine, 64*(2), 206–21. https://journals.lww.com/psychosomaticmedicine/Fulltext/2002/03000/History_of_Psycho_Oncology__Overcoming_Attitudinal.4.aspx

Hou, N., Zhang, X., Zhao, L., Zhao, X., Li, Z., Song, T., & Huang, C. (2013). A novel chronic stress-induced shift in the Th1 to Th2 response promotes colon cancer growth. *Biochemical and Biophysical Research Communications, 439*(4), 471–6. https://doi.org/https://doi.org/10.1016/j.bbrc.2013.08.101

Huh, J. Y., Park, Y. J., Ham, M., & Kim, J. B. (2014). Crosstalk between adipocytes and immune cells in adipose tissue inflammation and metabolic dysregulation in obesity. *Molecules and Cells, 37*(5), 365–71. https://doi.org/10.14348/molcells.2014.0074

Kaufmann, I., Eisner, C., Richter, P., Huge, V., Beyer, A., Chouker, A., ... Thiel, M. (2007). Lymphocyte subsets and the role of Th1/Th2 balance in stressed chronic pain patients. *Neuroimmunomodulation, 14*(5), 272–80. https://doi.org/10.1159/000115041

Kiecolt-Glaser, J. K., Robles, T. F., Heffner, K. L., Loving, T. J., & Glaser, R. (2002). Psycho-oncology and cancer: Psychoneuroimmunology and cancer. *Annals of Oncology, 13*, 165–9. https://doi.org/https://doi.org/10.1093/annonc/mdf655

Mantovani, A., Allavena, P., Sica, A., & Balkwill, F. (2008). Cancer-related inflammation. *Nature, 454*(7203), 436–44. https://doi.org/10.1038/nature07205

McEwen, B. S., Biron, C. A., Brunson, K. W., Bulloch, K., Chambers, W. H., Dhabhar, F. S., ... Weiss, J. M. (1997). The role of adrenocorticoids as modulators of immune function in health and disease: neural, endocrine and immune interactions. *Brain Research Reviews, 23*(1), 79–133. https://doi.org/https://doi.org/10.1016/S0165-0173(96)00012-4

Myint, A.-M., Leonard, B. E., Steinbusch, H. W. M., & Kim, Y.-K. (2005). Th1, Th2, and Th3 cytokine alterations in major depression. *Journal of Affective Disorders, 88*(2), 167–73. https://doi.org/https://doi.org/10.1016/j.jad.2005.07.008

Ostrand-Rosenberg, S. (2008). Immune surveillance: A balance between protumor and antitumor immunity. *Current Opinion in Genetics & Development*, *18*(1), 11–18. https://doi.org/https://doi.org/10.1016/j.gde.2007.12.007

Palli, D., Masala, G., Mariani-Costantini, R., Zanna, I., Saieva, C., Sera, F., … Ottini, L. (2004). A gene-environment interaction between occupation and BRCA1/BRCA2 mutations in male breast cancer? *European Journal of Cancer*, *40*(16), 2474–9. https://doi.org/https://doi.org/10.1016/j.ejca.2004.07.012

Reiche, E. M. V., Nunes, S. O. V., & Morimoto, H. K. (2004). Stress, depression, the immune system, and cancer. *The Lancet Oncology*, *5*(10), 617–25. https://doi.org/https://doi.org/10.1016/S1470-2045(04)01597-9

Song, M., Lee, K.-M., & Kang, D. (2011). Breast cancer prevention based on gene–environment interaction. *Molecular Carcinogenesis*, *50*(4), 280–90. https://doi.org/https://doi.org/10.1002/mc.20639

Touvier, M., Fezeu, L., Ahluwalia, N., Julia, C., Charnaux, N., Sutton, A., … Czernichow, S. (2013). Association between prediagnostic biomarkers of inflammation and endothelial function and cancer risk: A nested case-control study. *American Journal of Epidemiology*, *177*(1), 3–13. https://doi.org/10.1093/aje/kws359

Trayhurn, P. (2005). Endocrine and signalling role of adipose tissue: New perspectives on fat. *Acta Physiologica Scandinavica*, *184*(4), 285–93. https://doi.org/https://doi.org/10.1111/j.1365-201X.2005.01468.x

Turnbull, A. V., & Rivier, C. L. (1999). Regulation of the Hypothalamic-Pituitary-Adrenal Axis by cytokines: Actions and mechanisms of action. *Physiological Reviews*, *79*(1), 1–71. https://doi.org/10.1152/physrev.1999.79.1.1

Vanderpump, M. P. J. (2011). The epidemiology of thyroid disease. *British Medical Bulletin*, *99*(1), 39–51. https://doi.org/10.1093/bmb/ldr030

Vieira-Potter, V. J. (2014). Inflammation and macrophage modulation in adipose tissues. *Cellular Microbiology*, *16*(10), 1484–92. https://doi.org/https://doi.org/10.1111/cmi.12336

Zhong, Q., Peng, H.-L., Zhao, X., Zhang, L., & Hwang, W.-T. (2015). Effects of BRCA1- and BRCA2-related mutations on ovarian and breast cancer survival: A meta-analysis. *Clinical Cancer Research*, *21*(1), 211–220. https://doi.org/10.1158/1078-0432. Ccr-14-1816

6
STRESS AT THE PERSON LEVEL

INTRODUCTION

Stress has been mentioned in more or less every chapter of this book so far, so it is high time that we look at it in more detail. This chapter will cover what stress is, what it means to individuals psychologically and socially, and how it has an impact on health. Both biological and behavioural mechanisms are used to illustrate the impact of stress on a variety of metrics of health at the cellular and person levels. Modulators such as appraisal and coping are used to demonstrate the subjectivity of stress, and this is then related to personal trait factors (like optimism) that play a part in the physiological experience of stress. We will take a look at some of the dynamics of stress and explore different types of stress (both good and bad). Finally, we will consider how stress is buffered by social support, one of the most important things that stands between stress and damage to our health.

Learning Outcomes

- Define stress and its implications for health.
- Understand the importance of psychological factors to the experience of stress and coping.
- Describe different coping styles, how they may be employed during stressful experiences, and how these can have positive and negative outcomes.
- Appreciate the importance of social support in the psychological and biological experience of stress.

WHAT IS STRESS?

We all instinctively know what stress is because we all experience it, but stress itself can be hard to define. What might be paralysingly stressful to me may not even register on your stressometer and vice versa. Stress is very subjective. It is subjective between people, with people rating similar events quite differently, but it is also subjective within people. Think back to the second-to-last most stressful thing you experienced in your life. You may have thought 'that was *the* most stressful thing I have ever been through!', and you were absolutely right. However, the next time you experienced something horribly stressful, you thought exactly the same thing about that, and all of a sudden what used to be 'the most stressful thing' is now just a number in a long hit list of horrible experiences. Stress is in the eye of the beholder, but that is not to say that we cannot try to define it.

In terms of creating a definition of stress, many researchers have sought to adequately summarise stress in a way that can encompass the wide subjectivity of experience but still remain meaningful. Hans Selye, the godfather of stress, defined stress as 'The nonspecific response of the body to any demand made upon it' (Selye, 1976). Whilst this was a good attempt at explaining stress, we know now that the stress response is actually very specific. Moreover, we also know that stress is more than just demands made upon the body. In fact, more often than not in our modern lives, our stress is more about demands made upon our emotions and minds rather than upon our bodies. A lot of researchers have tried to describe precisely what stress is, but I think most of us now agree that it is a physical, emotional, and psychological state resulting from a discrepancy between what is being demanded of us (physically, emotionally, cognitively) and the corresponding resources we have (or feel we have) to be able to cope with that demand. The nature of the stressor can vary in terms of its severity, the extent to which it threatens which elements of a person's life, its predictability or controllability, and how long it may last. Equally, the emotions that may come with those events can vary as well. Some may induce fear, some anger, and some just a sustained feeling of worry and anxiety. Because stress is so subjective, whether a situation or event is determined to be stressful is down to the individual appraisal of the person experiencing it.

There have been three main ways that scholars have tried to define stress: as a response (i.e., an internal response to an external cue, designed to keep us alive), as a stimulus (i.e., the thing that instigates the internal response to action), and finally as a transaction (i.e., a dynamic process of appraisal that determines the salience of a stressor). The first theory was focused very centrally on the internal processes initiated during the stress response – the physiological and psychological responses to threat. The second was more focused on the thing causing the stress, with the idea that some things 'just are' stressful to whomever may encounter them. These two theories, whilst partly true, are quite insufficient given the varying degree between and within people that something that causes stress is determined to be stressful. The final model, the Transactional Model of Stress (later updated to be the Transactional Model of Stress and Coping) developed by Richard Lazarus and Susan Folkman (1984) is perhaps the best way of considering the nature of stress with the required subjectivity of understanding that situations and circumstances may vary. Essentially, this model dictates that we appraise a potentially stressful situation in two ways. First, we must determine whether it is a threat to us: what degree of harm could it cause us? What aspects of my life/welfare or the lives/welfare of the people or things I love does it threaten? If we determine here that the thing is not *that* worrisome, then we do not become stressed. If, on the other hand, we determine that this thing is in some way a threat, we undergo another stage of appraisal: can I cope? Do I have the resources available (or can I get the resources) needed to manage the stress this will cause? If we get through this stage and realise that actually we do have the resources to cope (whatever they may be) then this too is not considered to be too threatening. If, however, we determine that this stressor exceeds our resources to cope, this is when we experience stress. We will consider coping later in this chapter, as it is clearly an important element in not only what stress may result in, but also in the way that we determine something to be stressful.

One final note on defining stress is about valence. We tend to commonly talk about stress in very negative ways. We don't like it. It makes us feel bad and we cannot wait to get past it. However, stress is also sometimes useful. It teaches us about our boundaries and limits, as well as how we can smash through them and stay on our feet. The adage of *what doesn't kill you makes you stronger* very much works for the psychological experience of stress. We adapt and grow around the things that challenge us, and our experiences (and our ability to cope with them) can be a tremendous source of empowerment if we are able to focus on our resilience and inner strength. This type of stress is referred to as **eustress** (as opposed to distress), and it can be tremendously important in allowing us to grow psychologically. Think back to one of those times when you had 'the worst' experience of stress you had ever had. When you think about it now, do you feel pride that you were able to overcome it or otherwise get through it? Relief even? So much of these tests to our capabilities can be positive sooner or later. Physiologically, however, the story is a little different. Or, at least, the story is a little different now. Back when these responses first evolved it may well have been the case that as our stress responses were used and resolved we may have strengthened certain aspects of our bodies. Nowadays, that is not usually the way our stress works.

STRESS TYPOLOGIES

When we try to categorise stress, we can think of a variety of different ways of doing this. We could categorise it according to what is under threat (e.g., is it financial stress, relationship stress, or work stress?). We could also consider to what extent it may infiltrate the person's life (e.g., does it impact our working life, our home life, or everything?). Each of these, however, is also very subjective. In psychological theory and research, we tend to categorise stress in two main ways: acute and chronic. **Acute stress** is usually something quite episodic. It could last for a minute, a day, or even a year, but we would know at some point that it will end. It could be a minor hassle, or something that turns your entire life upside down. It could be getting stuck in a traffic jam on the way to work, having to sit an exam, or even having to write a book because you had a conversation with a publisher and things quickly got wildly out of hand. The key to acute stress is that it is short-term – you know that it will end and may even know when it will end. **Chronic stress**, on the other hand, is a stressful situation that we can't necessarily see the end of. It could be something associated with a long-term change to your lifestyle or welfare, or it could be the loss of someone or something that could be permanent. Examples of chronic stress that are used widely in this field of research are things like bereavement, job loss and unemployment, or caring for a sick, elderly, or disabled relative. These are referred to as 'models' of chronic stress, and whilst none are perfect (in that each one will be experienced very differently by different people) they are the closest things we have to what could be termed 'universally' stressful experiences (i.e., put pretty much anyone in that situation and they will be very stressed). Both types of stress can and are used in research to make sense of the ways that psychological experiences and situations can impact our health, and there have been decades of research carried out to make sense of the ways that these experiences get under our skin, and the person-to-person variation in these mechanisms that means that some will be more vulnerable than others to these experiences.

THE BIOLOGY OF STRESS

In Chapter 5, we looked at the hormonal stress axis as a way of describing endocrine function and communication. This was a very brief introduction to the physiology of stress, so here we will look at that in more detail. The physiological stress response is ancient in evolutionary terms, and we share it with pretty much all other vertebrate animals. It is perfectly designed to give us a bit of physical advantage in times of critical threat. The premise is quite simple: ramp up everything you need for peak physical exertion. Your body does this in two ways, it will selectively augment our ability to exert (through allowing faster and fuller blood flow, mobilising molecules for metabolic energy, and giving a boost to our brain to make split second decisions), and depress non-essential systems to allow energy and molecular support to be diverted to where it is needed at that stage. As outlined in Chapter 2, this is the sympathetic nervous system (SNS) in activation. If we are fighting or running away, we need our muscles and our brains to be prioritised for blood flow that will be carrying oxygen and nutrients, so our hearts beat faster, our vascular tone (the tension of our blood vessels) is optimised to create a balance between volume and pressure, our airways dilate to allow us to absorb more oxygen, and our livers and fat stores dump glucose into our bloodstream. The pupils also dilate to allow as much visual information in as possible so that we can make snap decisions during our fighting or running away. Some other minor tweaks that are made are small boosts to both adaptive and innate (humoural and cellular) immunity, including the mobilisation of blood-clotting factors in case we are injured. Almost all the other changes made by the SNS at this stage are to divert energy away from 'non-essential' systems and processes, to push everything we've got into our physical efforts of survival. Our digestive system is slowed down, any processes involved in bone maintenance or growth grind to a halt, and our sex hormone signalling is dampened. So at the time of fight or flight, we are pushing our cardiovascular systems to their limit, mobilising energy to feed our muscles, brains, and hearts, providing a safety net of clotting factors in case we are injured, and basically quietening everything else down to support this huge effort. This is a perfectly balanced system if we need to fight or run away, and it has without doubt ensured the survival of our, and many other, species. The problem is, though, that we don't often need to fight or run away anymore. We considered this briefly in Chapter 1, but will go into this in more detail now.

One thing you may be wondering about at this stage is why this still happens when we don't really need it so much. Well, the thing is we *do* actually still need it quite a lot, but perhaps in different ways. If you suddenly need to jump out of the way of a car coming towards you, or need to drop everything and run to that meeting or that class you forgot about, or need to deadlift that heavy box that you accidentally just set down on your toes – all of these can utilise your fight-or-flight response. The way we can make sense of what might happen to someone if they did not have a good fight-or-flight response is by observing what happens to people who have diseases and disorders of these systems. There are some diseases that affect certain systems in the body, meaning a physiological stress response cannot be created, such as Addison's disease (characterised by under-production of cortisol and aldosterone). People with Addison's disease can still *feel* stressed, but if they put their bodies in stressful situations then they cannot mount an appropriate physiological response to cope with it. Imagine trying to run for a bus without increasing your heart rate, blood pressure, or available energy in your bloodstream – what do you think would happen? In the case of Addison's disease, it can cause a state of *adrenal crisis*, which requires urgent medication. So, as much as the fight-or-flight response may not be perfectly attuned to our modern way of living, it is still essential and still serves a purpose. The real problem we encounter is that we don't enact the behaviours necessary to de-escalate that SNS response. The parasympathetic nervous system will kick in to undo all those actions (and send us back into *rest and digest* mode) if we physically exert ourselves. That is the way this whole system has been evolved to work: we experience stress, we prepare to deal with it, we deal with it by exerting ourselves, our stress response subsides, and we return to baseline. What has changed with our modern lives is that we do not do the physical exertion part. More often than not, we get stressed at computers, behind the wheel of the car, sitting down in conversation with someone, or otherwise in a very sedentary state. It is less that our bodies are out of step with our lives, and more that our lives are out of step with our bodies.

Along with not adequately using (or resolving) our fight-or-flight response, we also tend to activate our stress responses too frequently, and for far too long. Humans also have the unique ability to set off the stress response ourselves. How many times have you lain in bed at night thinking about all the things you have to worry about? That awkward conversation with the person you were trying to impress. The exam or the deadline you have coming up soon. The family event that you're secretly dreading. It could even be just reliving some embarrassing or stressful events you have already been through in your long distant past. As if this wasn't enough, we also like to go out of our way to make ourselves stressed too. We may watch horror films, go on roller-coaster rides, participate in open mic events or other types of performance, or – worse still – we may sign up for some sort of networking event. We tend to live our lives lurching from one stressful situation to the next, and in this way even acute stressors, if serially encountered and not physiologically resolved, can cause problems for our health. When chronically turning on stress responses and not resolving them adequately we are ignoring the need to de-escalate these physiological cascades, and causing a serious amount of wear-and-tear. This wear-and-tear is referred to as **allostatic load**, and it is a significant problem for our health.

Allostatic Load

Allostasis refers to the careful balance of each of our bodily systems. You may have heard of *homeostasis* before, which is the ability to ensure we retain a good balance of things that we need (hydration, blood sugar etc.). Allostasis is about ensuring that our systems are working in a good balance. As we have already seen, the various systems we have are intimately entwined, and often share the same hardware/software to operate. Allostasis is the ability for flexibility and function in each of our systems to keep us working at our optimal levels, and adapting to our environments efficiently (McEwen, 1998). The fight-or-flight response is essentially allostatic because it is tinkering with a variety of systems in the body (immune, endocrine, digestive, cardiovascular). This is allostasis in its basic sense – the ability to regulate a variety of different processes using a variety of different pathways with some processes being ramped up and others slowed down. If the stress response goes on for too long and is not in some way resolved, some systems that are dampened remain so in favour of more 'essential' systems for that context (i.e., stress). Professors Bruce McEwen and Elliot Stellar (1993) proposed that ongoing allostasis could cause *allostatic load* (sometimes referred to as allostatic overload also) – where a constant demand on bodily systems causes internal competition for resources, and reduces the ability of the individual to cope either psychologically or physically with new demands. Professor Robert Sapolsky describes allostasis as being like two elephants on a seesaw – it may be in balance, but so much weight on either side will cause something to break eventually (leading to allostatic load). The more the elephants lurch up and down on the seesaw, the more damage is done to the seesaw itself and to the infrastructures around it that are affected by its movement. It is an excellent analogy. Another type of allostatic load has been characterised – Type 2 – where overload occurs due to subtle but persistent social conflict/disturbance. They don't necessarily require very strong responses like major trauma, but over time can cause a great deal of damage (McEwen & Wingfield, 2003). The types of stressors in this second category can be more damaging because they can sneak up on us without us consciously knowing how much damage they cause.

Key Questions

Some people may be more vulnerable to allostatic load than others - that could be due to a variety of factors. What biopsychosocial factors do you think might explain variance in allostatic load?

- Allostatic load can be initiated from more than just stress. Any time we are creating an over-exertion of the balance of our bodily systems we are potentially putting ourselves into allostatic load.
- What sorts of things might these be? (Think: behaviours, lifestyles)
- When in our lifetimes might these occur?

The perspective used to explain allostatic load relies on looking at the body as a whole made from smaller systems. To quantify allostatic load, we have to examine the way multiple systems are working to adequately determine if someone is or is not experiencing it. Rather than just focusing on whether or not someone under stress develops an illness, looking at multiple biological markers of physiological functioning can tell you more about the internal state and its vulnerability to illness (McEwen & Seeman, 1999). Measuring the function of the HPA axis (by looking at stress hormones like **cortisol** or **dehydroepiandrosterone**), the SNS (with **adrenaline, noradrenaline**), the cardiovascular system (using blood pressure, heart rate, or **heart rate variability**), and metabolic markers (waist-to-hip ratio, ratio of low-density to high-density lipoprotein) can tell us not just about potential chemical mediators to disease, but also about likely contributors to pathology. This perspective allows us to see and understand not just what happens when we are stressed and that this affects our health, but also the underlying mechanisms for it. Allostatic load and the impact it has on multiple systems is one of the key ways in which we can make sense of the multiple impacts on health that occur through each of the aspects on the health onion, such as socio-economic status, social relationships, lifestyles, work factors, genetics, gender, and ethnicity (Beckie, 2012). We can also make sense of the impact of life course events on health through allostatic load, within observable pathways from adverse childhood experiences right up to the way that we age over our adulthood having an impact on allostatic load and its subsequent impact on our health (Guidi et al., 2021).

STRESS AND BEHAVIOUR

Whilst most of this chapter so far has focused on the biological aspects of stress, remember that it's not just biological changes that impact health. Stress is an excellent example of biobehavioural influence on health in terms of how our behaviour may adapt in the face of it. When something makes us stressed, we may be more likely to adopt negative health behaviours (such as eating unhealthy foods, or using alcohol or tobacco) and less likely to engage in positive health behaviours (such as exercise and getting enough sleep), so there is a double effect on our health from that perspective. The lack of physical activity during times of stress is a real big hitter because this is actually what we are designed to do when our stress response initiates, and it is the one thing that will allow the resolution of the physiological stress response and the re-initiation of parasympathetic activity. There are a lot of cultural and social factors wound up in the way that we respond to stress behaviourally, and whilst they can differ from community to community, and may change with generational trends, we as humans are all pretty united in these responses being less than ideal for our physical health.

Generally speaking, our behavioural responses to stress could be considered to be as a result of stress (for example, being able to exercise less because you are so busy working towards an assessment, or losing sleep because you are worrying), or could be a response designed to cope with the impact of stress (for example, self-medicating with tobacco, alcohol, or other substances, or engaging in unhealthy/unwise behaviours to distract yourself from the stress). There is also the nature of the stressor to consider when it comes to impact on behaviour. If someone is stressed because they are in debt, or because they otherwise cannot afford to pay their bills, the resulting impact on behaviour may not be a direct result of the stress, it could be a consequence of the thing causing stress itself. The links between stress and behaviour become even more complicated when you consider that over time stress can have an impact on overall mental health as well, impacting our motivational states and attitudes towards staying healthy. Just as there are layered biopsychosocial influences on health, there are layered biopsychosocial influences on behaviour too. It makes things very complicated, but that's because people are complicated. Chapter 7 will consider this a little bit further when it comes to thinking about stress at the group/population level. Diving into these complicated intersections really requires an entire book dedicated to it, so for now I have included some recommended reading at the end of this chapter if you would like to learn more about this fascinating area. To get a feel for how complex and nuanced the relationships between stress and behaviour can be, have a go at the next activity.

Key Questions

Try to use the Health Onion in a different way now, and consider what influences each of the layers may have on our behaviour. Choose one type of health behaviour (this could be positive or negative), and consider how someone's behaviour may change in response to an acute stressor (e.g., an exam period, or a house move). This could be in consideration of our emotional responses to the behaviour, or our attitudes to the behaviour, but it could also be about the accessibility/availability of the behaviour in general. Try to think within and across cultures as well.

- Consider what impact the stressor itself may have on the behaviour.
- Consider what impact coping with the stressor may have on the behaviour.
- Are there types of people that may be more or less likely to engage or not engage in this behaviour in response to that stressor?

STRESS MODIFIERS: APPRAISAL AND COPING

I have already hinted in previous sections of this chapter about a very important aspect of stress and health: coping. **Coping** is very important because it is the way we manage stress, and it can impact our behaviour, our thoughts and feelings, and our overall responses to the stress we encounter (both psychologically and biologically). It is yet another area of the fascinating field of stress that could have (and has had) an entire book written about it. How we cope (or do not cope) with stressful circumstances can have a huge impact on both our mental and physical health. The coping method itself can also have a direct impact on health, as discussed in the last section. If we choose to use alcohol to cope with our problems, this has direct consequences for our cellular and systems-level physical health, and will likely impact our mental health over time as well. It may even permeate into our social health, degrading our relationships with others and making a bad situation even worse. There are many different types of coping, and generally speaking we will all adopt different types of these coping styles in different ways depending on different stressors. Before we dive into coping styles in more detail, try the next exercise to see how you might cope with some of these stressful scenarios.

Key Questions

Consider the following stressful scenarios and how you might cope with the stress you experience from them. Perhaps you have already encountered some of these and can reflect on how you dealt with them at the time and think about whether you would still use the same method of coping if you encountered them again, or whether you would adopt a different strategy.

1 Moving house
2 Sitting an exam that carries 100% of the course credit
3 Losing your job
4 Being diagnosed with a chronic health condition

- What types of behaviours do you/would you engage with in dealing with these stressors?
- Are they all the same, or do you use different tactics for different stressor types?
- Do you use one way of coping, or do you employ lots of different ways of coping?

Carrying out that activity will have hopefully shown you that you have used (or would use) a variety of different methods to cope with stress. There are some types of stressors that we meet head on – we will seek out information about them, take active steps to confront them (or perhaps break them down into smaller, less intimidating components), and ensure we are as prepared as we can be to deal with them. This is referred to as *problem-focused coping*. Another way of coping can be to deal with the emotional fallout of the stress – to attend to our feelings about the stressor, to manage our emotional pain or distress that will result from experiencing that stressor. That is referred to as *emotion-focused coping*. Whether or not we adopt problem-focused or emotion-focused coping will depend on a myriad of personal factors that will be decided by your individual personality, your culture, your upbringing, and your available resources, but may also be dependent on the type of stressor. As well as where our efforts are focused (the problem itself or our emotional responses to it), we can also consider coping in terms of its style, in whether it is avoidant (i.e., if we do our best to avoid both the problem and its emotional consequences) or adaptive (i.e., if we choose to confront the problem and/or its emotional consequences). In considering styles, we can see that certain behaviours that we may turn to in stressful scenarios can be a mixture of both focus and style. To take one of the examples of the exercise, receiving a diagnosis of a chronic medical condition, we can choose problem-focused coping that is both adaptive (e.g., researching the medical condition, connecting with others with a similar diagnosis for informational support) and avoidant (e.g., not exercising to avoid pain or flare-ups of symptoms). We could also choose an emotion-focused coping strategy that is either adaptive (e.g., we talk about how we feel to a counsellor or close friend) or avoidant (e.g., we start to eat more comforting food in greater excess to deal with our feelings of stress). We can break this down further by also considering that coping strategies might be cognitive or behavioural. We may choose to tackle a problem by researching our problem and gaining information (a cognitive, problem-focused, adaptive style), by engaging in exercise (a behavioural, emotion-focused, adaptive style), by some 'mind over matter' technique (a cognitive, emotion-focused, avoidant style), by consulting an expert (a behavioural, problem-focused, adaptive style), or by using drugs or alcohol (a behavioural, emotion-focused, avoidant style). What is most likely is that we will engage in a few different ways of coping, and some of these will be positive and some will be negative. In this way, if the negative means of coping tends to be preferentially engaged, then we may have far worse outcomes, and the opposite may be true for preferential use of positive coping mechanisms. How we may choose to deal with a certain stressor can vary from person to person, and from time to time. It will depend on what else we are dealing with at the time (rarely does any stressful life event emerge on its own, or simply impact one aspect of life), and how we feel about the stressor and its level of potential threat to ourselves, our welfare, or the welfare of those we value.

Considering how relative our coping is to both ourselves and the nature of the stressor that we are confronting, it has been difficult to develop suitable models for coping that can consider the huge number of factors that are likely to be involved. Lazarus and Folkman (1984) have also developed a transactional model of coping, which critically also incorporates the capacity for positive emotions to result from our stress and coping experience, such as finding a new or renewed meaning to life. This model is very helpful when considering some of the complex and life-changing stressors that can occur, that are rarely straightforward and rarely result in one emotional response. However, this model does little to account for some of the more complex environmental factors that are associated with our ability to cope, and our adoption of particular coping styles. There is likely a great deal of interplay between both the person's individual appraisal of the stressful situation and the resources they may draw from in their environment at any one time. To expand on this further, sometimes things are stressful *because* of our context – in other words, they would not be stressful (or perhaps as stressful) if our situation were different. For example, if you lose your wallet with all of your important personal effects such as bank cards, driving license and so forth – how much more stressful would this be if you were to do so in another country, where you do not speak the language very well, where the legal and practical systems may be unfamiliar, and where you have not yet established a social support network? The context of the stressor can be just as important as our personal appraisal in determining both how stressful something is and how we cope with it. Another model that attempts to account for this complexity comes from Rudolf Moos (1984), who is credited as the first scholar to attempt to incorporate the intricacies of our social environment into a model of coping. This model views coping not just as a transaction between person and stressor, but also their social and physical environment, and a consideration of their current status of health and wellbeing (see Figure 6.1).

The model looks quite complex, but if we are looking to consider broader contextual factors into our understanding of how someone will cope with any given stressor at any

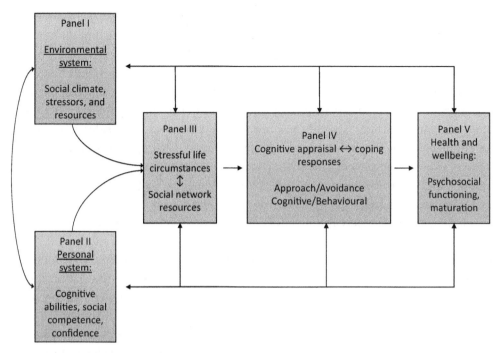

Figure 6.1   Moos' (1984) Framework of context and coping
Source: Author's own drawing, with permission of John Wiley & Sons

given time, there are a variety of elements that will be involved and that will influence each other. Panels I and II provide the contextual element of the coping framework, where our personal and environmental systems are important in deciding the way that we will cope. Each of the factors within these domains will vary throughout someone's life, even if the same type of stressor is experienced more than once. Consider how you have experienced moving house. If this has been more than once, you will have been at different life stages, with different personal competencies, and there will have been different contextual reasons around that house move. Panel III considers the interplay between the other stressful experiences that may be going on at the time, as well as the availability of a support network (more on social support soon). Panel IV is our Lazarus & Folkman style appraisal element, that there will be an appraisal of the stressor and our perceived ability to cope with it. Finally, Panel V is about our current health and wellbeing, and how those factors will influence our experience of the stressor and our ability to cope with it, as well as being directly influenced by the stressor and our coping, recognising that the relationship between health and wellbeing and stress and coping is reciprocal. Each of the panels plays a part in the overall ability for the person to cope, but they also influence each other. The consideration of environment and context with this model is very important not just because our context can change, but also because not everyone is the same, nor do they live in the same context. This model has also been highlighted as an important step towards considering a culturally relevant and appropriate consideration of coping, where our personal cultures (made up of any of the micro, meso, and macro layers that we considered in Chapter 3) will be hugely varied from person to person, from nation to nation. Culture is a complex factor to consider and will likely have an impact on each and every one of the considerations within that model, which is why it has been argued that – as a consideration – it sits around the entire model, influencing each of the individual components as well as their interplay (Chun et al., 2006). Two basic concepts within culture are the two dominant types of social interrelation: collectivism and individualism. Collectivism is the concept that we are all connected, that we as individuals in our society are interdependent with one another, and our society is dependent on reciprocity and mutual effort. Individualist cultures are more centred on the concept of being independent and looking after ourselves, that we must be responsible for ourselves, our actions, and the consequences of those actions. They are somewhat diametrically opposed, but they exist on a continuum, with micro, meso, and macro cultures sitting somewhere along that spectrum. You will also have personal variation within those cultures, with individuals that exist in individualist societies that take on a more collectivist personal philosophy and vice versa. Culture is incredibly complicated, but it is important to be considered. I can only scratch the surface in this chapter, so I have added some important and interesting further reading options at the end that will help to unravel some of these complexities.

Optimism: the Double-Edged Sword

One seemingly positive way of coping with stressful situations is through **optimism**. If we are generally more optimistic, we may be more likely to frame stress in a less negative way (so it could be appraised as more of a challenge than a threat), meaning we may not suffer the stronger ill effects of stress (Baumgartner et al., 2018). If we are more optimistic about the future, we may also be more likely to take control of our health, make better health behaviour choices, and be higher in self-efficacy when it comes to stressful situations (Schwarzer & Fuchs, 1996). People with an optimistic outlook tend to frame stress in either a situational way (e.g., 'This situation is terrible, but others are not'), a temporary way (e.g., 'this won't last'), or an external way (e.g., 'it's the situation, not me'). Compared with those who are pessimistic, optimists tend to have longer, healthier lives (Lee et al., 2019). Optimists tend to have lower levels of inflammation, will physiologically respond to stress more conservatively (e.g., lower blood pressure spikes), and are much less likely to die from cardiovascular events such as myocardial infarction (Baumgartner et al., 2018; Everson et al., 1996; Roy et al., 2010). Optimism appears to impact individuals' coping mechanisms, with positive associations between optimism and more 'approach'-oriented types of coping (or adaptive coping), and negative associations with avoidant coping styles (Nes & Segerstrom, 2006). Research with HIV patients has also found that optimism is associated with more proactive behaviour and lower levels of depression, overall being associated with a slower decline in key T-cells associated with HIV disease progression as well as with a lower HIV viral load (Ironson et al., 2005). Optimism is also associated with more active coping strategies such as positive reappraisal, which has, in turn, been associated with better immune outcomes as well (Koh et al., 2006). This all sounds like an all-round win for optimism. Unfortunately, the case for optimism is a little more complicated.

Unrealistic optimism, where someone always assumes good outcomes will happen, may not actually be all that helpful when it comes to stress and health. Optimistic bias – the mistaken belief that chances of negative events are lower, or chances of positive events are higher than most people's – can influence people to engage in *less* positive health behaviours and to take more risks. Weinstein (1982) asked students to rate how likely it would be that they would develop a health condition (e.g., substance dependence disorder, developing cardiovascular disease, cancer, and other chronic health conditions) to investigate how prevalent optimistic bias was in this cohort of young people with their whole lives ahead of them. The majority believed they were 'much less likely' than their peers to develop the health problems, and those that were high in optimistic bias were far less worried about the risk of these issues and considered each of the outcomes less severe than those with less optimistic bias. This has been seen in other samples, with a review of a substantial amount of literature looking at a wide variety of other health conditions (e.g., HIV, substance abuse etc.) (Helweg-Larsen & Shepperd, 2001).

If being overly optimistic is bad – is it more advantageous to be less optimistic? Optimists tend to have better moods, and this alone is beneficial for health (Wenglert & Rosén, 1995). On top of this, optimists have been shown to have better immune function, and to help sustain immune function under stress (Segerstrom & Sephton, 2010). In law students, those who were more optimistic about their future academic success had far fewer immune decrements during the stressful period of exam time (Segerstrom et al., 1998). Optimism is associated with lower cortisol, and in women has been associated with markers of inflammation like **C-Reactive Protein** (Steptoe et al., 2007). As well as having different physiological reactions to stress, optimists tend to employ different coping strategies in times of stress, which – as we have seen above – can be positive and negative. Optimists are more likely to try to actively change stressful events, or engage in proactive problem-focused coping, whereas pessimists are more likely to passively disengage during times of stress and will ruminate a lot more (Carver & Connor-Smith, 2010). Rumination has also been linked to excessive self-criticism, a past history and/or tendency towards depression, and an over-reliance on others (Spasojević & Alloy, 2001). Overall, there is good evidence to suggest that optimism can protect our health provided that it is not unrealistic and is deployed in the right scenario. In a brilliant article summarising what was known of the field at the time, Professor Suzanne Segerstrom examined the literature on optimism and immune responses, finding that optimism was associated with better immune outcomes when the stressor itself was relatively simplistic, short-lived, or otherwise controllable, but could be damaging for those types of stressors that are more complex, chronic, and uncontrollable (Segerstrom, 2005).

SOCIAL SUPPORT

I will conclude this chapter with one last, but very significant, consideration for understanding stress: **social support**. One of the biggest names in stress research, Professor Sheldon Cohen, posited social support as a key player in the stress/health relationship, coining the term the *Stress Buffering Hypothesis* (Cohen & Wills, 1985). Social support is supposed to have benefits to health via three main pathways: behaviourally (by encouraging and supporting good health behaviours), psychologically (by helping to reframe stress appraisals and manage emotions), and via cellular mechanisms (both immune and endocrine) (Uchino et al., 2012). Social support is all about the *quality* of your relationships rather than the quantity – you can have hundreds of friends, but they may not be able to provide the support that you need. Social support can provide a variety of benefits in dealing with stress, and – in a similar manner to coping – can be associated with confronting the stressor, or dealing with the emotional fallout. Social support can provide validation, encouragement, more positive perceptions of self-efficacy, and reassurance. Sometimes social support can provide more tangible means of support as well, in providing information or perhaps financial support. Critically, social support is in the eye of the beholder, with many studies that consider it using a measure of perceived social support, rather than some objective measure of the number of social contacts, the frequency of social interaction, or some other observer measure of the quality of a support network. Social support can come from friends, family members, colleagues, romantic partners, pets, or even people you have never met before. As a social species, we are innately geared to be empathetic to others, and many of us that feel that empathy towards others choose to display it by the offering of support, either 'moral support' through statements of validation and encouragement, or more physical means of support by standing up for and standing by those that need our help.

Social support falls into three domains: informational, emotional, and instrumental (Taylor, 2011). Informational support is as it sounds – a type of support that helps in providing information. This could be in terms of novel information about the problem you are facing, advice about a course of action, or simply a different perspective that will assist in breaking down the components of the stressor to understand how to overcome it. Emotional support is that type of support that helps us to feel that we are heard, that others understand our feelings, that our feelings are not 'wrong', and that despite how much we may be struggling, we have those around us to give us love and encouragement. Instrumental support is a more tangible means of support, which could be in the form of financial aid, the loaning of a physical resource such as a car, or the offer of a place to stay. Further, we don't actually have to physically receive these types of support to benefit – just knowing that such support is available should it be needed is enough for us to feel supported and cared for (Taylor, 2011). Each of these types of support will offer either direct means to cope with the stressor (for example through providing material benefits or guidance), or indirect means to cope by attending to the emotional aspects of stress (through offering positive social interaction or feedback, for example). Much like the way in which we cope, the way in which we seek support from others is culturally relevant, with deeply complex cultural expectations and norms for both support seeking and support offering (Chen et al., 2012; Kim et al., 2008; Taylor et al., 2004).

Social support is a well-established buffer to psychosocial stress, with a wealth of evidence demonstrating its ability to counter the most harmful effects of stress (like depression) from a variety of different domains in life, such as work stress (La Rocco et al., 1980), academic study stress (Wang et al., 2014), financial stress (Peirce et al., 1996), involuntary job loss (Canavan et al., 2021), and divorce (Kołodziej-Zaleska & Przybyła-Basista, 2016) amongst many others. Conversely, we can also see the impact of losing a social support network, as has been demonstrated in migration in both those that emigrate and those left behind (Lu, 2012). On the cellular level, social support is associated with lower levels of inflammation (Uchino et al., 2018), stronger immune responses to vaccination (Gallagher et al., 2008), lower cortisol reactivity after acute lab-elicited stress (Heinrichs et al., 2003), and lower cortisol in general life stress (Rosal et al., 2004).

We also know that social support is highly beneficial to those coping with major health issues, such as the experience of significant health events or the diagnosis of a chronic or terminal health condition. There is a huge amount of literature that evidences the benefits of social support in both psychological and physical health outcomes for those that experience myocardial infarction (heart attack) (Mookadam & Arthur, 2004), as well as those who are diagnosed with HIV (Nott et al., 1995), breast cancer (Nausheen et al., 2009), Type 2 Diabetes (van Dam et al., 2005), multiple sclerosis (Briones-Buixassa et al., 2015), and chronic obstructive pulmonary disorder (Barton et al., 2015), and those who suffer chronic pain (Che et al., 2018), to provide a handful of examples. This is an important consideration, as many health issues can carry with them significant psychological difficulties. Moos and Schaefer (1984) describe health changes as a crisis that can impact a variety of different domains. There are changes to identity, where we suddenly go from 'healthy' to 'unhealthy', we may be physically away from our homes or normal living location if we are bed-bound or hospitalised, we may lose our independence, we may lose contact with our social support network (particularly if we lose our independence), and we may have to re-evaluate a once relatively known future. The adjustment to chronic illness or life-changing diagnoses is a huge field in health psychology, and there is a lot of evidence for the role of social support in helping to adjust and make positive changes thereafter. Having considered how social support can help mediate stress at the (inter)personal level, we will go on, in Chapter 7, to consider how loneliness, which is in part an absence of a support network, has strong associations with stress.

Learning Outcomes Summary

- Define stress and its implications for health.

We have looked at different stress typologies and have examined different mechanisms by which stress can impact health.

- Understand the importance of psychological factors to the experience of stress and coping.

We have looked at psychological and behavioural factors in both the experience of stress, and as a result of trying to cope with stress. We have explored some of the ways in which psychological and behavioural factors in coping with stress may make health outcomes worse.

- Describe different coping styles, how they may be employed during stressful experiences, and how these can have positive and negative outcomes.

We have explored a variety of different types of stress and coping models and have looked at how they can help us understand some of the varying ways we may deal with stressful experiences. Optimism was used as a case study for how individual factors can relate to both stress and coping, and their impact on health.

- Appreciate the importance of social support in the psychological and biological experience of stress.

We have looked at types of social support, what they offer to us psychologically, and how it can help to support our health. We have looked at the specific examples of receiving a diagnosis of a chronic health issue, as well as social support in cellular markers of health.

FURTHER READING

Anisman, H. (2014). *An introduction to stress and health*. Sage.
An excellent book entirely dedicated to the health impacts of stress. Chapter 2 (coping), Chapter 3 (hormonal changes due to stress), Chapter 5 (immunological changes due to stress), and Chapter 6 (stress, immunity, and disease) are particularly useful.

Dhabhar, F. S. (2009). Enhancing versus suppressive effects of stress on immune function: Implications for immunoprotection and immunopathology. *Neuroimmunomodulation*, *16*(5), 300–17.
A great overview of the different ways that acute and chronic stress affect our immune function.

Juster, R. P., McEwen, B. S., & Lupien, S. J. (2010). Allostatic load biomarkers of chronic stress and impact on health and cognition. *Neuroscience & Biobehavioral Reviews*, *35*(1), 2–16.
A wonderful and informative review paper written by some of the biggest names in the field. This paper will walk you through what allostatic load means, and how it has been used in research to understand the implications of stress for health.

McEwen, B. S., & Lasley, E. N. (2002). *The end of stress as we know it*. Joseph Henry Press.
An excellent book written by one of the biggest names in stress research, Bruce McEwen.

Stephens, R. (2015). *Black sheep: The hidden benefits of being bad*. John Murray.
A very entertaining and well-informed book on some of the more controversial areas of life. The chapter on stress (Chapter 6) is particularly relevant here, but the whole book is a great read.

Uchino, B. N. (2006). Social support and health: A review of physiological processes potentially underlying links to disease outcomes. *Journal of Behavioral Medicine*, *29*(4), 377–87.
An excellent article summarising the various mechanisms by which social support has been evidenced to support health.

Wong, P. T., Lonner, W. J. & Wong, L. C. (2006). *Handbook of multicultural perspectives on stress and coping*. New York: Springer.
This edited volume provides a variety of perspectives on the multicultural aspects of coping, both on the individual and collective levels. There are some excellent chapters here that consider elements of culture (e.g., collectivist versus individualist) and how these filter down to personal choices in coping styles.

REFERENCES

Barton, C., Effing, T. W., & Cafarella, P. (2015). Social support and social networks in COPD: A scoping review. *COPD: Journal of Chronic Obstructive Pulmonary Disease, 12*(6), 690–702. https://doi.org/10.3109/15412555.2015.1008691

Baumgartner, J. N., Schneider, T. R., & Capiola, A. (2018). Investigating the relationship between optimism and stress responses: A biopsychosocial perspective. *Personality and Individual Differences, 129*, 114–18. https://doi.org/https://doi.org/10.1016/j.paid.2018.03.021

Beckie, T. M. (2012). A systematic review of allostatic load, health, and health disparities. *Biological Research for Nursing, 14*(4), 311–46. https://doi.org/10.1177/1099800412455688

Briones-Buixassa, L., Milà, R., Mª Aragonès, J., Bufill, E., Olaya, B., & Arrufat, F. X. (2015). Stress and multiple sclerosis: A systematic review considering potential moderating and mediating factors and methods of assessing stress. *Health Psychology Open, 2*(2), 2055102915612271. https://doi.org/10.1177/2055102915612271

Canavan, M., Gallo, W. T., & Marshall, G. L. (2021). The moderating effect of social support and social integration on the relationship between involuntary job loss and health. *Journal of Applied Gerontology, 40*(10), 1272–9. https://doi.org/10.1177/07334648209210

Carver, C. S., & Connor-Smith, J. (2010). Personality and coping. *Annual Review of Psychology, 61*, 679–704. https://doi.org/10.1146/annurev.psych.093008.100352

Che, X., Cash, R., Ng, S. K., Fitzgerald, P., & Fitzgibbon, B. M. (2018). A systematic review of the processes underlying the main and the buffering effect of social support on the experience of pain. *The Clinical Journal of Pain, 34*(11), 1061–76.

Chen, J. M., Kim, H. S., Mojaverian, T., & Morling, B. (2012). Culture and social support provision: Who gives what and why. *Personality and Social Psychology Bulletin, 38*(1), 3–13.

Chun, C.-A., Moos, R. H., & Cronkite, R. C. (2006). Culture: A fundamental context for the stress and coping paradigm. In P. T. P. Wong & L. C. J. Wong (eds.), *Handbook of Multicultural Perspectives on Stress and Coping* (pp. 29–53). Springer: US. https://doi.org/10.1007/0-387-26238-5_2

Cohen, S., & Wills, T. A. (1985). Stress, social support, and the buffering hypothesis. *Psychological Bulletin, 98*(2), 310.

Everson, S. A., Goldberg, D. E., Kaplan, G. A., Cohen, R. D., Pukkala, E., Tuomilehto, J., & Salonen, J. T. (1996). Hopelessness and risk of mortality and incidence of myocardial infarction and cancer. *Psychosomatic Medicine, 58*(2), 113–21. https://journals.lww.com/psychosomaticmedicine/Fulltext/1996/03000/Hopelessness_and_Risk_of_Mortality_and_Incidence.3.aspx

Gallagher, S., Phillips, A. C., Ferraro, A. J., Drayson, M. T., & Carroll, D. (2008). Social support is positively associated with the immunoglobulin M response to vaccination with pneumococcal polysaccharides. *Biological Psychology, 78*(2), 211–15. https://doi.org/https://doi.org/10.1016/j.biopsycho.2008.01.001

Guidi, J., Lucente, M., Sonino, N., & Fava, G. A. (2021). Allostatic load and its impact on health: A systematic review. *Psychotherapy and Psychosomatics, 90*(1), 11–27. https://doi.org/10.1159/000510696

Heinrichs, M., Baumgartner, T., Kirschbaum, C., & Ehlert, U. (2003). Social support and oxytocin interact to suppress cortisol and subjective responses to psychosocial stress. *Biological Psychiatry, 54*(12), 1389–98. https://doi.org/https://doi.org/10.1016/S0006-3223(03)00465-7

Helweg-Larsen, M., & Shepperd, J. A. (2001). Do moderators of the optimistic bias affect personal or target risk estimates? A review of the literature. *Personality and Social Psychology Review, 5*(1), 74–95. https://doi.org/10.1207/s15327957pspr0501_5

Ironson, G., Balbin, E., Stuetzle, R., Fletcher, M. A., O'Cleirigh, C., Laurenceau, J. P., Schneiderman, N., & Solomon, G. (2005). Dispositional optimism and the mechanisms by which it predicts slower disease progression in HIV: Proactive behavior, avoidant coping, and depression. *International Journal of Behavioral Medicine, 12*(2), 86–97. https://doi.org/10.1207/s15327558ijbm1202_6

Kim, H. S., Sherman, D. K., & Taylor, S. E. (2008). Culture and social support. *American Psychologist, 63*(6), 518. https://doi.org/10.1037/0003-066X

Koh, K. B., Choe, E., Song, J. E., & Lee, E. H. (2006). Effect of coping on endocrinoimmune functions in different stress situations. *Psychiatry Research, 143*(2–3), 223–34.

Kołodziej-Zaleska, A., & Przybyła-Basista, H. (2016). Psychological well-being of individuals after divorce: The role of social support. *Current Issues in Personality Psychology, 4*(4), 206–16. https://doi.org/10.5114/cipp.2016.62940

La Rocco, J. M., House, J. S., & French Jr, J. R. (1980). Social support, occupational stress, and health. *Journal of Health and Social Behavior, 21*(3), 202–18.

Lazarus, R. S., & Folkman, S. (1984). *Stress, appraisal, and coping.* Springer Publishing Company.

Lee, L. O., James, P., Zevon, E. S., Kim, E. S., Trudel-Fitzgerald, C., Spiro, A., Grodstein, F., & Kubzansky, L. D. (2019). Optimism is associated with exceptional longevity in 2 epidemiologic cohorts of men and women. *Proceedings of the National Academy of Sciences, 116*(37), 18357–62. https://doi.org/doi:10.1073/pnas.1900712116

Lu, Y. (2012). Household migration, social support, and psychosocial health: The perspective from migrant-sending areas. *Social Science & Medicine, 74*(2), 135–42. https://doi.org/https://doi.org/10.1016/j.socscimed.2011.10.020

McEwen, B. S. (1998). Stress, adaptation, and disease: Allostasis and allostatic load. *Annals of the New York Academy of Sciences, 840*(1), 33–44. https://doi.org/https://doi.org/10.1111/j.1749-6632.1998.tb09546.x

McEwen, B. S., & Seeman, T. (1999). Protective and damaging effects of mediators of stress: Elaborating and testing the concepts of allostasis and allostatic load. *Annals of the New York Academy of Sciences, 896*(1), 30–47. https://doi.org/https://doi.org/10.1111/j.1749-6632.1999.tb08103.x

McEwen, B. S., & Stellar, E. (1993). Stress and the individual: Mechanisms leading to disease. *Archives of Internal Medicine, 153*(18), 2093–101. https://doi.org/10.1001/archinte.1993.00410180039004

McEwen, B. S., & Wingfield, J. C. (2003). The concept of allostasis in biology and biomedicine. *Hormones and Behavior, 43*(1), 2–15. https://doi.org/https://doi.org/10.1016/S0018-506X(02)00024-7

Mookadam, F., & Arthur, H. M. (2004). Social support and its relationship to morbidity and mortality after acute myocardial infarction: Systematic overview. *Archives of Internal Medicine, 164*(14), 1514–18. https://doi.org/10.1001/archinte.164.14.1514

Moos, R. H. (1984). Context and coping: Toward a unifying conceptual framework. *American Journal of Community Psychology, 12*(1), 5–36. https://doi.org/https://doi.org/10.1007/BF00896933

Moos, R. H., & Schaefer, J. A. (1984). The crisis of physical illness. In R. H. Moos (ed.), *Coping with Physical Illness* (pp. 3–25). Springer.

Nausheen, B., Gidron, Y., Peveler, R., & Moss-Morris, R. (2009). Social support and cancer progression: A systematic review. *Journal of Psychosomatic Research, 67*(5), 403–15. https://doi.org/https://doi.org/10.1016/j.jpsychores.2008.12.012

Nes, L. S., & Segerstrom, S. C. (2006). Dispositional optimism and coping: A meta-analytic review. *Personality and Social Psychology Review, 10*(3), 235–51. https://doi.org/10.1207/s15327957pspr1003_3

Nott, K. H., Vedhara, K., & Power, M. J. (1995). The role of social support in HIV infection. *Psychological Medicine, 25*(5), 971–83. https://doi.org/10.1017/S0033291700037466

Peirce, R. S., Frone, M. R., Russell, M., & Cooper, M. L. (1996). Financial stress, social support, and alcohol involvement: A longitudinal test of the buffering hypothesis in a general population survey. *Health Psychology, 15*(1), 38.

Rosal, M. C., King, J., Ma, Y., & Reed, G. W. (2004). Stress, social support, and cortisol: Inverse associations? *Behavioral Medicine, 30*(1), 11–22. https://doi.org/10.3200/BMED.30.1.11-22

Roy, B., Diez-Roux, A. V., Seeman, T., Ranjit, N., Shea, S., & Cushman, M. (2010). Association of optimism and pessimism with inflammation and hemostasis in the Multi-Ethnic Study of Atherosclerosis (MESA). *Psychosomatic Medicine, 72*(2), 134–40. https://doi.org/10.1097/PSY.0b013e3181cb981b

Schwarzer, R., & Fuchs, R. (1996). Self-efficacy and health behaviours. In M. Conner & P. Norman (eds.), *Predicting Health Behavior: Research and Practice with Social Cognition Models* 163–96. Open University Press.

Segerstrom, S. C. (2005). Optimism and immunity: Do positive thoughts always lead to positive effects? *Brain, Behavior, and Immunity, 19*(3), 195–200. https://doi.org/https://doi.org/10.1016/j.bbi.2004.08.003

Segerstrom, S. C., & Sephton, S. E. (2010). Optimistic expectancies and cell-mediated immunity: The role of positive affect. *Psychological Science, 21*(3), 448–55. https://doi.org/10.1177/0956797610362061

Segerstrom, S. C., Taylor, S. E., Kemeny, M. E., & Fahey, J. L. (1998). Optimism is associated with mood, coping, and immune change in response to stress. *Journal of Personality and Social Psychology, 74*(6), 1646.

Selye, H. (1976). Stress without distress. In G. Serban (ed.), *Psychopathology of Human Adaptation* (pp. 137–46). Springer US. https://doi.org/10.1007/978-1-4684-2238-2_9

Spasojević, J., & Alloy, L. B. (2001). Rumination as a common mechanism relating depressive risk factors to depression. *Emotion, 1*(1), 25.

Steptoe, A., O'Donnell, K., Badrick, E., Kumari, M., & Marmot, M. (2007). Neuroendocrine and inflammatory factors associated with positive affect in healthy men and women: The Whitehall II Study. *American Journal of Epidemiology, 167*(1), 96–102. https://doi.org/10.1093/aje/kwm252

Taylor, S. E. (2011). Social support: A review. In H. S. Friedman (ed.), *The Oxford Handbook of Health Psychology* (pp. 190–214). Oxford University Press.

Taylor, S. E., Sherman, D. K., Kim, H. S., Jarcho, J., Takagi, K., & Dunagan, M. S. (2004). Culture and social support: Who seeks it and why? *Journal of Personality and Social Psychology, 87*(3), 354. https://doi.org/10.1037/0022-3514.87.3.354

Uchino, B. N., Trettevik, R., Kent de Grey, R. G., Cronan, S., Hogan, J., & Baucom, B. R. (2018). Social support, social integration, and inflammatory cytokines: A meta-analysis. *Health Psychology, 37*(5), 462.

Uchino, B. N., Vaughn, A. A., Carlisle, M., & Birmingham, W. (2012). Social support and immunity. In *The Oxford Handbook of Psychoneuroimmunology* (pp. 214–33). Oxford University Press. https://doi.org/10.1093/oxfordhb/9780195394399.013.0012

van Dam, H. A., van der Horst, F. G., Knoops, L., Ryckman, R. M., Crebolder, H. F. J. M., & van den Borne, B. H. W. (2005). Social support in diabetes: A systematic review of controlled intervention studies. *Patient Education and Counseling, 59*(1), 1–12. https://doi.org/10.1016/j.pec.2004.11.001

Wang, X., Cai, L., Qian, J., & Peng, J. (2014). Social support moderates stress effects on depression. *International Journal of Mental Health Systems, 8*(1), 41. https://doi.org/10.1186/1752-4458-8-41

Weinstein, N. D. (1982). Unrealistic optimism about susceptibility to health problems. *Journal of Behavioral Medicine, 5*(4), 441–60. https://doi.org/10.1007/BF00845372

Wenglert, L., & Rosén, A.-S. (1995). Optimism, self-esteem, mood and subjective health. *Personality and Individual Differences, 18*(5), 653–61. https://doi.org/https://doi.org/10.1016/0191-8869(94)00193-V

7
STRESS AT POPULATION LEVEL

INTRODUCTION

In Chapter 6 we looked at stress in its most individual sense, in terms of what happens when we get stressed, but also what may mitigate some of the more serious effects of stress. This chapter focuses on conditions that can make groups of people more vulnerable to stress. We will use four case studies: loneliness, unemployment, ageing, and caregiving. We will also look at the ways these types of population-level stressors can intersect in those who may experience them simultaneously, and what impact this has on mental and physical health. We end the chapter considering how a whole-population stressor (the Covid-19 pandemic) has had an impact on groups already experiencing one of these group-scale stressors.

Learning Outcomes

- Understand what types of stress can be experienced at the population level.
- Describe the impact of this stress on individuals and groups.
- Understand the compounding of stressors in stressed groups.

WHAT IS MEANT BY 'POPULATION-LEVEL STRESS'?

Some events can be so significant that they cause stress in entire populations. Terrorist attacks, natural disasters, pandemics – these are all examples of incidents that can cause trauma to huge numbers of people. We have already discussed the impact of several population stressors on aspects of health via intergenerational trauma. We have also discussed some social factors that relate to specific populations that cause multiple stress situations (e.g., racism, indigenous and ethnic minority status, refugee status). These are all important aspects to consider for this chapter as well – remember that we never belong to just one group, we are constellations of group membership or group identity (referred to as **intersectionality**), and each of those identities have biopsychosocial health impacts on them. Also remember those factors that were discussed in the previous chapter about how stress may be buffered or otherwise modulated by personal factors such as coping and social support. These are important considerations when we consider stress at the society level too.

LONELINESS

We left Chapter 6 considering the impact that social support has on buffering against the harmful effects of stress. I mentioned in this chapter that loneliness is – in some ways – the inverse of social support. Loneliness is much greater than that, however, and there are very many sections of our communities who are more vulnerable to it, and its subsequent effects on health and wellbeing. Loneliness is a growing concern in health literature, and in our society. It is generally described as a discrepancy between someone's actual and desired levels of social connection (Vanhalst et al., 2012). It is distinct from merely lacking social support because you can still have social connections and social support but feel lonely (Hawkley & Cacioppo, 2010). It is said to be the consequence of the sociality of our species, and our innate need to belong (Baumeister & Leary, 1995). Before we continue onto the specific health outcomes associated with loneliness, have a go at the next activity to think about why loneliness is such an issue, and who may be most vulnerable.

Key Questions

With the ever-increasing sophistication of technology, and the number of technological infrastructures to support connection, it would be reasonable to think that loneliness should be decreasing. However, robust evidence suggests that loneliness is increasing rather than decreasing (Buecker et al., 2021).

- Why might we be getting lonelier?
- What sorts of groups might experience loneliness?
- Are there differences between countries and cultures in who may be more vulnerable to loneliness?
- What psychological and social mechanisms do you think might explain the link between loneliness and health?

Loneliness has been associated with a variety of health outcomes, both on the cellular level and when considering specific health outcomes like the incidence of disease and mortality. On the cellular level, it is associated with increased inflammation in response to acute stress (Jaremka, Fagundes, Peng, et al., 2013), cortisol dysregulation (Doane & Adam, 2010), shorter telomere length (Wilson et al., 2018), and oxidative stress (Li & Xia, 2020). On the system level, it is associated with impaired immune responses after vaccination (Pressman et al., 2005), immune dysregulation (Jaremka, Fagundes, Glaser, et al., 2013), and elevated blood pressure (Hawkley et al., 2006). For overall health and disease outcomes, loneliness has been associated with the incidence of coronary heart disease and other cardiovascular diseases (Valtorta et al., 2016), cancer mortality (Kraav et al., 2021), Type 2 diabetes incidence (Hackett et al., 2020), prevalence of acute and chronic pain (Allen et al., 2020), and all-cause mortality (Rico-Uribe et al., 2018).

Loneliness is being used here as an example of a factor that can be additional to the experiences of certain social groups, but also as an independent factor relating to health in and of itself. If we are a member of a group that is in the minority in our society, we may be more likely to feel lonely as we do not have others we can relate to, so we will have loneliness to contend with along with the other social stressors that come along with being in a minority (such as prejudice and stigma). This has been evidenced in sexuality and gender-identity minority groups (Eres et al., 2021), and in ethnic minorities in some countries (Victor et al., 2012). Even if our group is not a minority, if our group is marginalised by society in favour of others then this can also increase loneliness. A good example of this is seen in the elderly, and we will be looking at that in more detail later in this chapter. However, remember that anyone can be vulnerable to loneliness regardless of their group identities or life stage.

UNEMPLOYMENT

A good example of a population of people that experience chronic stress is those that are unemployed. The unemployed are not a defined social group that may share a similar identity – they can be from any community, any group, and at any life stage. Unemployment is considered to be a good 'model' of chronic stress, meaning an example of chronic stress that is relatively robust across people. It is a type of chronic stress because it has no defined end point, and the impact it has on someone will seep through to almost every domain of their life. Unemployment is stressful in a number of ways, but critically because it deprives individuals of what are termed the 'latent and manifest' benefits of employment (Jahoda, 1981). Manifest benefits from employment are things like financial stability (or at least further opportunity for financial stability), health-benefitting perks such as health insurance, and social status. The financial stress of being unemployed will pervade all elements of our health. The stress itself will impact our health, but the poverty that may result from unemployment impacts a variety of other aspects as well, including our access to good food, our ability to reach or access our healthcare providers, our ability to access our social support networks if they are far away, and generally reducing our freedom and autonomy. Social status is an important aspect of employment because unemployment is often a very stigmatised status. In many cultures, one of the first things we may ask someone when we meet them is 'what do you do?', because we wish to understand someone else's place in society (and relative to ourselves, in cases of commonalities or interests). Being unemployed, in this way, is to therefore lack a social 'slot' in which you can be put. The latent benefits of employment tend to be more subtle, but are still incredibly important when it comes to stress and health. The structure of a daily routine is hugely important, and something that is very much lost when unemployed. Similarly, the feeling of purpose, of contributing to something, and achieving goals. Employment also provides a social support network, as we will very often have a group of colleagues with whom we can discuss problems that they can relate to. We will also have a shared culture and sense of identity within a workplace. There are obviously some exceptions to this, as some roles may be very solitary, or may be based on an ever-changing team of colleagues, and in these cases, this can be a particular type of work stressor. In addition to missing out on these benefits of employment, the stress incurred through unemployment can also be associated with poor health outcomes if the person dealing with the stress does so in unhealthy ways. We may be less able to continue positive health behaviours like taking regular exercise if this costs money, and we may be isolated from a social support network (and will have lost a social support network if we have lost our job as well). Unemployment effectively takes away something positive regarding our health and can replace it with something negative. To bring in our consideration of loneliness here, a large-scale meta-analysis has found a strong association between unemployment and loneliness, sometimes in a bi-directional fashion, meaning that as much as unemployment may cause loneliness, loneliness may also cause unemployment (Morrish & Medina-Lara, 2021). This is an important consideration when bringing this all together to consider how this may affect someone's health, as loneliness is hard for people to break free from, and must be doubly so if they are unemployed without the opportunity for regular social connections at work.

Unemployment is associated with lower levels of happiness, life satisfaction, self-esteem, and psychological wellbeing (Paul & Moser, 2009), as well as increased risk of suicide (Garcy & Vågerö, 2013), increased depression and mortality (Wanberg, 2012), increased risk of all-cause mortality and negative health behaviours (Roelfs et al., 2011), and dysregulation of the physiological stress response (Gallagher et al., 2016; Sumner & Gallagher, 2017). Much of this evidence, however, has been gathered when comparing those who are unemployed to those who are employed, which may not always be a fair comparison. We have already seen in the previous paragraph how some types of work may be uniquely stressful (in the case of those roles where work may be more solitary, or involve irregular contact with changing colleagues), but there has been a growing trend in the employment market over the last decade or so, which is also impacting work-based stress: temporary employment. For some, temporary employment is exactly what they want – something to tide them over during their studies, for example, or something on a more casual and flexible basis. For others, however, being employed on a temporary contract can be tremendously stressful, particularly if it is a 'zero hours' type contract, where you are not guaranteed a minimum amount of work (and therefore a minimum amount of income). To understand more about this, my colleagues and I decided to use some population-level data from the UK to understand whether unemployment was consistently associated with poorer outcomes when compared to different profiles of employment (Sumner et al., 2020). We split our sample to compare those who were unemployed with those who were permanently employed, temporarily employed, and self-employed. We used the Understanding Society (University of Essex & Institute for Social and Economic Research, 2022) dataset, a UK household survey that has been running for nearly two decades. This longitudinal study collected blood samples from its participants in 2010–13, which coincided with a period of economic recession in the UK, and a rise in both unemployment and temporary employment. We chose to look at two blood markers of inflammation, C-Reactive Protein (CRP) and **Fibrinogen**. Both of these are markers for inflammation, and are both released in times of stress, but they also serve other functions in the body such as clotting (in the case of Fibrinogen) and the clearance of invading pathogens (CRP). After controlling for a variety of important health-impacting factors (such as smoking, alcohol consumption, education level, partnership status, subjective financial status, medication use, chronic illness status, adiposity, sex, and age) we found that when comparing unemployed to the whole employed group, Fibrinogen was significantly higher in those who were unemployed (indicating higher stress, higher inflammation, and poorer health outcomes).[1] However, when we compared all four employment profiles, there was only a significant difference between the unemployed and those on permanent contracts or self-employed. Those with temporary contracts were no better off than those who were unemployed (in terms of their Fibrinogen levels, at least).

Key Questions

We just saw in the previous section that being unemployed is associated with a huge number of stressful factors that will influence our health. There is very conclusive evidence of the negative impacts of unemployment on mental and physical health, but our recent work has also now suggested it may not be that simple. Have a think now about the potential stresses and strains of being temporarily employed, and how those stresses and strains (and their various associated health outcomes) may compare with being unemployed.

- Why might having a temporary employment contract be stressful?
- What does it mean if our temporarily employed individuals have similar health profiles to the unemployed?
- Might this affect some more than others?

OLDER PEOPLE

We as a species are, on average, getting older. Courtesy of infinitely improved healthcare, and (in some cases) falling fertility rate (that is, the number of babies we are producing, not literally how fertile humans are), many countries are seeing growing elderly populations. When we look at median age (the 'middle' number of an age range, where there are the same number of people above that as below), very many countries across the world have seen a steady increase of this in recent decades (Roser & Ortiz-Ospina,

---

1 We did not, however, find any significant differences for CRP in any of our analyses-a finding that puzzles us and other users of these data to this day. We have provided some thoughts on why this may be in the paper.

2022a). Japan, for example, has had a rise of median age from about 22 in 1950 to 48 in 2020, China from 24 to 39, Brazil from 19 to 33, and India from 21 to 28. We looked a bit at how older age is associated with key changes to health in Chapter 4. Our immune systems and endocrine systems age (immunosenescence and endocrinosenescence, respectively), and as they and the rest of the systems in our bodies age, we become more vulnerable to infection, less likely to bounce back robustly after injury, and we commence a period of decline from the peak performance of our former adult years. As medicine is getting better at fighting diseases, we are living longer lives. The ability to radically extend life expectancy through advances in healthcare has been a monumental achievement for humanity, but it (as all things do) has come at a price. We now have many more people living far longer, and as a result we are seeing many more people experiencing chronic illness and the heavy life-quality burden of age-related diseases and disorders. Nearly a quarter of global disease burden is found in our populations of older people, and whilst this is proportionately higher in high-income countries, the burden of cost in terms of **disability-adjusted life years** is greater in lower-income countries (Prince et al., 2015).

As with many aspects of society-level stress, the degree to which your group membership is stressful will depend on your society, and how much your group is catered for, supported, or otherwise included in policy and infrastructure. Some cultures place great importance on supporting and caring for the elderly, others do not. In Chapter 6, we considered the aspects of the continuum of collectivist-individualist cultures, and – broadly speaking – those cultures that are more collectivist tend to include and consider the elderly far greater in both personal and public care than those in individualist cultures. However, the cultural complexities of elder care are a lot more convoluted than that, and there are some important factors to consider in the experience of the elderly as to how stressful their being elderly may be, and how this may ultimately impact their health. I mentioned in Chapter 4 that the consideration of ageing as a health priority was so important that the United Nations (UN) had established an international action plan on ageing (the Madrid International Action Plan on Aging: United Nations, 2022). This plan was established in 2002 in recognition of the need to establish more equal and just consideration and support of the elderly, to ensure their inclusion in policies that are designed to support the health and wellbeing of citizens across the world. I had the opportunity to contribute to a report on the implementation of this plan in Eastern Europe and Central Asia (a designation provided by the UN for the purposes of the report) after 15 years with another group of colleagues (Zaidi et al., 2017). The development of this report was a real eye-opener for me not just in terms of the very many ways in which the elderly may be socially disadvantaged, and how this will impact their health, but also in how this varies incredibly between the very diverse nations and cultures within this cluster.

Key Questions

Using the health onion, and considering all you have learned so far in this book, have a think now about how being elderly in your society may impact your health. Think beyond biological factors, and consider the social, political, and structural aspects of your society and what your future health may look like as a result. Do you think these issues would be the same in other countries?

- Think about spaces and places, like shops, healthcare facilities, and the required transport to get there.
- Think about people and professions - what might you need to access or gain support with as you age?
- Think about laws and policies - how might these protect you or disadvantage you as you get older?

There are many aspects of daily life to consider that may make old age particularly stressful. We have discussed the impact of discrimination in other senses elsewhere so far, but what about discrimination against the elderly? In some countries that we examined, there were no laws protecting the elderly against abuse either privately at home or in institutions. Poverty tends to be a highly magnified issue in older age (particularly for women), and there is a huge variation between nations in financial support from the state in old age (both in terms of when someone may be eligible, and how much they may be provided). Much as we may consider the financial restrictions in place from unemployment, this also applies in old age. If we have less financial freedom this can impact our ability to get to where we need to be for healthcare appointments, or even to carry out basic functions such as grocery shopping. This is compounded even further if we also happen to be physically less capable and less mobile due to ageing. In some of the countries we examined, there is a high proportion of elderly people in very rural areas that may have had to travel very far indeed to receive medical care. If you are unable to drive (either due to poor health or poverty, or both), you will be even further disadvantaged in being able to look after yourself and your health. As we get older, our physiology changes, and there is a huge variation in the provision of specialist gerontological services between nations, in terms of both access and availability. Another important aspect of cultural differences in the experience of ageing is the availability of informal caring, which may typically be delivered by a family member. There are nations where there is little or no financial support for carers, and there may be little legislative protection for those whose lives are impacted by caring responsibilities (more on this later). Loneliness is also a very common factor in those who are in their advanced years, meaning that you can add all of the other health factors associated with loneliness on top of these factors as well (Hawkley & Cacioppo, 2007). Available data show self-reported loneliness in older people to be as high as 65% in Greece, 48% in Israel, and 47% in Italy, ranging to as low as 30% in Sweden, 26% in Switzerland, and 25% in Denmark (Roser & Ortiz-Ospina, 2022b). As astonishingly high as some of those levels are, even the lowest levels recorded show that a quarter of older people feel alone, which is a very large proportion. Ageing is a vastly under-considered factor across many nations, and we could all do better by putting ourselves in the shoes of our 80-year-old selves and seeing whether our societies are doing what they should for those who have contributed so richly to them across their lifetimes.

CARING

Being a carer is a complex role. It is full of benefits, but also full of stress. Caring is when someone provides support and assistance to another who may have a chronic health condition, or be elderly or disabled. Many people are what are referred to as 'sandwich' carers, in that they have the caregiving role of being a parent and also provide care to another person, who may be their parent or other relative. Caregiving is another one of the 'models' of chronic stress that has been used in health research for many years. In a similar fashion to unemployment (but in different ways), it is deemed a chronic stressor because it has no determinable end point (and if there is an end point, that may come in the form of the loss of the care recipient, and so not an end to distress), and will impact many different domains of someone's life. It is difficult to adequately assess the level of caring that is undertaken because it is, by its very nature, informal and inconsistently officially reported. The organisation Carers Worldwide (2022) estimate that (based on available data from Europe) there may be about 20% of the population providing care to another relative (aside from the traditional means of caring of a parent for their healthy or typically developing child), equating to over 273 million people, with the vast majority (estimated at 84%) of these being women. Nearly all (92%) worry about money as a result of their caring role, the majority (82%) report having significant mental health issues such as anxiety and depression, and nearly half (48%) worry about their own physical health. So caring is no small issue, and as with unemployment, older age, and loneliness, the status of being a carer can intersect with other group memberships or identities that put someone at a higher vulnerability for marginalisation, stigma, or other social disadvantage.

Caregiving is such a reliable model for chronic stress that it has been used in research for a long time to understand its health consequences. Researchers have examined the impact of caring for another in every generation: above (of a parent or other relative in that tier), parallel (of a spouse or partner), and below (of a child with disabilities, atypical development, or significant health impairment). There are a few mechanisms by which caregiving has an impact on health and wellbeing, both immunological and endocrinological. Informal caring is associated with reduced lymphocyte function (Bauer et al., 2000), the balance of T-cells (helpers versus killers: Benaroya-Milshtein et al., 2014), reduced antibody response to vaccines (Gallagher et al., 2009), reduced salivary antibodies (Gallagher et al., 2008), increased inflammation (Gouin et al., 2016), and sympathetic and endocrine dysregulation (Lovell & Wetherell, 2011). Having such a huge number of the population also responsible for providing informal care means they are a section of the population that deserves particular attention. The impact of giving care on health and wellbeing has been well-documented, and is evidenced from subjective wellbeing right through to cellular measures of health and mortality (Pinquart & Sörensen, 2007). Much like the health dynamics of unemployment, as more research has been conducted it has become clear that it is not as simple as 'caring equals stress, equals poor health'; there are other nuances in the caring experience that may modulate the impact on the carer's health. Some of the impacts of caregiving on health are attributable to specific contexts within caregiving, either in terms of the conduct of the care recipient, the characteristics of the carer, or the interpersonal dynamics between both. Some important aspects here are: challenging behaviour of the care recipient (Pinquart & Sörensen, 2007); the age and sex of the caregiver, along with the specific relationship to the care recipient (Vitaliano et al., 2003); associated marital strain (Kang & Marks, 2016); care recipient personality factors (Riffin et al., 2012); and the existence of other stressors such as financial strain (Do et al., 2014).

Given the prevalence of informal caring, and the increase in the 'sandwich generation' of caring (i.e., caring for individuals in the generational tier both below and above), the potential health impacts of caring constitute a significant public health concern. This also means that when there are other public health concerns at play this may compound the health impact on these individuals. Looking at the Covid-19 pandemic, now is the time to start considering this as it has been (and continues to be) a significant factor in the health of populations across the world. Before I go on to discuss some important and interesting work that has been undertaken to look at the added impact of the pandemic on the health and wellbeing of carers, go through the next brief exercise to think about this for yourselves.

Key Questions

Thinking about the pandemic - what do you think this might mean for those people caring?

- What additional stressors does this cause?
- Are there some people that may be more affected than others?
- Are there policies that may have made these stressors worse, or taken some of the stress away?
- What impact might all this have had in addition to the existing strain of caring?

Bringing together the threads of loneliness and caring, and using the Understanding Society dataset once more, Professors Stephen Gallagher and Mark Wetherell (two excellent names in psychobiology, with extensive back catalogues of fascinating research) sought to understand the impact of the Covid-19 pandemic on carers. The advantage of using this dataset is that the data are collected in waves across time. The last study I mentioned where colleagues and I looked at different profiles of unemployment was over one time point, because blood samples were only taken once at that point in the study's history when we undertook our analysis. This study, however, used the survey data from 2017–19 as their pre-Covid levels and data collected in April 2020 in the first few months of the pandemic in the UK, where some of the strictest stay-at-home orders were passed to minimise the potential for community spread of the disease. Recognising that the instructions to remain at home may place an additional stress burden on those who were caring, they were interested to see whether levels of depression and loneliness may have increased because of these safeguards. As would be reasonably expected, levels of depression were higher during the pandemic than pre-pandemic levels, but at both time points, those who were carers reported higher levels of depression than those who were not. On top of this, those who were also self-reporting as lonely were almost four times more likely to be depressed, with those reporting that they 'never' felt lonely relatively robustly protected against depression. This highlights the importance of loneliness as a factor that can radically increase the impact of other stressful circumstances, and have a profound impact on population health and wellbeing. So, add something else into the mix (like a pandemic, with its associated restrictions on mobility, socialisation, and activity), and it can make an already stressful situation a whole lot more stressful. There were likely other factors at play in these experiences as well. Those caring for others were also having to cope with the very real possibility of bringing the virus to those they were caring for, and many people that are cared for are at heightened risk for severe disease, either because of their age or because of underlying health vulnerabilities. Add in loneliness, which here was marginally decreased (7.1%, down from 7.5%) in non-carers, and marginally increased (8.2%, up from 8.0%) in carers between the pre-pandemic and beginning pandemic levels, and this can make a huge difference to an entire population of people who are already vulnerable to experiencing extreme, prolonged stress, and the physiological health consequences that result from that.

Learning Outcomes Summary

- Understand what types of stress can be experienced at the population level.

We have looked at three different populations of people (the unemployed, those who are ageing, and those who are carers), and also looked at a subjective status (loneliness) that can create a population in itself or add to other populations in determining health outcomes.

- Describe the impact of this stress on individuals and groups.

We have looked at the various mechanisms responsible for some of the health outcomes notable in these populations. These have been at the cellular (i.e., immunological and endocrinological) and the system (i.e., cardiovascular system) levels.

- Understand the compounding of stressors in stressed groups.

Using loneliness as an example of how a common additional factor may add to other group-level factors to influence health, we have seen that many of these groups have their health impacts greatly added to by loneliness. Not only this, we have also seen that many of these groups may be, by virtue of their group membership, more likely to be lonely.

FURTHER READING

Alexander, J. C., Eyerman, R., Giesen, B., Smelser, N. J., & Sztompka, P. (2004). *Cultural trauma and collective identity*. University of California Press.
This is a wonderful book that goes into some of the more in-depth nuances around culture. Its focus is on trauma rather than stress, but it uses some important examples of traumatic situations that sit at a cultural level, how these are processed, and how they echo through generations.

Cacioppo, J. T., & Patrick, W. (2008). *Loneliness: Human nature and the need for social connection*. WW Norton & Company.
John Cacioppo is one of the biggest contributors to the field of loneliness and health. This book gives a comprehensive but accessible overview to the field, and is beautifully written too.

Murthy, V. H. (2020). *Together: Loneliness, health and what happens when we find connection*. Profile Books.
Vivek Murthy was the Surgeon General of the United States under the presidencies of Barak Obama and, after a period of being relieved of the role, Joe Biden. This book is a comprehensive and thoughtful piece on how loneliness is creeping ever further into our lives and societies, how it is affecting our health and wellbeing, and what we can do about it.

REFERENCES

Allen, S. F., Gilbody, S., Atkin, K., & van der Feltz-Cornelis, C. (2020). The associations between loneliness, social exclusion and pain in the general population: A N=502,528 cross-sectional UK Biobank study. *Journal of Psychiatric Research, 130*, 68–74. https://doi.org/https://doi.org/10.1016/j.jpsychires.2020.06.028

Bauer, M. E., Vedhara, K., Perks, P., Wilcock, G. K., Lightman, S. L., & Shanks, N. (2000). Chronic stress in caregivers of dementia patients is associated with reduced lymphocyte sensitivity to glucocorticoids. *Journal of Neuroimmunology, 103*(1), 84–92. https://doi.org/10.1016/S0165-5728(99)00228-3

Baumeister, R. F., & Leary, M. R. (1995). The need to belong: Desire for interpersonal attachments as a fundamental human motivation. *Psychological Bulletin, 117*(3), 497–529.

Benaroya-Milshtein, N., Apter, A., Yaniv, I., Yuval, O., Stern, B., Bengal, Y., … Valevski, A. (2014). Neuroimmunological function in parents of children suffering from cancer. *Journal of Neural Transmission, 121*(3), 299–306. https://doi.org/10.1007/s00702-013-1098-6

Buecker, S., Mund, M., Chwastek, S., Sostmann, M., & Luhmann, M. (2021). Is loneliness in emerging adults increasing over time? A preregistered cross-temporal meta-analysis and systematic review. *Psychological Bulletin, 147*(8), 787.

Carers Worldwide. (2022). *Global carer data and statistics*. Retrieved 16 Aug 2022 from https://carersworldwide.org/about-us/carers-issue/

Do, E. K., Cohen, S. A., & Brown, M. J. (2014). Socioeconomic and demographic factors modify the association between informal caregiving and health in the Sandwich Generation. *BMC Public Health, 14*(1), 362. https://doi.org/10.1186/1471-2458-14-362

Doane, L. D., & Adam, E. K. (2010). Loneliness and cortisol: Momentary, day-to-day, and trait associations. *Psychoneuroendocrinology, 35*(3), 430–41. https://doi.org/https://doi.org/10.1016/j.psyneuen.2009.08.005

Eres, R., Postolovski, N., Thielking, M., & Lim, M. H. (2021). Loneliness, mental health, and social health indicators in LGBTQIA+ Australians. *American Journal of Orthopsychiatry, 91*(3), 358.

Gallagher, S., Phillips, A. C., Drayson, M. T., & Carroll, D. (2009). Caregiving for children with developmental disabilities is associated with a poor antibody response to influenza vaccination. *Psychosomatic Medicine, 71*(3), 341–4. https://doi.org/10.1097/PSY.0b013e31819d1910

Gallagher, S., Phillips, A. C., Evans, P., Der, G., Hunt, K., & Carroll, D. (2008). Caregiving is associated with low secretion rates of immunoglobulin A in saliva. *Brain, Behavior, and Immunity, 22*(4), 565–72. https://doi.org/https://doi.org/10.1016/j.bbi.2007.11.007

Gallagher, S., Sumner, R. C., Muldoon, O. T., Creaven, A.-M., & Hannigan, A. (2016). Unemployment is associated with lower cortisol awakening and blunted dehydroepiandrosterone responses. *Psychoneuroendocrinology, 69*, 41–9. https://doi.org/https://doi.org/10.1016/j.psyneuen.2016.03.011

Garcy, A. M., & Vågerö, D. (2013). Unemployment and suicide during and after a deep recession: A longitudinal study of 3.4 million Swedish men and women. *American Journal of Public Health, 103*(6), 1031–8. https://doi.org/10.2105/ajph.2013.301210

Gouin, J.-P., da Estrela, C., Desmarais, K., & Barker, E. T. (2016). The impact of formal and informal support on health in the context of caregiving stress. *Family Relations, 65*(1), 191–206. https://doi.org/https://doi.org/10.1111/fare.12183

Hackett, R. A., Hudson, J. L., & Chilcot, J. (2020). Loneliness and type 2 diabetes incidence: Findings from the English Longitudinal Study of Ageing. *Diabetologia, 63*(11), 2329–38. https://doi.org/10.1007/s00125-020-05258-6

Hawkley, L. C., & Cacioppo, J. T. (2007). Aging and loneliness: Downhill quickly? *Current Directions in Psychological Science, 16*(4), 187–91. https://doi.org/10.1111/j.1467-8721.2007.00501.x

Hawkley, L. C., & Cacioppo, J. T. (2010). Loneliness matters: A theoretical and empirical review of consequences and mechanisms. *Annals of Behavioral Medicine, 40*(2), 218–27. https://doi.org/10.1007/s12160-010-9210-8

Hawkley, L. C., Masi, C. M., Berry, J. D., & Cacioppo, J. T. (2006). Loneliness is a unique predictor of age-related differences in systolic blood pressure. *Psychology and Aging, 21*(1), 152–64. https://www.jstor.org/stable/20183194

Jahoda, M. (1981). Work, employment, and unemployment: Values, theories, and approaches in social research. *American Psychologist, 36*(2), 184.

Jaremka, L. M., Fagundes, C. P., Glaser, R., Bennett, J. M., Malarkey, W. B., & Kiecolt-Glaser, J. K. (2013). Loneliness predicts pain, depression, and fatigue: Understanding the role of immune dysregulation. *Psychoneuroendocrinology, 38*(8), 1310–17. https://doi.org/https://doi.org/10.1016/j.psyneuen.2012.11.016

Jaremka, L. M., Fagundes, C. P., Peng, J., Bennett, J. M., Glaser, R., Malarkey, W. B., & Kiecolt-Glaser, J. K. (2013). Loneliness promotes inflammation during acute stress. *Psychological Science, 24*(7), 1089–97. https://doi.org/10.1177/0956797612464059

Kang, S., & Marks, N. F. (2016). Marital strain exacerbates health risks of filial caregiving: Evidence from the 2005 National Survey of Midlife in the United States. *Journal of Family Issues, 37*(8), 1123–50. https://doi.org/10.1177/0192513x14526392

Kraav, S.-L., Awoyemi, O., Junttila, N., Vornanen, R., Kauhanen, J., Toikko, T., … Tolmunen, T. (2021). The effects of loneliness and social isolation on all-cause, injury, cancer, and CVD mortality in a cohort of middle-aged Finnish men: A prospective study. *Aging & Mental Health, 25*(12), 2219–28. https://doi.org/10.1080/13607863.2020.1830945

Li, H., & Xia, N. (2020). The role of oxidative stress in cardiovascular disease caused by social isolation and loneliness. *Redox Biology, 37*, 101585. https://doi.org/https://doi.org/10.1016/j.redox.2020.101585

Lovell, B., & Wetherell, M. A. (2011). The cost of caregiving: Endocrine and immune implications in elderly and non elderly caregivers. *Neuroscience & Biobehavioral Reviews, 35*(6), 1342–52. https://doi.org/https://doi.org/10.1016/j.neubiorev.2011.02.007

Morrish, N., & Medina-Lara, A. (2021). Does unemployment lead to greater levels of loneliness? A systematic review. *Social Science & Medicine, 287*, 114339. https://doi.org/https://doi.org/10.1016/j.socscimed.2021.114339

Paul, K. I., & Moser, K. (2009). Unemployment impairs mental health: Meta-analyses. *Journal of Vocational Behavior, 74*(3), 264–82. https://doi.org/https://doi.org/10.1016/j.jvb.2009.01.001

Pinquart, M., & Sörensen, S. (2007). Correlates of physical health of informal caregivers: A meta-analysis. *The Journals of Gerontology: Series B, 62*(2), P126–P137. https://doi.org/10.1093/geronb/62.2.P126

Pressman, S. D., Cohen, S., Miller, G. E., Barkin, A., Rabin, B. S., & Treanor, J. J. (2005). Loneliness, social network size, and immune response to influenza vaccination in college freshmen. *Health Psychology, 24*(3), 297.

Prince, M. J., Wu, F., Guo, Y., Gutierrez Robledo, L. M., O'Donnell, M., Sullivan, R., & Yusuf, S. (2015). The burden of disease in older people and implications for health policy and practice. *The Lancet, 385*(9967), 549–62. https://doi.org/https://doi.org/10.1016/S0140-6736(14)61347-7

Rico-Uribe, L. A., Caballero, F. F., Martín-María, N., Cabello, M., Ayuso-Mateos, J. L., & Miret, M. (2018). Association of loneliness with all-cause mortality: A meta-analysis. *PLOS ONE, 13*(1), e0190033. https://doi.org/10.1371/journal.pone.0190033

Riffin, C., Löckenhoff, C. E., Pillemer, K., Friedman, B., & Costa, P. T., Jr. (2012). Care recipient agreeableness is associated with caregiver subjective physical health status. *The Journals of Gerontology: Series B, 68*(6), 927–30. https://doi.org/10.1093/geronb/gbs114

Roelfs, D. J., Shor, E., Davidson, K. W., & Schwartz, J. E. (2011). Losing life and livelihood: A systematic review and meta-analysis of unemployment and all-cause mortality. *Social Science & Medicine, 72*(6), 840–54. https://doi.org/https://doi.org/10.1016/j.socscimed.2011.01.005

Roser, M., & Ortiz-Ospina, E. (2022a). *Median age, 1950 to 2020*. Retrieved 16 Aug. 2022 from https://ourworldindata.org/age-structure

Roser, M., & Ortiz-Ospina, E. (2022b). *Self-reported loneliness among older adults*. OurWorldInData.org. Retrieved 16 Aug 2022 from https://ourworldindata.org/social-connections-and-loneliness

Sumner, R. C., Bennett, R., Creaven, A.-M., & Gallagher, S. (2020). Unemployment, employment precarity, and inflammation. *Brain, Behavior, and Immunity, 83*, 303–308. https://doi.org/https://doi.org/10.1016/j.bbi.2019.10.013

Sumner, R. C., & Gallagher, S. (2017). Unemployment as a chronic stressor: A systematic review of cortisol studies. *Psychology & Health, 32*(3), 289–311. https://doi.org/10.1080/08870446.2016.1247841

United Nations. (2022). *Madrid Plan of Action and its Implementation*. Retrieved 30 Sep 2022 from www.un.org/development/desa/ageing/madrid-plan-of-action-and-its-implementation.html

University of Essex, & Institute for Social and Economic Research. (2022). *Understanding Society: Waves 1–11, 2009–2020 and Harmonised BHPS: Waves 1–18, 1991–2009* UK Data Service. https://doi.org/http://doi.org/10.5255/UKDA-SN-6614-17

Valtorta, N. K., Kanaan, M., Gilbody, S., Ronzi, S., & Hanratty, B. (2016). Loneliness and social isolation as risk factors for coronary heart disease and stroke: Systematic review and meta-analysis of longitudinal observational studies. *Heart, 102*(13), 1009–16. https://doi.org/10.1136/heartjnl-2015-308790

Vanhalst, J., Luyckx, K., Raes, F., & Goossens, L. (2012). Loneliness and depressive symptoms: The mediating and moderating role of uncontrollable ruminative thoughts. *The Journal of Psychology, 146*(1–2), 259–76. https://doi.org/10.1080/00223980.2011.555433

Victor, C. R., Burholt, V., & Martin, W. (2012). Loneliness and ethnic minority elders in Great Britain: An exploratory study. *Journal of Cross-Cultural Gerontology, 27*(1), 65–78. https://doi.org/10.1007/s10823-012-9161-6

Vitaliano, P. P., Zhang, J., & Scanlan, J. M. (2003). Is caregiving hazardous to one's physical health? A meta-analysis. *Psychological Bulletin, 129*(6), 946.

Wanberg, C. R. (2012). The individual experience of unemployment. *Annual Review of Psychology, 63*(1), 369–96.

Wilson, S. J., Woody, A., Padin, A. C., Lin, J., Malarkey, W. B., & Kiecolt-Glaser, J. K. (2018). Loneliness and telomere length: Immune and parasympathetic function in associations with accelerated aging. *Annals of Behavioral Medicine, 53*(6), 541–50. https://doi.org/10.1093/abm/kay064

Zaidi, A., Bennett, R., & Sumner, R. C. (2017). *The Madrid International Plan of Action on Ageing: Where is Eastern Europe and Central Asia region fifteen years later?* https://eeca.unfpa.org/en/publications/madrid-international-plan-action-ageing

8
EPIDEMIOLOGICAL PERSPECTIVES: PUBLIC HEALTH

INTRODUCTION

This chapter is designed to introduce you to the field of public health, and how public health and epidemiology are intertwined. There will be an introduction to the area of health promotion, including perspectives on how health promotion is achieved effectively, for whom, and in what conditions. We will draw on some of the themes from Chapters 3 and 7 by looking at the UN **Sustainable Development Goals** to understand population-level wellbeing, with health being a core component, but also a product of all other components. The Global Charter for the Public's Health is discussed, along with public health theory, and current trends. The aim of this chapter is to introduce you (if you are not already familiar with it) to the field of public health as a discipline, which is an important part of the complex and multidisciplinary perspective required of the contemporary health practitioner.

Learning Outcomes

- Understand what public health and epidemiology are.
- Appreciate the ways in which public health and epidemiology feed into each other.
- Critique the impact of public health in the context of policy.

EPIDEMIOLOGY AND PUBLIC HEALTH

Epidemiology is the study of how often diseases occur in different groups of people and why. Epidemiological information is used to plan and evaluate strategies to prevent illness and as a guide to the management of patients in whom disease has already developed. **Public health** is the science of protecting and improving the health of people and their communities. This work is achieved by promoting healthy lifestyles, researching disease and injury prevention, and detecting, preventing and responding to infectious diseases. So, epidemiology provides information for public health, and public health provides solutions for the problems identified by epidemiology. There is also a branch of health psychology that is concerned with public health, reasonably called **public health psychology**. This is focused on health promotion and prevention at the population level more than the individual level. Here, health is seen as an outcome of social, economic, and political aspects of peoples' lives. There are several perspectives that are particular to public health psychology, perhaps the most primary being that individual-level intervention is insufficient to tackle widespread public health issues (Albee & Fryer, 2003). Public health psychology sees primary prevention of health issues as the key to bringing about better health in the population. Here, prevention is often targeted at the group or community level, which can often make it more difficult to define and evidence than individual-level intervention. It is a very interdisciplinary area of health psychology, requiring research and knowledge from epidemiology, health communication, public health, health economics, and medical sociology and anthropology.

An important aspect of the interconnection between public health and epidemiology is what is referred to as **translational research**. This is effectively epidemiological research that is directly put into public health practice, and then hopefully back into research once more. It is the product of the unique interplay between these two disciplines, and is a wonderful example of how multidisciplinary work is not only important, but is actually critical to achieving the grand outcomes we hope for in health research, such as preventing disease and saving lives. This type of research is proposed to have five different phases (see Table 8.1), and epidemiology has a role to play in each of these.

This rather nicely linear phase timetable is usually in reality a lot messier, with iterative cycles of discovery (from epidemiology) into practice (public health), leading to further discovery (epidemiology), leading to further practice (public health), and so on. An important element in this type of research is the involvement with the community in its design, development, and implementation. This is particularly important in understanding the needs and requirements of specific communities, and how these are influenced by the systems within which those communities live (more on this later in this chapter, and in Chapter 9). The involvement of the community in the research and development process is important for two main reasons. First, it allows researchers the opportunity to speak to people 'on the ground' who understand how their health operates in their context and who understand the challenges faced by people like them and have insight into how those challenges may be addressed. This will make the outcome of the practice or intervention both more effective, as it is tailored very specifically to its target group, and more authentic because it has been developed with the help of people with lived experience, who know the barriers and facilitators to engaging with whatever practice or intervention is being attempted. This is a win–win, but it is something that we as researchers can and should do a lot more of, and can and should do better, to ensure we are serving our communities equally and effectively. Second, by involving communities in our research we are also demonstrating transparency and engagement; a difference between *doing to/for* and *doing with*. Whilst researchers and practitioners can do all the reading in the world to develop their informed opinions about public health strategies, this is no replacement for the knowledge that comes with lived experience. By *working with* instead of *doing to* or *for*, researchers and practitioners can build trust and a more collaborative relationship with the public they serve. This type of approach is referred to as *coproduction* or *codevelopment* or *cocreation*, and is a part of community-based participatory research.

Table 8.1 Translational research phases

T0: *Description and discovery*: describing patterns of health and disease by person, place, and time; observational studies to identify potential 'causes' of health outcomes.

T1: *From discovery to application (e.g., tests, interventions)*: clinical and population studies to further characterise discoveries from T0 and identify potential interventions to improve health.

T2: *From application to evidence-based guidelines*: observational and experimental studies to assess the efficacy of an intervention to inform guidelines and recommendations.

T3: *From guidelines to practice*: studies to assess the implementation and uptake of guidelines (e.g., identifying barriers to uptake).

T4: *From practice to health outcomes*: evaluation studies to assess the effectiveness of interventions (e.g., a screening programme) in practice.

Source: Khoury et al. (2010)

The translational research perspective is quite different when compared to a more traditional epidemiology research approach, where our research may be discretely packaged and have an end point that is defined by gathering the results of our study, whatever that may be. The point of translational research is that it is not fixed, and does not necessarily ever end. The health of the public will change over time with cultural shifts, technological and medical advances, fluctuations in the economy, and other influences (such as we have seen with the pandemic). The 'outcome' with translational research is not merely to assess the impact of an intervention or new mode of practice, but to focus on whether or not this improves the health of the public, and whether it continues to. There is also a slightly different approach in translational research to evidence synthesis as well. Systematic reviews and meta-analyses are said to be 'top tier' evidence because they draw together and summarise available research on one topic or another. However, the general focus for these syntheses tends to be on outcomes (e.g., 'is this drug effective in treating breast cancer?'). The emphasis for translational research here is to take a more nuanced approach, to still ask those 'big questions', but to incorporate a greater understanding of the context with those questions. This may mean that evidence syntheses are less able to rely on these more systematic approaches, as they seek to incorporate knowledge garnered through multiple methods and through the lenses of multiple disciplines, but this provides a richer and more complex body of evidence to feed into practice. The spirit of translational research, and where it sits at the intersection between epidemiology and public health, is very much the spirit of what I have been trying to outline in this book. It is a more integrated and nuanced approach to health, that will have no full and final answers on what does or does not work because it recognises that the contexts in which we live and in which our health operates are changeable and dynamic. Table 8.2 outlines some of the key differences between translational research and more traditional means of research. The framework the translational perspective was drawn from was developed by Professor David Ogilvie and colleagues (2009).

PUBLIC HEALTH

Public health can be described as the role of the state in providing services and general protection of health to the population (particularly the workforce). Public health as we know it started in the late 19th and early 20th centuries. All industrialised nations now provide some guaranteed level of education, healthcare, and housing/income support, although this varies massively from country to country. Our health and wellbeing are

Table 8.2 Comparing traditional epidemiological research to translational research

Traditional epidemiological research	Translational research
Implements an intervention/practice, tests whether that intervention has had an effect.	Implements an intervention/practice, tests whether that has improved overall population health.
Uses health surveillance to understand health risks or issues in populations and groups.	Combines health surveillance with an understanding of social determinants of health (at the group/population level) and modifiable risk factors (at the person level).
Uses evidence synthesis practices (i.e., systematic reviews and meta-analyses) to understand the combined evidence for the effect of an intervention/practice.	Uses evidence synthesis practices to understand the combined evidence integrating evidence from broader disciplines with more complex and nuanced outcomes. Less 'hard' outcomes achieved here, but more practical and real-world evidence that can be fed into practice.
Linear framework of evidence → implementation → outcome.	Recognises the iterative and bidirectional relationship between epidemiology and public health, contributing to a feedback loop between evidence-based practice and practice-based evidence.

improved not just by being able to access healthcare and public health support, but by simply knowing it is there if we/our friends/families/loved ones need it. Public services are also an important expression of prosociality and solidarity – that we are prepared to look after all, no matter who they are or where they come from. I tell my students every time I give a lecture that touches on public health or socialist models of healthcare how extraordinarily lucky we are in the UK to have our NHS (National Health Service). It is not perfect, nor is any other model of healthcare, but any healthcare provision that is free at the point of service is an extraordinarily special thing and must be protected (and respected) at all costs. Before considering what public health is today, it is perhaps helpful to consider some of the historical approaches to health and public health to see how public health practices have evolved in line with both technological advances and epidemiological evidence.

The History of Health and Illness

Much of how we understand historical conceptualisations of health and disease is reliant upon documentary evidence, of which most tend to exist from Western cultures. That is not to say that non-Western cultures do not also have very rich and fascinating histories of health and medicine, in fact a lot of our modern understanding of medicine was heavily influenced by the scientific advances made by Islamic medicine in the intervening period between Greek and Roman scholarship and the Renaissance. However, it is harder to place these in a timeline due to the perishing (and often destruction) of documentary evidence through the colonialist gentrification perpetrated on these nations by our ancestors and those of other European countries. I have included some excellent references for a more comprehensive overview of the development of global medicine at the end of this chapter. For understanding the development of Western medicine, and the conceptualisation of health and disease, there is no better (and no further) historical example than those preserved from Ancient Greece. At this time, illness was considered to be due to dysfunction of bodily systems. The prevailing philosophy on the human body was that our minds and bodies were one and the same, and completely inseparable (a perspective referred to as *monism*). Subsequently, some like Plato (who lived somewhere across the fourth and third centuries BCE) broke away from this, preferring the idea that the mind or spirit was distinct from the physical body (referred to as *dualism*). Hippocrates (a contemporary of Plato, and considered the father of medicine) made the radical suggestion that disease occurred in the body through processes independent of the mind. The Hippocratic school of medicine proposed the idea of 'humours': blood, black bile, yellow bile, phlegm (referred to as *humoral theory*, and is where we get the term 'humoral immunity'), and thought diseases were a result of an imbalance in the humours. This remained a dominant theory for quite some time – picked up again by Galen in circa 2 CE, who then demonstrated that disease occurs in specific places in the body.

Following the collapse of the Roman empire in 5 CE, the advancement of knowledge in Europe slowed considerably, and we lose the excellently specific and comprehensive recording of societal changes and traditions (hence the term 'the Dark Ages'). The understanding of what caused ill health regressed from organic causes to being the subject of evil spirits or punishment by God. There was an overall shift back to a very religious framework for health, a shift back to monism, and also treatment of health issues (such as the use of torture to drive away demons). Healers were commonly priests; medical knowledge was the purview of the church. From here, dissection of humans and animals was forbidden, which then slowed further progress of understanding the causes of health considerably. Meanwhile, it should be noted that scholarship in the areas of medicine and science continued significantly in other regions of the world, particularly the Middle East, where knowledge in pharmacy and surgery continued to accumulate. The next big shift in what we understand Western medicine to be came from the Renaissance, with much of the knowledge from Islamic medicine being incorporated into this movement as soon as cultural changes in how medicine and medical techniques were viewed permitted. Renaissance means 'rebirth' – this was a time of re-engagement with science and knowledge, leading to a scientific revolution in the 1600s. Thoughts about the body and mind were once more reoriented to dualism by thinkers such as René Descartes who now proposed that the mind and body were completely separate, but that they were able to communicate through the pineal gland. The body began to be viewed as a physical machine, paving the way for once more considering ill health to be a malfunction of various aspects of the body. Dissection was made legal again with the change of social tone initiated by the likes of Descartes, who proposed that at death the soul left the body, and animals had no soul at all, so there was no fear of sacrilege or sin. This led to a massive acceleration of knowledge accompanied by a massive acceleration of technology and techniques in medicine. Microscopy was developed in the late 1600s (van Leeuwenhoek), allowing us to be able to look at cells and microbes previously never seen. Advanced methods of autopsy were developed in the 17th–18th centuries from Giovanni Battista Morgagni – considered the father of pathology – which led ultimately to the rejection of humoral theory. So, at this stage, Western medicine was beginning to understand that ill health was the result of changed or decreased function in certain systems, and that this could be remedied by intervention that would act on those systems. Public health was not really a thing at this point, but there was understanding that certain diseases could spread through communities, and the development of our understanding of health and medicine continued in a steady trajectory.

The Sanitary Movement Era

In the first half of the 19th century, the link between cleanliness and health became closer, and the first 'movement' of public health was born. The *Miasma Theory* of health became the prevailing line of understanding on how ill health is caused. It was thought that decomposing organic matter creates odours and particles in the air (*miasma*) that are harmful to health, evidencing an understanding that disease can spread through undetectable particles. The association made between decomposing organic matter and ill health had been colloquially made so far back it extends beyond the reach of our physical documentation, with our ancestral societies separating housing from sewage, and ensuring of the proper treatment of our dead (through burning or burying). Accordingly, public health issues were mostly concentrated on sanitation, with a focus on disease prevention across the whole population. Sanitation at this stage was not new, with most human settlements being situated near abundant sources of fresh water, and also archaeological evidence of sanitation infrastructures that can be found in many sites attributable to the Roman Empire as well as from the Indus Valley in what is now the Punjab region of Pakistan and Northern India, which far predates any other examples of physical sanitation infrastructure. However, at this point sanitation took a further step – not just to ensuring fresh water for consumption and hygienic disposal of sewage, but also general cleanliness of all things in our living spaces, from food to furnishings, and of ourselves. Reforms to policy in line with this movement brought about huge improvements in public health, even though the underlying theory wasn't correct. At this stage, epidemiology, as a means of understanding causes of diseases in the population, was a core part of public health – public health practitioners were involved in population-wide health improvements.

Germ Theory Era

In the late 19th to early 20th centuries bacteria were discovered, and were beginning to be understood to contribute to disease. This superseded the miasma theory with the understanding that it was not some sort of vapour that caused ill health, but identifiable microbes that could invade and infect. This paved the way for the development of vaccinations and lab-based diagnostics, and advancements ran in parallel with the continual development of laboratory technology and methods, which were driven by this new understanding. The paradigm shifted from looking at population-based health to more individual-based understandings of health, with a focus on disease pathology and treatment of individuals. This era saw the rise of medical-industrial growth, with the mass marketisation of immunisations and drug treatments. The philosophy of this time (if you can call it that) was very in line with the medical model – that patients are victims, and health is an individually oriented aspect of life. Here, as we saw with the regression during the Dark Ages, epidemiology was more a by-product rather than a focus because medicine was more focused on individuals rather than populations.

Chronic Disease Era

From the mid-20th century, after the growth of immunisations and effective medical treatment, infectious disease was starting to become less of a key concern to public health. Correspondingly, the emphasis on germ theory also declined and was replaced with the 'risk factor' or 'black box' paradigm. The 'black box' paradigm refers to being able to use epidemiological methods to examine associations between risk factors and health outcomes without necessarily tracing the precise mechanism by which those associations occur. You can think of it as simply reading Chapter 3 and ignoring Chapters 1 and 2 from this book. The 'black box' is, therefore, the void in knowledge or understanding between cause and effect. The fundamental premise at this time was that chronic disease was multi-causal, and could not be attributed to a specific factor.

There was a shifted emphasis to multi-professional approaches to health, and health was discussed as being influenced at the population (or specific group) level. Chronic disease epidemiology tended to focus on individual health behaviours rather than looking at wider social aspects.

Current Trends in Public Health

Public health theory is now polarising to a certain extent. On one side, there is a move to the micro level (molecular and genetic epidemiology) and the other very much macro (social epidemiology). Recent innovations and rapid improvements in biotechnology have altered the way that disease is understood at the very mechanistic cellular level, allowing these differing (but complementary) perspectives to develop significantly.

Social epidemiological theories include psychosocial, social production of disease/ political economy of health, and ecosocial (Krieger, 2014). These theories attempt to provide reasons for the social inequalities in health and disease distribution. All agree that health and disease are the consequence of social, political, environmental, financial, and demographic causes, but they differ in terms of what weight they place on each of those areas in terms of their contribution to health and illness. Broadly speaking, psychosocial and social production of disease/political economy of health paradigms focus more on the external determinants of health, whereas ecosocial also considers the contribution of biological (internal) factors.

Health Promotion Approaches from Modern Public Health

Broadly speaking, there are three main approaches to tackling public health issues in today's incarnation of public health as a discipline and practice.

The behaviour change approach: this is all about encouraging individuals to change their behaviours (either stopping bad ones or increasing good ones). The alteration of thinking processes (beliefs, attitudes etc.) is thought of as being the central focus. A lot of the work in this area is very much at the core of health psychology as a discipline, with behaviour change being uniquely advised from a psychology perspective, but there are important considerations to be made from sociology and anthropology as well, understanding that 'individual' behaviour is never entirely created in a vacuum of existence, and that we are always a product of our cultures and societies.

The self-empowerment approach: this argues that health promotion is best tackled by improving individual self-efficacy and agency. Increases in self-empowerment are proposed to influence decision making – and it occurs through engagement with effective health-related activities at either individual or community level. The focus here is less on trying to effect change, and more about trying to help people feel more in control of their lives and feel empowered to make changes if that is what they wish to do.

The collective action approach: This is sometimes referred to as community development approach. Emphasis is on the relationship between the individual and their social context – improve the self by improving the context. This is the more critical-social approach. Ideally, public health is a combination of all three.

WHY WE NEED PUBLIC HEALTH NOW MORE THAN EVER

I will take the example here of the UK, because that is the nation I know best seeing as it is where I have lived for most of my life. Having previously extolled the virtues of our priceless and wonderful NHS, the UK as it stands in 2022 (to me) is broken. Funding cuts made to health and social care services in the last decade have meant real reductions in public health initiatives such as Sure Start (centres to provide support and advice on child and family health, parenting, and other matters critical to supporting children), health visitors, stop-smoking services, and sexual health clinics. Some key public health indicators are beginning to worsen in the UK. For example, some sexually transmitted infections are rising, and the number of deaths due to drug poisoning has reached a record high (The King's Fund, 2022). The gap in life expectancy between the least and most deprived areas in England has widened to 9.3 years for males and 7.4 for females; the gap in healthy life expectancy is even greater at 19.1 years and 18.8 years respectively. This has been mostly attributed to key policy changes in the UK in recent years, some of which will be elaborated on later in this chapter. In 2013, the government decided to restructure the way that public health is managed in the UK, moving it away from NHS responsibility to local authorities. Alongside this responsibility, local authorities also actually inherited the provision of services for certain areas such as sexual health and drug and alcohol dependency. They were also made responsible for environmental health protection, meaning they would be at the forefront of tackling infectious disease outbreaks, and incidents related to environmental health hazards like chemical leaks and radiation. Whilst this was an awkward transition, it is largely common sense as the local authorities tend to deal with the structural issues in communities that are often associated with public health issues (like education, housing etc.), and these will differ from region to region. However, the way that local authorities are constituted and funded in the UK is far from equal, with (very frequently) those with more numerous and complex issues often receiving proportionately far less than those with less complex issues. Of course, it can be said that perhaps some of the lack of funding is because the issues are more numerous and complex, but it can also be true that with insufficient funding to stem these problems, they will necessarily become more numerous and complex. It is a case of the rich getting richer and the poor getting poorer, and that will not change unless the system is changed. Sadly, the Covid-19 pandemic has greatly worsened these disparities, and it will take decades for the balance to be redressed, provided there is sufficient social and political will to redress it.

GLOBAL PUBLIC HEALTH: THE UN SDGs AND THE GLOBAL CHARTER

So far in this chapter, we have looked at some of the health inequalities present in the UK. A key tenet of public health is to reduce health inequalities in a population. To reduce health inequalities, public health must aim to promote good health in all – and this can be done in a variety of ways. We tend to think of public health as being a national concern, but it is also considered in the international context by the World Health Organization (WHO), the UN, the Global Health Council, and private organisations like the Bill & Melinda Gates Foundation. Public health knowledge and priorities are then actively applied within individual countries in different settings and contexts according to what is needed. Global health priorities are not always the same in all countries, and how they are tackled is often highly individual to each country depending on the culture, the reasons behind health issues, and the motivations for change.

In 2015, the United Nations member states adopted the 2030 Agenda for Sustainable Development, which sets out the 17 Sustainable Development Goals (SDGs) (United Nations, 2022). This framework is designed to provide a 'shared blueprint for peace and prosperity for people and the planet, now and into the future' (2022). The goals (Figure 8.1) are designed to be adopted by all nations, both those developed and those still developing, with the understanding that our planet's resources are finite, our populations are expanding, and the increasing number of global problems (pandemics being a fine example of this) cannot be solved with individual responses, but require a shared commitment and strategy to move forward without leaving anyone behind.

You will see that each of these goals pertains to different aspects of human and planetary existence. There is a specific goal for good health and wellbeing (SDG3), but consider the other goals in this list and how they too contribute to human health

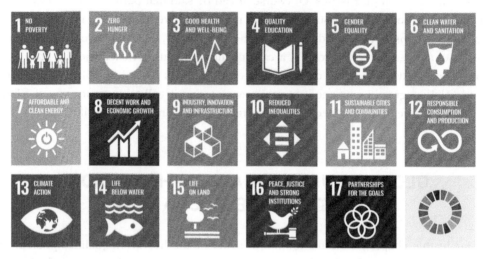

Figure 8.1 The United Nations Sustainable Development Goals. Image reproduced with kind permission from the UN SDG permissions office.[1] Find out more at: www.un.org/sustainabledevelopment/

and wellbeing. The whole point of the SDGs is to ensure equal and fair opportunities for all, and in that way all the goals will support good health and wellbeing. So, whilst the SDGs are not – in their truest sense – a public health initiative or formulation, they undoubtedly go towards serving a very ambitious and truly global sense of public health.

A more central public health initiative comes from the World Federation of Public Health Associations (WFPHA) developed with the World Health Organization in 2016. The Global Charter for the Public's Health serves as a framework with which public health professionals and organisations can build the capacity to develop policy, prompt systemic change, and advocate for improved health. It was developed with the recognition that whilst individual countries require robust public health systems, there is a need to consider public health on a global scale given our interconnected societies, and to provide a benchmark for good practice that can be implemented by those nations seeking to develop their public health provision. The main objectives of the charter (Figure 8.2) link in with the SDGs, and provide a framework for more collaborative working across and between organisations, and involving end-user stakeholders (i.e.,

---

1 The content of this publication has not been approved by the United Nations and does not reflect the views of the United Nations or its officials or Member States.

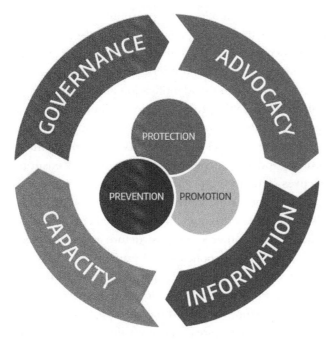

Figure 8.2 The Global Charter for the Public's Health. Image reproduced with kind permission of the World Federation of Public Health Associations (WFPHA): https://www.wfpha.org/.

the public). Many of the key components are not just about providing a service, but also about ensuring best practice is reinforced through research and development, and that this is shared through the network of organisations that sign the charter (see Table 8.3).

Within its framework, the Charter establishes the functions of information, capacity, effective advocacy, and good governance in promoting public health, increasing health security, and fulfilling the human right to health. The framework has at its core the

Table 8.3 The Global Charter for the Public's Health objectives

Encourage work between non-governmental organizations (NGOs), universities, civil society members, governments, and corporations.

Strengthen health systems' ability to implement universal health coverage through promoting global health security and sustainable, fair health outcomes.

Plan and implement strategies for better health outcomes globally.

Support economic growth and the post-2015 Sustainable Development Goals (SDGs).

Provide a flexible framework for tools that can be applied in different health and income settings.

Reinforce effective leadership and governance to encourage public health capacity building and improve the quality of health systems.

Ensure a comprehensive approach to tackling the threats to health everywhere.

Source: www.wfpha.org

central tenets of protection, promotion, and prevention, deemed 'services'. Protection is about providing services that control communicable disease, provide health impact assessments, consider occupational and environmental health, emergency and disaster preparedness, and consider national and international health regulation and coordination. Promotion is concerned with the identification and addressing of social and environmental determinants of health, promoting health literacy and positive behaviours, and reducing inequalities. Prevention focuses on embedding high-quality preventive care and interventions at each level of health service, implementing vaccination programmes, supporting good management of healthcare, and ensuring person-centred healthcare perspectives. Around these services are the charter 'functions': governance, capacity, advocacy, and information. Governance is concerned with all the policy-level functions of public health, the development and implementation of public health policies and other policies across other key infrastructure areas that support good health, sufficient funding to support such policies, and transparency in their implementation. Capacity is concerned with ensuring an adequately staffed and suitably skilled workforce, which includes planning, personal development and training, standards for practice, and sufficient infrastructure to support the workforce. Advocacy is about ensuring quality, ethical leadership that inspires and motivates solidarity and care for all, that engages with communities and the voluntary sectors, and pushes for fairer and more equal access and provision of critical services that support health. Finally, Information focuses on more of the academic side of public health, the monitoring, evaluation, and continuous improvement of services aimed at supporting public health, and the generation of practice-based evidence that will feed into evidence-based practice. The Charter has been adopted by many nations across the world, and there are some excellent case studies of the difference it has made to public health policies, available on the WFPHA website.

EPIDEMIOLOGY, PUBLIC HEALTH, AND THE CELL-TO-SOCIETY PERSPECTIVE

Having had a look at what epidemiology and public health are, and seen how public health works, it is now time to look at how public health perspectives can inform our understanding of health on the cell-to-society level. You will have seen so far that much of public health functions on the society level, that we consider populations of people, and attempt to implement policy, interventions, and health promotion to entire communities. It is likely that you will have witnessed much of public health in action throughout the pandemic, with most countries across the world implementing national policy and intervention to prevent the spread of Covid-19 to advise and encourage good health behaviours to ensure personal and community safety, and to implement mass vaccination programmes on a scale not seen in living memory. Public health is of course about all of these things, but it is also about understanding more about vulnerabilities, and about which groups may require more support to engage in certain health behaviours, may be more vulnerable to certain conditions, or may require uniquely tailored interventions as they may be underserved through mainstream public health awareness programmes. As much as public health and epidemiology perspectives focus on the macro, they can also tell us a great deal about the micro through detailed health surveillance and complex methods to understand risk and vulnerability. Some of these methods were discussed in Chapter 3 along with an introduction to the excellent work of Prof Sir Michael Marmot. We will now be looking at his work in more detail as a case study of how epidemiology and public health perspectives have allowed us to understand more not just about populations, but also about people.

The Marmot Review (2010)

In 2010, the UK government commissioned Professor Sir Michael Marmot to head up a review into health inequalities across England. The review made a strongly evidenced case that health inequalities have social determinants, and that health and wellbeing were just as important measures for the success of society as economic growth (Marmot, 2010). This review was the first to definitively outline the social gradient to health in England, and kick-started everything we know now about social determinants of health at both the individual and population levels. It was also the first time that any official documentation had been produced to suggest that economic growth was *not* the key marker of the success of a country. In addition, it was the first official report to suggest that health inequalities and climate change must be tackled together.

The report highlighted that health inequalities are a direct result of social inequalities. All those aspects of the health onion that you have been using as a tool to interrogate the cell, person, and society levels of health – they are all involved. The report concluded that monumental societal change was required, that it was simply not enough to focus on those who were most disadvantaged, that because the inequalities faced by so many lay at the most fundamental and structural levels, that wholesale change in policy culture was needed. This is very much the critical health psychology perspective – that our health and wellbeing are the products of the systems and structures within which we live, and that individual-level health requires systems-level change. Importantly, the report also introduced the life course perspective, highlighting the importance of health outcomes at the prenatal stages right up to very old age. All those factors highlighted in Chapters 3 to 4 in this book are included within the findings of the report, although the mechanisms by which some of the relationships occur were beyond the scope of that colossal piece of work. It is an excellent example of how we can observe the cell-to-society perspective at its most zoomed-out level, and how that information can then be used to understand the mechanisms at the most zoomed-in level.

Whilst there has been plenty of research that has understood the impacts of poverty or social marginalisation on individuals, this report was a real step change in understanding how these factors mushroom up into entire populations. It is the cell-to-society and then back again, effectively. The report highlighted the fact that our life expectancy could vary hugely depending on where we are born (remember that this is within one nation as well), and that the responsibility for this lies throughout the many layers of systems within which people sit (interpersonal, community, local authority, and national legislative systems). From this work, there were several very clear policy implications and directives made that would hopefully address some of the health inequalities that were observed as a result of this audit of public health. The main overarching aim was that health and wellbeing could and should be improved for all, and that tackling health inequalities through legislative action would achieve this. Critically, it highlighted that the cost of intervening effectively was drastically lower than the costs of not intervening at all.

The Marmot Review 10 Years On

Despite both its commissioning and its findings creating a real change in discourse around public health in England, the years that were to follow have really been the test of the impact of the findings. A subsequent report led by Prof Sir Michael Marmot has detailed where that landmark report has led in terms of policy and the health of the nation (Marmot et al., 2020). After the Marmot Review was published, the UK government of 2010 accepted all recommendations of the review aside from one: ensuring a healthy standard of living for all.

Since this time, successive governments have not prioritised action on health inequalities and many, but not all, policies in health and social determinant areas have run counter to the Marmot Review's recommendations. There has been no new national health inequalities strategy and little priority given to social determinants of health towards supporting greater equity in health. More encouragingly, many other organisations, particularly local government, have adopted and adapted the approaches and recommendations advocated in the 2010 Marmot Review. NHS England and Public Health England both have the stated aim and ambition to reduce health inequalities.

The report found that increases in life expectancy have slowed since 2010, with the slowdown greatest in more deprived areas of the country, and the UK seeing lower rates of life expectancy increases compared with most European and other high-income countries. Despite the warnings of the initial report, inequalities in life expectancy have increased since 2010, especially for women. There is a strong relationship between deprivation measured at the small area level and healthy life expectancy at birth. The poorer the area, the worse the health. The report also detailed that there was a social gradient in the proportion of life spent in ill health evidenced in the data, with those in poorer areas spending more of their shorter lives in ill health. Overall, healthy life expectancy has declined for women since 2010 and the percentage of life spent in ill health has increased for both men and women. It is a sad report to read, and shows that despite the very clear warnings provided in 2010, and the clear directions provided on how to steer away from the current trajectory, conditions in England have become more unequal, not less. This is a very hard part of research that advocates for those who need it most. We may do the research, provide compelling and painful evidence, even produce neatly packaged roadmaps out of the situation with costings and projections, but sometimes we cannot make those who must act do so. It is something I have experienced in my career, particularly recently in work that has been advocating for frontline workers during Covid-19, and it is painful and frustrating. That does not mean that it should not be done, however. If anything (in my opinion) it means that we should just shout louder.

Key Questions

Perhaps the previous section of this book has left you feeling hopeless and downhearted about the capacity of health practitioners to effect change. Perhaps it has inspired you to think about how your research or practice could make a difference in the future. I hope it is the latter. The next chapter is all about policy and how this impacts health, but before you go into that I want you to have a think about your role as a professional, whether that is a health psychologist, a nurse, a public health practitioner, or someone in another area of health and wellbeing, and consider where you sit on the evidence-practice spectrum, and what you would like your work to stand for in the future.

- What can we, as health professionals, do to improve public health?
- What if this is in the context of government policy that doesn't listen to the advice it, itself, has commissioned?
- Is it as simple as party politics - or are there more factors at play?

Learning Outcomes Summary

- Understand what public health and epidemiology are.

We have looked at both definitions of public health and epidemiology, as well as some of the practices and theories of work in these areas.

- Appreciate the ways in which public health and epidemiology feed into each other.

Using the perspective of translational research, we have seen how epidemiology and public health are complementary halves of a complex and nuanced whole when it comes to understanding health in our changing world.

- Critique the impact of public health in the context of policy.

We have looked at the Marmot Review and its outcomes. Through the activity at the end of the chapter you will have considered what role health practitioners have in the informing of policy.

FURTHER READING

CDC Foundation – What is Public Health?
There are a variety of useful resources available here, including a quick What is Public Health quiz: www.cdcfoundation.org/what-public-health

Coggon, D., Barker, D., & Rose, G. (2009). *Epidemiology for the Uninitiated*. John Wiley & Sons.
This is a great entry-level text that will give you a comprehensive overview of epidemiology. There is an online version available at www.bmj.com/about-bmj/resources-readers/publications/epidemiology-uninitiated.

Ebrahimnejad, H. (ed.) (2009). *The Development of Modern Medicine in Non-Western Countries: Historical Perspectives*. Routledge.
This book provides a very thorough (and brutally honest) perspective on the development of modern medicine from a non-Western perspective. There is a detailed account of how the abhorrent conduct of colonial Europe influenced the medicine traditions of a variety of nations across the world, bringing through the interweaving of these traditions into how medicine is practised today.

Nutbeam, D. (2000). Health literacy as a public health goal: A challenge for contemporary health education and communication strategies into the 21st century. *Health Promotion International, 15*(3), 259–67.
This article gives an excellent overview of one component of public health, health literacy, and its importance as a priority in achieving some of our greatest aims in public health.

REFERENCES

Albee, G., & Fryer, D. (2003). Praxis: Towards a public health psychology. *Journal of Community & Applied Social Psychology*, *13*(1), 71–5.

Khoury, M. J., Gwinn, M., & Ioannidis, J. P. A. (2010). The emergence of translational epidemiology: From scientific discovery to population health impact. *American Journal of Epidemiology*, *172*(5), 517–24. https://doi.org/10.1093/aje/kwq211

Krieger, N. (2014). Got theory? On the 21st c. CE rise of explicit use of epidemiologic theories of disease distribution: A review and ecosocial analysis. *Current Epidemiology Reports*, *1*(1), 45–56. https://doi.org/10.1007/s40471-013-0001-1

Marmot, M. (2013). *Fair society, healthy lives* Fair society, healthy lives, 1–74. The Marmot Review.

Marmot, M., Allen, J., Boyce, T., Goldblatt, P., & Morrison, J. (2020). *Health equity in England: The Marmot Review 10 years on*. www.health.org.uk/publications/reports/the-marmot-review-10-years-on

Ogilvie, D., Craig, P., Griffin, S., Macintyre, S., & Wareham, N. J. (2009). A translational framework for public health research. *BMC Public Health*, *9*(1), 116. https://doi.org/10.1186/1471-2458-9-116

The King's Fund. (2022). *Public health: Our position*. Retrieved 16 Aug 2022 from www.kingsfund.org.uk/projects/positions/public-health

United Nations. (2022). *The 17 Goals*. Retrieved 16 Aug 2022 from https://sdgs.un.org/goals

9

THE SOCIAL DETERMINANTS OF PUBLIC HEALTH

INTRODUCTION

This chapter is going to use some of the knowledge from the last chapter, but look at specific case studies from public policy to understand top-down health influence. In the last chapter, the example of the Marmot Review of 2010 was given to introduce the concept of the social gradient to health on the population level. Social issues are key drivers of health inequalities, and many social issues are not purely interpersonal from the sense of communities and groups; many can be the subject of policies and leadership. This chapter is going to look specifically at areas of public policy and how they have an impact on public health, and where social inequalities in these areas may exist. I have chosen three case studies that align to the UN Sustainable Development Goals: transport (SDG12: Responsible consumption and production); education (SDG4: Quality education); and housing (SDG11: Sustainable cities and communities), but it is worth noting that all of these case studies also touch on other goals (particularly SDG9: Industry, innovation, and infrastructure; and SDG10: Reduced inequalities). The examples used in this chapter are centred on the UK because this is the nation with which I am most familiar, but also (as in Chapters 3 and 8), it is a country of curious parallels, being both a global financial superpower (although this status is now arguably changing) and a nation of increasing inequality. The combined knowledge from this chapter and the last will provide you with an integrated overview of the complex interplay between person-level and system-level factors in health. We will look at the case studies to illustrate the impact of public health policy on populations, individuals, and cellular-level health. Each case study discusses why that policy is a public health issue (even though each policy being focused on is not explicitly about health), including the impact on people and groups, how this particular area can help or harm health, social factors associated with each component, and how public policy then impacts health outcomes. It is also useful to consider how some of the topics that were discussed in Chapter 3, particularly the elements introduced in the section on social exclusion, will be relevant to each of these policy case studies. In this way, you should be able to get an appreciation of the institutional level of social exclusion that exists in societies, and of how this filters down to people and groups of peoples to impact their health. Each section also closes with specific notes on policy and the various factors that may influence and be influenced by policy.

TRANSPORT

Policy relating to transport will have both direct and indirect impacts on public health. There are many different elements associated with transport policy and how that then relates to health, spanning the spectrum of private to public transport. Regulations on the availability of cycle lanes, the requirements for vehicle safety, the control of emissions, the amount of public (or private) money spent on maintaining and expanding transport infrastructures, even the regulations surrounding noise pollution made by traffic can all have direct and indirect consequences for health and wellbeing. Decisions on funding associated with public transport will have an impact on its accessibility, and therefore individuals' abilities to get to healthcare settings, or even get to large supermarkets to buy food. Control of safety elements, such as the legal requirement for safety belt or crash helmet use (and their quality), crash testing and general safety standards of modes of transport, the legal limit for alcohol consumption before driving, the proximity of pollution-heavy transport hubs such as airports to living areas, the width of cycle lanes, the maximum capacity for trains and buses, the control of harmful particulate emissions from vehicles, and minimum quality standards for vehicle parts (both in their production and general operation) will all have an impact on the health of drivers, pedestrians, cyclists, and transport users. There are also public health issues associated with transport that are important for policy, such as encouraging active transport, like cycling or walking, to increase fitness and decrease pollution. There are many countries where active transport is culturally well-embedded, and there are countries where towns and cities are so centrally designed around cars that active transport is dangerous. Socially, access to transport can be a means to decrease loneliness, facilitate employment, and provide independence. This can be hugely important for specific populations, particularly those outlined in Chapter 7, who may be less independently mobile due to either having less disposable income or being physically less capable. Such access can be to the extent of the availability of public transport, in terms of how many locations a network will serve, the frequency and safety of service, and the variety of different methods, but also the accessibility, including the price and whether it can be accessed by those that require support with their mobility. So, there are impacts on physical health, mental health, and general quality of life that come from policy associated with transport.

The policy that goes into transportation is also a delicate balance. Many economies rely on taxation of vehicles and road users in order to maintain the physical infrastructures that are available. Some provide public transportation centrally and therefore need to also front the cost of provisioning and maintaining these services. Another important consideration is that most countries have politicians to whom donations are given by interested parties to protect their interests, something that will apply to any area of policy. Even in the nations where political corruption is reportedly well-monitored, there are always party supporters that will have their own interests, and will seek to have those interests preserved via their donations. It is a sad fact that some of the largest political donors worldwide are those from fossil fuel companies, and they will repeatedly invest in those politicians that vote against more environmentally sound policies (Goldberg et al., 2020; Open Secrets, 2022). It will be very hard to make progress towards cleaner and greener modes of transport whilst the interests of fossil fuel companies are being protected by those deciding whether to invest capital in public transport, improving active transport highways, facilitating planning for cleaner air in towns and cities, or whether to continue facilitating private, non-renewable fuel transportation.

Transport as a Health Danger

Transportation poses many risks to health. There are the risks to our health from being a transport user (a driver or a passenger), risks as a pedestrian, and risks from just living or working in an area where we are exposed to emissions. It is likely you will have seen messaging around wearing seatbelts, looking twice before crossing the road, not venturing onto train tracks, or making sure you wear a cycle helmet – transportation is a dangerous thing. Very obvious physical danger with transport can be encountered at all levels of policymaking, from how high pavement kerbs should be to barriers surrounding rail infrastructure. Safety is another area very well related to health in public transport, such as how many people can safely be allowed into cars/buses/train carriages. There are also other impacts of transportation on poorer health, particularly from emissions making the air we breathe toxic, and also in the degradation of the living conditions of our planet. Emissions from fossil fuels into our living environments are damaging at almost every stage of life, but very much more so in our early stages, with observable impacts on foetal development, birth outcomes, and infant and child health

(Perera & Nadeau, 2022). We also have emissions from road-wear of tyres, which can be inhaled but also settle into the soil and waters in our environment (Baensch-Baltruschat et al., 2020). Air pollution is associated with the occurrence of many health conditions across the lifespan, such as childhood asthma (Patel & Miller, 2009), diabetes (Thiering & Heinrich, 2015), Alzheimer's disease (Fu & Yung, 2020), cardiovascular disease (Rajagopalan et al., 2018), and cancer (Turner et al., 2020) through many of the cellular mechanisms described in Chapter 1. Air pollution is associated with so many serious health outcomes that it is estimated to lead to 3.3 million premature deaths every year across the world (Lelieveld et al., 2015). Climate change and global heating are driven massively by the consumption of fossil fuels (Johnsson et al., 2019), which are abundant in transportation. Climate change impacts our health in a huge number of very worrying ways, from the increase of extreme weather events, which can cause ill health and death, to the depletion of our natural resources from flooding and drought, meaning crops fail and important animal species collapse. These are all important threats to global health, and they are all – somewhat absurdly – still being driven by us even though we are fully aware of what is going on.

Transport as a Health Facilitator

Personal transport allows great autonomy, providing people with the means to go where they want, when they want. In the absence of personal transport, public transport can also improve a variety of health outcomes by facilitating trips for healthcare, such as visiting hospitals and doctors, as well as being able to obtain prescriptions from pharmacies. For some, access to public transport is the only means of getting anywhere they need to be, particularly those in rural areas, those who are unemployed or with financial difficulties, and those who are physically less mobile, or in old age. Public transport use can also be a good means to increase mobility in those who are otherwise sedentary, with more activity being recorded by public transport users due to needing to walk to bus stops and train stations (Rissel et al., 2012). Having nearby public transport links also facilitates employment, with those areas with better public transport having higher employment rates, which then provides all the other health benefits that employment brings as well (Saif et al., 2019). Active transport can be a means of encouraging physical activity as well as driving down pollution, which helps the health of all. A review of the evidence has shown that the strongest associations between active transport (to work or school) are seen for cardiovascular health, with associations for cancer and mental health having weaker associations (Xu et al., 2013). There are economic benefits for areas that encourage active transport also, with decreases in accidents and injuries resulting in estimated savings that run to tens of millions of euros over time (Pérez et al., 2017).

Social Factors and Transport

There is a social gradient to transport use – with those on the lower end of the socio-economic spectrum needing to rely on public transport, or in some cases being priced out of it altogether. As is the case with many choices that need to be made by those with less disposable income, the short-term cost benefit of cheaper cars is usually also more liable to longer-term costs through repairs, and may not be as safe. With the rising trend for active/eco-friendly transport, even bicycles are becoming too expensive for many. The higher up the socio-economic scale you are, the more likely you are to be able to travel in greater luxury, with greater safety and greater freedom, and often at greater economic, social, and environmental cost (Wiedmann et al., 2020). Some trends for how we get around are changing over time, particularly with the emergence of prestige electric or hybrid vehicles, and a generational shift in attitude is being seen in some countries, with reduced car ownership and usage in younger generations (Zhang & Li, 2022).

In the global North, the status symbol of the 2010s onwards is the sports utility vehicle (SUV) – with increasingly bigger sizes. In the UK alone, the sales of SUVs have outstripped electric car sales 37 to 1 since 2017, with purchases mostly being in urban areas where they are least suited to the infrastructure. The blame for this rise in the UK has been attributed to the marketing around these types of vehicles, with the assertion that their use in urban settings is both desirable and safe (with themes of 'dominating the road' and 'protecting your family') despite the environmental impacts (New Weather Institute, 2021). Their rise in popularity has been named as the second biggest cause of emission rises globally (IEA [International Energy Agency], 2019), with CO_2 emissions 25% higher than those of a medium sized car. They are also a health danger in terms of accidents and crashes, being both extremely heavy and positioned higher, thereby obstructing the view of those in normal vehicles, and also striking pedestrians at centre mass, damaging vital organs, rather than lower in the body. In a pedestrian accident, children under 18 are eight times more likely to die if struck by a large vehicle such as an SUV, and adults are four times as likely to (Edwards & Leonard, 2022). Whilst seeming safer (and being advertised as such), SUVs are 11 times more likely to roll in a crash (El-Menyar et al., 2014), meaning more serious injuries for the passengers inside, and potentially others too (Daly et al., 2006). What does seem to matter is what you are driving, with those crashes with another vehicle where you are in the SUV being associated with better outcomes, but those where you are in a normal car being associated with worse (Jehle et al., 2021) – so the marketing around safety may be true in this sense (if we take the higher likelihood of rolling out of the equation), but only in the same way as trying to assert that you should bring a gun to a knife fight. Consequently, those with more money can afford to buy cars that cause more health damage both environmentally and physically.

Key Questions

- What sorts of policies and regulations are made in your country to tackle these problems?
  - Locally
  - Nationally
- Do these changes leave anyone behind?
- What can we do to level the playing field for transport and public health?
- What are the alternatives?

Potential Targets for Policy

It is clear from the available evidence that promoting active transport (i.e., walking, cycling) would have far-ranging benefits for health both directly and because of the associated impact on the environment. Public transport comes a close second to this, with excellent benefits to health both directly in encouraging more activity, but also indirectly by supporting social connection and healthcare utilisation, as well as being associated with employment. Counter to this, reducing motor vehicle transport (both passengers and goods) will reduce accidents and improve air quality, but this may be hampered by the influence of fossil fuel companies and their financial support for political decision makers as well as their large budgets for advertising and influencing. We also need to see better communication between the public ministries of countries to promote cross talk between departments of transport and health. If transport is not considered a public health issue, the benefits of supporting more positive modes of transportation will be even further watered down. However, there is the question here of how we make the trade-off between disincentivising the use of cars (particularly those that pollute) and pricing some people out of the market, ultimately decreasing social mobility. It is not an easy question to answer. It makes good sense, however, to ensure that public transport is at least equivocal in cost (if not cheaper) than private transport. In the UK, rail travel, which is necessary for long journeys, often far exceeds the price you would pay in the equivalent distance in fuel for your car, which makes the choice straightforward for many.

EDUCATION

Education is absolutely a critical element in public health. From having an equitable start in life, and therefore equitable opportunities when it comes to the job market, and the impact that will have on your finances, to more subtle considerations such as providing knowledge about what does and does not support good health, education is very strongly associated with health outcomes. Just as there are inequalities in health, there are inequalities in education – and they are both often cumulative and coincident. Your education is often very much dictated by where you live (certainly up until you are 18), which is in turn dictated by your family income (also a predictor of reaching higher education), and they are both influenced by local employment prospects (which may also be linked to education level and prosperity). So, in yet another unfortunate case of 'the rich get richer, and the poor get poorer', your level of education, and therefore your outcomes associated with that (including your health), is based on the socio-economic status and education level of your family (whose own status was dictated to a large degree by theirs), with status being reinforced from generation to generation in the absence of meaningful policies for social mobility (Willson & Shuey, 2018). The good thing is, however, that education is something that can be changed – we can improve educational access and quality for the public, therefore improving their health trajectories, so it is an ideal area to examine in the context of public health. There is no single point of an educational pathway that is more important than another for longer-term outcomes, but obviously if there are falls at earlier hurdles, this has longer-term impact.

Education as a Health Inequality

In 2016, the Early Intervention Foundation estimated that the national cost of 'late intervention' (the acute, statutory and essential benefits and services that are required when children and young people experience significant difficulties in life that might have been prevented) was £16.6 billion (Early Intervention Foundation, 2016). The 2010 Marmot Review concluded that reducing inequalities in early years experiences should be a priority for reducing inequalities in multiple desirable outcomes, including health (Marmot, 2010). Since the Marmot Review, austerity in the UK has seen rising child poverty and the closure of children's centres, as well as declines in education funding. In a large-scale analysis spanning 20 years across 26 OECD (Organisation for Economic Co-operation and Development[1])

---

1 A collaborative organisation of 38 countries founded to stimulate trade and economic development. Member states currently include Austria, Belgium, Canada, Denmark, France, Germany, Greece, Iceland, Ireland, Italy, Luxembourg, the Netherlands, Norway, Portugal, Spain, Sweden, Switzerland, Turkey, the United Kingdom, and the United States.

member states, better education was consistently associated with less disease and longer lifespans, particularly tertiary-level (university) education, which predicted higher levels of child vaccination, infant mortality, and life expectancy (Raghupathi & Raghupathi, 2020). Education level is so consistently associated with health that it is often used as a control variable in studies seeking to understand the relationships between social and psychological factors and particular health outcomes. If we do not control for educational level in our analyses, our findings could very easily be attributable to the education–health gradient and may not at all be associated with what we are really interested in understanding. Of course, level of education is still an unequal measure. Schools and universities are all different: they provide different qualities of education and different resources and supports, and carry different statuses in the job market. Someone with an undergraduate degree from a prestigious university may well be prioritised for a work role over someone with a postgraduate degree from a university considered less prestigious. This social currency from our educational institutions also provides other opportunities in life, with alumni networks and access to social circles that are otherwise impenetrable for those from other institutions, let alone those who have never had the opportunity to reach tertiary education.

For some, education is also limited depending on who you are. In some countries, even today, women and girls are denied the opportunity to access education both structurally, by policies from governments, and socially, by social gender norms, often requiring girls to remain home to support the running of the household. Even if women and girls are included in mainstream education by law, there are still sometimes differences in their quality of education that are influenced by social norms around gender, particularly around what some cultures determine to be more 'masculine' subjects, such as mathematics and the sciences. Similarly, in countries where all children are not just permitted to enter education, but where a minimum level of education is mandated, there are still inequalities across communities in terms of their equality of opportunity for participation in schooling, their chances of being excluded, and – occasionally – a clash between their culture and the expectations of the society in which their culture exists. An example of this in the UK comes from the equality of opportunity (or lack thereof) of educational access for people from Gypsy, Roma, Traveller, or Mincéir backgrounds. Despite education being fundamentally entrenched in UK law, these distinct groups (whilst being grouped together here, each of these nomadic heritages have distinct and diverse cultures and challenges in being included into settled communities) often face prejudice, misunderstanding, and social exclusion, meaning their educational attainment is significantly lower than other groups in the UK, limiting their options of progression onto tertiary education. The barriers that these communities face to any type of social participation are manifold for children and adults, but with many occurring so early in life this sets a tone that will continue throughout their lives. A good start, as we saw in Chapter 4, creates a good adulthood. A bad start can influence many different outcomes across time. I have included a report in the further reading section if you would like to learn more about the issues faced by these communities in the UK.

Education as a Means of Supporting Public Health

Schools have long been a mechanism of public health action specifically for children, with the nutritional supplementation (such as with milk provision), the supply of free school meals, and child health services being provided through education systems in many nations across the world. Not only is there direct health support in school systems, but also the capacity to learn about what being healthy means, a term referred to as *health literacy* (Nutbeam, 2000). Health literacy refers not just to the understanding of what health is and how it is made, but also to applying more abstract knowledge to understanding health and illness (such as political and economic changes). Health literacy is associated with both better overall health over time and more positive health behaviours, including having more agency in one's own health and having more collaborative relationships with healthcare providers (Paasche-Orlow & Wolf, 2007). Related to this is the concept of *scientific literacy*, which is the ability to consume and understand knowledge relating to science, including understanding scientific methodologies, limitations, and applications. We have seen some of the problems arising from poor scientific literacy in the ever-increasing emergence of misinformation that relate to public health measures (particularly vaccination), which are damaging to public health both in general terms (as in the case of longer-term population health strategies) and in responsive terms (as in the case of combatting emergent issues such as the Covid-19 pandemic). Of course, these issues are compounded by other societal problems (such as the deliberate spread of misinformation), but ensuring that our education systems support the ability to access and engage effectively with public health strategies and medical science throughout life should be a priority.

There is more to the relationship between education and health than health literacy, and from many years of data, including cross-cultural comparisons, the shared continuum of poorer to better education and poorer to better health is consistent. Using secondary population-level data from 11 European countries, Albert & Davia (2010) found that education is consistently a direct determinant of health. They found that secondary education is hugely associated with health in most cases (interestingly not in the UK or the Netherlands), and tertiary education in all cases. In the US, studies have shown that educational attainment is inversely related to physical disability in older age in both cross-sectional (Berkman & Gurland, 1998) and longitudinal studies (Liao et al., 1999). This has been echoed in studies in Finland (Rautio et al., 2001), Italy (Amaducci et al., 1998), and Spain (Béland & Zunzunegui, 1999). There is also evidence from

India to suggest 'upward transmission' of educational benefits to health, with children's education being associated with better old-age health in their parents (Thoma et al., 2021), meaning the benefits of good education are not just for the person receiving it. The field of adverse childhood experiences (ACEs; including lack of education) is a huge part of health research and ACEs are associated with many health and wellbeing outcomes across the life course (Felitti et al., 1998).

Key Questions

- What sorts of policies and regulations are made in your country to tackle these problems?
  - Locally
  - Nationally
- Do these changes leave anyone behind?
- What can we do to level the playing field for education and public health?
- What are the alternatives?

Potential Targets for Policy

From the available evidence, it is abundantly clear that education provides important opportunities to intervene in health (from the provision of nutritional supplementation and support), as well as the opportunity to develop health literacy. Educational attainment overall is associated with many different markers of health, and not just in those experiencing the education – they also transmit this to other generations. Education provides a variety of different opportunities in life that will all have different pathways to good health including social capital, good employment opportunities, and higher income. However, as we have seen, even in countries where education to a certain level is compulsory for all, there are still inequalities between groups and their ability to participate equitably in education. We can also observe the opposite relationship, where the lack of quality education is associated with lifelong health impact in comparison to those with it, so it can be truly considered a public health issue. Like all other areas of public policy, education requires sufficient investment from those who are responsible for leading nations, and there is clearly a requirement beyond just mandating education – there must be an effort to ensure inclusion and participation throughout communities to maximise the benefits derived from it for all. The evidence for upward transmission of health benefit from education would suggest that these benefits can be made at any time as well, and that they reach beyond the individual being educated.

HOUSING

Housing may seem like an odd aspect to focus on with regard to public health, but there are many facets to it that have implications for population health and wellbeing. We have already discussed how disease prevalence differs across the country, but it appears to be clustered in certain areas too. We can consider housing on the individual level, literally what the living conditions are in your house, but we can also consider it on the community level, where community planning and environmental health are dictated by your local government administration, and on a national level, where the guidance for minimum living standards in dwellings (both old and new, privately owned or rented) is created by policymakers. Each of these layers will have an influence over your individual living conditions, those of your community, and those of other people like you in your nation, and each of those influences will be associated with different types of health outcomes. In the UK, we have already seen that there are certain places where life expectancy and other health outcomes may be quite different, such as certain cities, but this extends beyond just town or city borders. The long-term limiting illness of women shows dense clustering in the North West, South Wales, and Northern parts of the map, with far more dense clustering above the North–South divide (Wiggins et al., 2002). Health is clearly experienced differently in different areas – but is this because certain individuals tend to live in certain places (*composition*), or is it the environment (*context*)?

Housing and Public Health

Teasing out the differences between compositional factors and contextual factors is extremely difficult when using population-level data, but there are certain statistical methods that allow the possibility of examining not just those that live in the same type of area, but also those living in similar spaces and using similar infrastructures (e.g., education, health services, transport etc.). This type of analysis can be made more difficult by the way that these areas are measured. Largely, census wards (administrative boundaries such as local authority areas) are commonly used. These physical/geographical boundaries don't always map onto the psychologically/socially defined communities that individuals have, but it is a good approximation (Campbell & McLean, 2002). There are also other factors to consider, including *selection* and *endogeneity*, which make examining the influence of community living standards and health very complicated (Kawachi & Subramanian, 2007). Endogeneity refers to the movement of people in order to better support their health. For example, you may have someone with a chronic lung condition choosing to move out of the city for better air quality. Selection refers to reverse causation of communities and health, where we may have more fast-food outlets in a particular area associated with obesity or diabetes, but it may be that the fast-food outlets are there because of a pre-existing demand, rather than them being the cause of the problem. With this in mind, I have tried to select an overview of neighbourhood-level health-outcome studies that use some of these more advanced methods to best account for the complexities involved in this type of analysis. Bear in mind that there is no perfect measure, but despite this there is a volume of evidence that supports neighbourhood factors in individual and community health outcomes.

Neighbourhoods

There are a variety of neighbourhood factors that we know have impacts in terms of health and wellbeing. In attempting to extricate the context from the composition, a critical review of the available data at the time suggested that neighbourhood-level variables are associated with health outcomes contextually (i.e., the social environment), with the adjustment for composition (i.e., individual measures such as socio-economic status), suggesting that our environments themselves and their social and physical characteristics may well be quite influential on our health even when we account for something as powerful as our socio-economic status (Pickett & Pearl, 2001). Neighbourhood poverty has been associated with poor general and mental health, and the relationship might be particularly strong for those who have individual poverty within those areas as well, who tend to cite more neighbourhood and financial problems (Stafford & Marmot, 2003). Local unemployment has been found to be associated with increased all-cause mortality, even when taking into account individual-level unemployment (Osler et al., 2003). On examining several datasets that evaluate mortality from cancer, heart disease, accidents, and suicide, the element of social capital (that is, the sociability of a neighbourhood) appears to be protective against each of these outcomes, even when controlling for other demographic factors well-established to predict these outcomes (Folland, 2007). Neighbourhood green space and nearby nature has very many associations with health outcomes, both physical and mental health, across the lifespan. There is a curvilinear relationship here, however, with the greatest benefits being observable at childhood and in old age (Douglas et al., 2017). The relationship between green space and health is a fascinating one, and has been the subject of a huge amount of work. Some colleagues and I have ventured into looking at this in more detail to understand the mechanisms, and we have been able to attribute these to three different exposure-type pathways ('being', 'doing', and 'living' in green space or nature), as well as some dynamic factors associated with the individual and the environment they interact with (Sumner et al., 2022a, 2022b). There are more neighbourhood factors that are associated with health – access to education and healthcare being two that have been discussed already in this chapter – but also the types of commerce available in neighbourhoods, such as the accessibility of supermarkets that supply fresh food, the presence and accessibility of bars and other places that serve alcohol, and the presence and accessibility of shops for gambling.

Housing and Health

Housing has direct impacts on health. In what is referred to as 'environmental health', our direct living environment either will be supportive of good health or may cause bad health. Whether our dwelling has sufficient basic amenities such as fresh water, sewerage, adequate aeration, electricity, and heating/air conditioning will directly influence our daily health. The type of house or dwelling in which we live can serve as a function of personal capital as well, with bigger houses with more amenities being available to those with more wealth, and the ownership of a dwelling often being associated with higher income also. Additionally, there are factors associated with the age of houses, and the quality with which they and their amenities were built, that have an impact on health too. Building materials like asbestos (Baumann et al., 2013), dampness and mould (Peat et al., 1998), sufficient ventilation (Fisk, 2018), and adequate natural lighting (Edwards & Torcellini, 2002) all impact health. Even furnishings can have an impact on health, with recent research showing an association between certain flame-retardant chemicals and the onset of diabetes (Lind & Lind, 2018). Indoor air quality can also be impacted by energy usage in dwellings, and residential energy-use emissions have been associated with a variety of different morbidities, including cardiovascular disease, cerebrovascular disease, and pulmonary (lung) diseases (Conibear et al., 2018).

Housing as a Health Hazard

There are other impacts of housing that can cause particular issues for health, particularly those seen recently in the UK. In 2017, 72 people were killed and a further 70 were seriously injured when the 24-storey Grenfell Tower block in London caught fire. What made this disaster so lethal was the cladding used on the outside of the building, which has since been assessed as being highly flammable as well as capable of emitting toxic smoke (McKenna et al., 2019), and should therefore never have been approved for use in housing. The tragedy of this situation showed that extreme emergency situations can also have very different outcomes if the way that our housing is built is not of a sufficiently high standard, but the lessons to be learned from this tragedy run deeper. This tower block also happened to be social housing (i.e., housing provided by the local council to those with restricted financial means), which some have suggested may be the reason the cladding was used in the first place, as it was cheaper than higher-specification (and, critically, safer) alternatives that may have been used had it not been a building for those in poverty. It has been suggested by many that this disaster was not just unavoidable, but was emblematic of the disparities and inequalities that are rife throughout the UK (Shildrick, 2018), a country that also happens to be one of the richest on the planet but is still subject to staggering inequality. Similar questions about the risks and damages that are disproportionately shouldered by those in poverty were also asked in the aftermath of the 2005 Hurricane Katrina in the United States, where whilst a hurricane could not have been foreseen, the impact this would have had on what was primarily a deprived and underserved community and locality, was (McKee, 2017). I have included further reading on the Grenfell disaster and the public health debate it has instigated in the UK at the end of this chapter.

Key Questions

- What sorts of policies and regulations are made in your country to tackle these problems?
  - Locally
  - Nationally
- Do these changes leave anyone behind?
- What can we do to level the playing field for housing and public health?
- What are the alternatives?

Potential Targets for Policy

Housing is a complicated and intricate public health issue. From the physical structures in which we live to the communities that they create, there are directly observable relationships between housing and human health and wellbeing. Governments, both central and local, are responsible for mandating minimum standards for housing quality, which has many impacts on health by determining our exposure to pollutants and toxins, and sheltering us from the harshest elements of our weather systems. Neighbourhoods as superordinate clusters of housing can be very facilitative of health and wellbeing, or they can negatively impact it also. As is the case with almost every element of public health, those who are in poverty or are otherwise underserved or socially marginalised are most vulnerable to the impact of their living conditions. Even those whose living conditions are directly under the remit of policymakers, such as those that require social housing, can suffer, where we should be able to see a direct and powerful example of how policy can protect the health of its populous through its impact on housing regulations. The evidence that our direct and local living environments can protect our health and support our social currency and capital would suggest that those policies that go to directing the physical infrastructures of our living environments should be an important element of public health. However – aside from the intervention of environmental health services – the link between housing arms of policy and public health is rarely very strong.

Learning Outcomes Summary

- Understand the interplay between social issues, policy, and how they impact health.

We have looked at three different case studies of policy and have seen how they have relationships to human health and wellbeing. We have also looked at some of the social inequalities each of those areas has, and how these modulate the relationships between these aspects and their health outcomes.

- Apply your interdisciplinary knowledge around health to broader socio-political issues.

Through the exercises, you should have been able to draw together some of your knowledge from the prior chapters in this book to make more sense of the cell-to-society factors that each of these policy areas will have on human health and wellbeing.

- Appreciate the complexity with which policy contributes to broader health outcomes.

We have looked at how – even in countries that are ruled by one government and have strong regulations for health and safety – inequalities, injustices, and disparities are common. Through the sections on relevant policy at the end of each of the case studies, you should have a deeper appreciation for the nuances of how policies affect health, and how external influences affect policies.

FURTHER READING

The Early Intervention Foundation website (www.eif.org) has a whole host of very useful and informative documents on supporting young people to minimise societal inequalities. Their work has focused on a variety of factors, including education, and they have produced some important reports regarding the impact of the Covid-19 pandemic on inequalities affecting young people.

The Indices of Deprivation explorer (http://dclgapps.communities.gov.uk/imd/iod_index.html) provides some very fine detail on the disparities between communities in both larger and smaller areas across England. Look and see how deep some of the differences are even within the same very small country. You can use the filters on the page to select health, income, employment, education, and other indices. Here, you can unfortunately also see how little has changed, and (in some cases) how it has got worse.

MacLeod, G. (2018). The Grenfell Tower atrocity: Exposing urban worlds of inequality, injustice, and an impaired democracy. *City, 22*(4), 460–89.
This is a deeper overview of the structural inequalities and societal injustices that have been highlighted since the disaster of Grenfell Tower.

Mulcahy, E., Baars, S., Bowen-Viner, K., & Menzies, L. (2017). The underrepresentation of Gypsy, Roma and Traveller pupils in higher education: A report on barriers from early years to secondary and beyond. London: King's College. https://www.cfey.org/wp-content/uploads/2017/07/KINGWIDE_28494_proof3.pdf
This report goes into some detail about the various barriers that groups from nomadic backgrounds face in the UK throughout their education.

Walsemann, K. M., Gee, G. C., & Ro, A. (2013). Educational attainment in the context of social inequality: New directions for research on education and health. *American Behavioral Scientist, 57*(8), 1082–1104.
A great overview of the link between education, social inequalities, and health.

REFERENCES

Albert, C., & Davia, M. A. (2010). Education is a key determinant of health in Europe: A comparative analysis of 11 countries. *Health Promotion International, 26*(2), 163–70. https://doi.org/10.1093/heapro/daq059

Amaducci, L., Maggi, S., Langlois, J., Minicuci, N., Baldereschi, M., Di Carlo, A., Grigoletto, F., & Group, I. L. S. o. A. (1998). Education and the risk of physical disability and mortality among men and women aged 65 to 84: The Italian longitudinal study on aging. *The Journals of Gerontology: Series A, 53A*(6), M484–90. https://doi.org/10.1093/gerona/53A.6.M484

Baensch-Baltruschat, B., Kocher, B., Stock, F., & Reifferscheid, G. (2020). Tyre and road wear particles (TRWP) – A review of generation, properties, emissions, human health risk, ecotoxicity, and fate in the environment. *Science of The Total Environment, 733*, 137823. https://doi.org/https://doi.org/10.1016/j.scitotenv.2020.137823

Baumann, F., Ambrosi, J.-P., & Carbone, M. (2013). Asbestos is not just asbestos: An unrecognised health hazard. *The Lancet Oncology, 14*(7), 576–8. https://doi.org/10.1016/S1470-2045(13)70257-2

Béland, F., & Zunzunegui, M. V. (1999). Predictors of functional status in older people living at home. *Age and Ageing, 28*(2), 153–9. https://doi.org/10.1093/ageing/28.2.153

Berkman, C. S., & Gurland, B. J. (1998). The relationship among income, other socioeconomic indicators, and functional level in older persons. *Journal of Aging and Health, 10*(1), 81–98. https://doi.org/10.1177/089826439801000105

Campbell, C., & McLean, C. (2002). Ethnic identities, social capital and health inequalities: factors shaping African-Caribbean participation in local community networks in the UK. *Social Science & Medicine, 55*(4), 643–57. https://doi.org/https://doi.org/10.1016/S0277-9536(01)00193-9

Conibear, L., Butt, E. W., Knote, C., Arnold, S. R., & Spracklen, D. V. (2018). Residential energy use emissions dominate health impacts from exposure to ambient particulate matter in India. *Nature Communications, 9*(1), 617. https://doi.org/10.1038/s41467-018-02986-7

Daly, L., Kallan, M. J., Arbogast, K. B., & Durbin, D. R. (2006). Risk of injury to child passengers in sport utility vehicles. *Pediatrics, 117*(1), 9–14. https://doi.org/10.1542/peds.2004-1364

Douglas, O., Lennon, M., & Scott, M. (2017). Green space benefits for health and well-being: A life-course approach for urban planning, design and management. *Cities, 66*, 53–62. https://doi.org/https://doi.org/10.1016/j.cities.2017.03.011

Early Intervention Foundation. (2016). *The cost of late intervention: EIF analysis 2016.* www.eif.org.uk/report/the-cost-of-late-intervention-eif-analysis-2016

Edwards, L., & Torcellini, P. (2002). *Literature review of the effects of natural light on building occupants.* www.nrel.gov/docs/fy02osti/30769.pdf

Edwards, M., & Leonard, D. (2022). Effects of large vehicles on pedestrian and pedal-cyclist injury severity. *Journal of Safety Research, 82*, 275–82. https://doi.org/https://doi.org/10.1016/j.jsr.2022.06.005

El-Menyar, A., Al-Thani, H., Tuma, M., Parchani, A., Abdulrahman, H., Peralta, R., Asim, M., Zarour, A., & Latifi, R. (2014). Epidemiology, causes and prevention of car rollover crashes with ejection. *Annals of Medical and Health Sciences Research, 4*(4), 495–502.

Felitti, V. J., Anda, R. F., Nordenberg, D., Williamson, D. F., Spitz, A. M., Edwards, V., Koss, M. P., & Marks, J. S. (1998). Relationship of childhood abuse and household dysfunction to many of the leading causes of death in adults: The adverse childhood experiences (ACE) study. *American Journal of Preventive Medicine, 14*(4), 245–58. https://doi.org/https://doi.org/10.1016/S0749-3797(98)00017-8

Fisk, W. J. (2018). How home ventilation rates affect health: A literature review. *Indoor Air, 28*(4), 473–87. https://doi.org/https://doi.org/10.1111/ina.12469

Folland, S. (2007). Does 'community social capital' contribute to population health? *Social Science & Medicine, 64*(11), 2342–54. https://doi.org/https://doi.org/10.1016/j.socscimed.2007.03.003

Fu, P., & Yung, K. K. L. (2020). Air pollution and Alzheimer's disease: A systematic review and meta-analysis. *Journal of Alzheimer's Disease, 77*, 701–14. https://doi.org/10.3233/JAD-200483

Goldberg, M. H., Marlon, J. R., Wang, X., van der Linden, S., & Leiserowitz, A. (2020). Oil and gas companies invest in legislators that vote against the environment. *Proceedings of the National Academy of Sciences, 117*(10), 5111–12. https://doi.org/10.1073/pnas.192217511

IEA (International Energy Agency). (2019). *Growing preference for SUVs challenges emissions reductions in passenger car market.* Retrieved 23 Aug 2022 from https://www.iea.org/commentaries/growing-preference-for-suvs-challenges-emissions-reductions-in-passenger-car-market

Jehle, D., Arslan, A., Doshi, C., & O'Brien, C. (2021). Car ratings take a back seat to vehicle type: Outcomes of SUV versus passenger car crashes. *HCA Healthcare Journal of Medicine, 2*(4), 9.

Johnsson, F., Kjärstad, J., & Rootzén, J. (2019). The threat to climate change mitigation posed by the abundance of fossil fuels. *Climate Policy, 19*(2), 258–74. https://doi.org/10.1080/14693062.2018.1483885

Kawachi, I., & Subramanian, S. V. (2007). Neighbourhood influences on health. *Journal of Epidemiology and Community Health, 61*(1), 3–4. http://dx.doi.org/10.1136/jech.2005.045203

Lelieveld, J., Evans, J. S., Fnais, M., Giannadaki, D., & Pozzer, A. (2015). The contribution of outdoor air pollution sources to premature mortality on a global scale. *Nature, 525*(7569), 367–71. https://doi.org/10.1038/nature15371

Liao, Y., McGee, D. L., Kaufman, J. S., Cao, G., & Cooper, R. S. (1999). Socioeconomic status and morbidity in the last years of life. *American Journal of Public Health, 89*(4), 569–72. https://doi.org/10.2105/ajph.89.4.569

Lind, P. M., & Lind, L. (2018). Endocrine-disrupting chemicals and risk of diabetes: An evidence-based review. *Diabetologia, 61*(7), 1495–1502. https://doi.org/10.1007/s00125-018-4621-3

Marmot, M. (2010). *Fair society, healthy lives* (Fair society, healthy lives: Strategic review of health inequalities in England post-2010, Issue. T. M. Review.

McKee, M. (2017). Grenfell Tower fire: Why we cannot ignore the political determinants of health. *BMJ, 357*, j2966. https://doi.org/10.1136/bmj.j2966

McKenna, S. T., Jones, N., Peck, G., Dickens, K., Pawelec, W., Oradei, S., Harris, S., Stec, A. A., & Hull, T. R. (2019). Fire behaviour of modern façade materials – Understanding the Grenfell Tower fire. *Journal of Hazardous Materials, 368*, 115–23. https://doi.org/https://doi.org/10.1016/j.jhazmat.2018.12.077

New Weather Institute. (2021). *Mindgames on wheels: How advertising sold promises of safety and superiority with SUVs.* https://static1.squarespace.com/static/

5ebd0080238e863d04911b51/t/6065dbeb73734b58372d797b/1617288180453/
Mindgames+On+Wheels+-+how+advertising+sold+false+promises+of+safety+and+super
iority+with+SUVs.pdf

Nutbeam, D. (2000). Health literacy as a public health goal: A challenge for contemporary
health education and communication strategies into the 21st century. *Health
Promotion International, 15*(3), 259–67. https://doi.org/10.1093/heapro/15.3.259

Open Secrets. (2022). *Top contributors 2021–2022: Oil & Gas.* Retrieved 23 Aug 2022
from www.opensecrets.org/industries/indus.php?ind=E01

Osler, M., Christensen, U., Lund, R., Gamborg, M., Godtfredsen, N., & Prescott, E. (2003).
High local unemployment and increased mortality in Danish adults: Results from a
prospective multilevel study. *Occupational and Environmental Medicine, 60*(11), e16.
https://doi.org/10.1136/oem.60.11.e16

Paasche-Orlow, M. K., & Wolf, M. S. (2007). The causal pathways linking health literacy to
health outcomes. *American Journal of Health Behavior, 31*(1), S19–S26. www.
ingentaconnect.com/content/png/ajhb/2007/00000031/a00100s1/art00004

Patel, M. M., & Miller, R. L. (2009). Air pollution and childhood asthma: Recent advances
and future directions. *Current Opinion in Pediatrics, 21*(2), 235. https://doi.
org/10.1097/MOP.0b013e3283267726

Peat, J. K., Dickerson, J., & Li, J. (1998). Effects of damp and mould in the home on
respiratory health: A review of the literature. *Allergy, 53*(2), 120–28. https://doi.org/
https://doi.org/10.1111/j.1398-9995.1998.tb03859.x

Perera, F., & Nadeau, K. (2022). Climate change, fossil-fuel pollution, and children's
health. *New England Journal of Medicine, 386*(24), 2303–14. https://doi.org/10.1056/
NEJMra2117706

Pérez, K., Olabarria, M., Rojas-Rueda, D., Santamariña-Rubio, E., Borrell, C., &
Nieuwenhuijsen, M. (2017). The health and economic benefits of active transport
policies in Barcelona. *Journal of Transport & Health, 4*, 316–24. https://doi.
org/10.1016/j.jth.2017.01.001

Pickett, K. E., & Pearl, M. (2001). Multilevel analyses of neighbourhood socioeconomic
context and health outcomes: A critical review. *Journal of Epidemiology and
Community Health, 55*(2), 111–22. https://doi.org/10.1136/jech.55.2.111

Raghupathi, V., & Raghupathi, W. (2020). The influence of education on health: An
empirical assessment of OECD countries for the period 1995–2015. *Archives of Public
Health, 78*(1), 20. https://doi.org/10.1186/s13690-020-00402-5

Rajagopalan, S., Al-Kindi, S. G., & Brook, R. D. (2018). Air pollution and cardiovascular
disease. *Journal of the American College of Cardiology, 72*(17), 2054–70. https://
doi.org/doi:10.1016/j.jacc.2018.07.099

Rautio, N., Heikkinen, E., & Heikkinen, R.-L. (2001). The association of socio-economic
factors with physical and mental capacity in elderly men and women. *Archives of
Gerontology and Geriatrics, 33*(2), 163–78. https://doi.org/https://doi.org/10.1016/
S0167-4943(01)00180-7

Rissel, C., Curac, N., Greenaway, M., & Bauman, A. (2012). Physical activity associated
with public transport use – a review and modelling of potential benefits. *International
Journal of Environmental Research and Public Health, 9*(7), 2454–78.

Saif, M. A., Zefreh, M. M., & Torok, A. (2019). Public transport accessibility: A literature review. *Periodica Polytechnica Transportation Engineering*, *47*(1), 36–43. https://doi.org/10.3311/PPtr.12072

Shildrick, T. (2018). Lessons from Grenfell: Poverty propaganda, stigma and class power. *The Sociological Review*, *66*(4), 783–98. https://doi.org/10.1177/0038026118777424

Stafford, M., & Marmot, M. (2003). Neighbourhood deprivation and health: Does it affect us all equally? *International Journal of Epidemiology*, *32*(3), 357–66. https://doi.org/10.1093/ije/dyg084

Sumner, R. C., Cassarino, M., Dockray, S., Setti, A., & Crone, D. M. (2022a). Moving towards a multidimensional dynamic approach to nature and health: A bioavailability perspective. *People and Nature*, *4*(1), 44–52. https://doi.org/https://doi.org/10.1002/pan3.10266

Sumner, R. C., Cassarino, M., Dockray, S., Setti, A., & Crone, D. M. (2022b). Moving towards a multidimensional dynamic approach to nature and health: A bioavailability perspective. Theoretical paper with full literature review. *PsyArXiv*. https://doi.org/https://doi.org/10.31234/osf.io/knw3e

Thiering, E., & Heinrich, J. (2015). Epidemiology of air pollution and diabetes. *Trends in Endocrinology & Metabolism*, *26*(7), 384–94. https://doi.org/https://doi.org/10.1016/j.tem.2015.05.002

Thoma, B., Sudharsanan, N., Karlsson, O., Joe, W., Subramanian, S. V., & De Neve, J.-W. (2021). Children's education and parental old-age health: Evidence from a population-based, nationally representative study in India. *Population Studies*, *75*(1), 51–66. https://doi.org/10.1080/00324728.2020.1775873

Turner, M. C., Andersen, Z. J., Baccarelli, A., Diver, W. R., Gapstur, S. M., Pope III, C. A., Prada, D., Samet, J., Thurston, G., & Cohen, A. (2020). Outdoor air pollution and cancer: An overview of the current evidence and public health recommendations. *CA: A Cancer Journal for Clinicians*, *70*(6), 460–79. https://doi.org/https://doi.org/10.3322/caac.21632

Wiedmann, T., Lenzen, M., Keyßer, L. T., & Steinberger, J. K. (2020). Scientists' warning on affluence. *Nature Communications*, *11*(1), 3107. https://doi.org/10.1038/s41467-020-16941-y

Wiggins, R. D., Joshi, H., Bartley, M., Gleave, S., Lynch, K., & Cullis, A. (2002). Place and personal circumstances in a multilevel account of women's long-term illness. *Social Science & Medicine*, *54*(5), 827–38. https://doi.org/https://doi.org/10.1016/S0277-9536(01)00112-5

Willson, A. E., & Shuey, K. M. (2018). A longitudinal analysis of the intergenerational transmission of health inequality. *The Journals of Gerontology: Series B*, *74*(1), 181–91. https://doi.org/10.1093/geronb/gby059

Xu, H., Wen, L. M., & Rissel, C. (2013). The relationships between active transport to work or school and cardiovascular health or body weight: A systematic review. *Asia Pacific Journal of Public Health*, *25*(4), 298–315. https://doi.org/10.1177/1010539513482965

Zhang, M., & Li, Y. (2022). Generational travel patterns in the United States: New insights from eight national travel surveys. *Transportation Research Part A: Policy and Practice*, *156*, 1–13. https://doi.org/https://doi.org/10.1016/j.tra.2021.12.002

10

APPLYING INTERDISCIPLINARY KNOWLEDGE TO NON-COMMUNICABLE DISEASE: THE CELL-TO-SOCIETY OF CARDIOVASCULAR DISEASE

INTRODUCTION

To bring together the learning from the book, this chapter focuses on applying the cell-to-society perspective to an example of a **non-communicable disease** (i.e., something you cannot catch from someone else). This chapter focuses on cardiovascular disease, but the principles here can easily be applied to other public health priorities, and you will be encouraged to try this yourself with activities throughout the chapter. We will start with an overview of cardiovascular disease, and its relevance as a public health priority, and then we will go through the cellular-, system-, and population-level approaches to cardiovascular morbidity and mortality. Cellular and system-level pathology is explored, along with biopsychosocial determinants at each of those levels. For the population-level approach, racism is discussed as a unique biopsychosocial modifier of morbidity and mortality. Demographics and lifestyles associated with cardiovascular disease are discussed with reference to group-level influence, and in terms of social gradients.

Learning Outcomes

- Apply the knowledge gained throughout the book to the example of cardiovascular disease.
- Understand how we can make sense of aetiology and susceptibility through the cell-to-society perspective.
- Discuss the interaction between the levels of cell-to-society health and its contribution to public health issues in non-communicable disease.

WHAT IS CARDIOVASCULAR DISEASE?

Cardiovascular disease (or diseases, really) is the name of the very many conditions that affect the heart (cardio) and the circulatory (vascular) systems. We do not 'catch' cardiovascular disease (CVD), which is why it is referred to as 'non-communicable', but it is very common and a significant global public health issue. CVDs are the leading causes of death worldwide, outpacing the second leading cause (cancer) by almost double (Roth et al., 2018). They are sometimes also included with cerebrovascular diseases (i.e., stroke) because of their shared pathology in the vascular system, as strokes and heart conditions can both be produced by similar underlying causes. This chapter will focus centrally on heart diseases, but it is useful to remember that the impact of some of the aetiology involved in these conditions also extends to other diseases. CVDs may be associated with the physical working of the heart itself, or the effective transportation of blood through the vascular system. These issues, in turn, can be caused by a variety of different underlying factors that may originate at cellular- or system-level and which affect groups at the population level.

The emergence of CVD as a leading cause of death globally is largely down to two factors that have occurred alongside each other over the last hundred years. First, humanity has got better at treating and preventing infectious disease, and at preventing death during childbirth. This has meant that we live much longer than we used to, which on the surface is of course a good thing, but our bodies are not meant to last forever. In living longer, there is more opportunity for wear and tear to occur, and for systems and processes to slow down. Second, our lifestyles have changed significantly. With the numerous advances in technology, and the social and cultural changes that happen alongside that, our lives are becoming more sedentary. Our work is largely characterised by sitting down for most of the day, as opposed to being manual and physical. We spend our leisure time sat down or otherwise relatively immobile as well, and we rely on sedentary modes of transport to get us to where we need to be. On top of this, our diets are now full of processed foods, preservative chemicals, and (for many) are very dense with carbohydrates and sugars. So, we live longer, but we use that time engaging in unhealthy behaviours, avoiding healthy ones, and loading our bodies up with inappropriate nutrients. Throw in a bit of stress for good measure (see Chapter 5), and we have a recipe for a body that is being poorly looked after, over-exerted in the incorrect ways (i.e., stress and nutritional overloading), and under-exerted in the correct ways (i.e., exercise and activity). All of these factors mean that our cardiovascular systems are aging along with us, but are being poorly looked after and sometimes ageing beyond us. We are adding more stress and strain to an under-cared-for system, and something eventually has to give. Imagine your body is a car – if you give it the wrong type of fuel it won't take long before this damages its internal machinery; similarly if you never carry out decent maintenance to ensure all the parts are working well, it won't be long before the car breaks down.

Types of Cardiovascular Disease

There are many different distinct pathologies that sit under the CVD umbrella. I will provide a few examples here for a brief overview of some different types of heart disease, mostly to illustrate how they can be caused by various malfunctions or dysfunctions in the system. Each of these different conditions will have different types of predisposing factors, and different elements of influence from the cellular to the population level. The conditions I have chosen are (to an extent) cumulative, in that where we start (atherosclerosis) is a precursor to the subsequent conditions, and these are good examples of heart diseases that often have complex and intersecting causes. This is not an exhaustive list, but it will hopefully familiarise you with a few different pathologies in this system and help you to understand how issues within a system may often have cumulative outcomes.

Atherosclerosis

Atherosclerosis is an interesting condition to start with because it is both a 'condition' (in that, once diagnosed, we seek to treat it) and a predisposing factor in other CVDs. It is effectively the reduced internal capacity of your arteries and veins due to the deposition of plaque (not like the stuff that develops on your teeth, but it is a similarly accumulating layer of deposited substances), which is formed from fats (lipids), **cholesterol**, cellular waste, and other blood-borne particles and substances. However, the plaques do not necessarily have to restrict blood flow in situ to cause a problem, just the presence of plaques means that future blockages may occur if any of them shear away from the lining of the blood vessel and may increase the likelihood of clots that will cause an obstruction. The deposition of these plaques also reduces the elasticity of your blood vessels, where having stiffer blood vessels (also caused by several cellular and system-level factors, including inflammation, hormonal factors, oxidative stress, and epigenetic changes) means they are less able to adapt to pressure put on the system in the case of exertion (which can come from physical exertion or from psychological exertion in the form of stress). Atherosclerosis can begin to develop as early as childhood; however, in most it starts to develop in adulthood and continues slowly. The build-up of this plaque tends to worsen over time, and as the internal lining of your blood vessels becomes more heavily layered, inflammation increases, which also then has the potential to make the plaque deposition worse. As the layers of these deposits (referred to as **atheroma**) in your blood vessels increase, the diameter of the vessel able to support your blood flow decreases (see Figure 10.1). Much like squeezing the end of a hosepipe, as our flow capacity is decreased, the pressure of the flow increases,

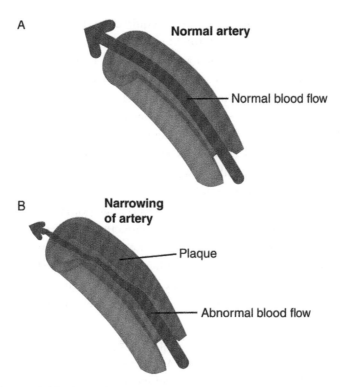

Figure 10.1   Atheroma in blood vessels

Source: Cook et al. (2019), *Essentials of Pathophysiology for Nursing Practice*, Sage

which is why atherosclerosis often leads to high blood pressure. Atherosclerosis can be difficult to observe (as we need to literally see the inside of the blood vessels), so very frequently indices of atherosclerosis likelihood are used, such as cholesterol levels and blood pressure. To treat atherosclerosis, patients are often recommended to change their diets to reduce cholesterol, to increase physical activity, reduce other health behaviours that may impact outcomes (such as smoking and drinking alcohol), and may also be prescribed medications that prevent clotting (to prevent blood vessel blockage), lower cholesterol, or lower blood pressure.

Ischemic Heart Disease: Angina and Myocardial Infarction

Ischemic[1] **heart disease** (IHD), sometimes also referred to as *coronary heart disease* or *coronary artery disease*, is a very common CVD across the world and is a cluster of related diseases that result from similar pathology. IHD starts off with atherosclerosis, but the conditions within this cluster are associated with the blockage of the blood vessels that feed the heart. These are not the blood vessels that transport blood to and from the heart around the body, but are the ones required by the heart to feed its muscles and keep it working (see Figure 10.2, the blood vessels that lie over the outside of the heart as opposed to those entering and exiting the heart). Early signs of IHD come in the form of **angina**, an IHD condition characterised by sharp and repetitive chest pains, usually accompanied by some other key symptoms such as dizziness, nausea, and fatigue. Angina is a warning sign of further IHD conditions to come because it is caused by the partial blockage of these blood vessels, leaving the tissue they are meant to feed in distress causing the pain. However, sometimes patients do not experience angina at all, and may develop more serious IHD without such warning. If the build-up of atherosclerosis is not treated, this can result in a complete blockage (or *occlusion*) of one of the blood vessels that feeds the heart muscles, causing a heart attack (*myocardial infarction*) and even the spontaneous cessation of the heartbeat altogether (*sudden cardiac death*). IHD can result from a slow progression over time as the plaques accumulate, but it can also happen quite quickly in the case of a bit of atheroma becoming dislodged and entering the bloodstream, or from a blood clot. Once a blockage occurs and the heart muscle is starved of blood, if the cells start to die due to this event, that is known as a heart

---

1 The term **ischemia** simply means that vital tissues are being deprived of oxygen and nutrients due to a blockage in blood supply. Another key outcome for CVD is **haemorrhage**, meaning we lose oxygen and nutrients due to a loss of blood supply usually from a bleed, which can be caused by a blood vessel rupturing because of a blockage, through trauma, or poor vessel wall integrity. You will come across both of these terms when looking further into both cardio- and cerebrovascular diseases.

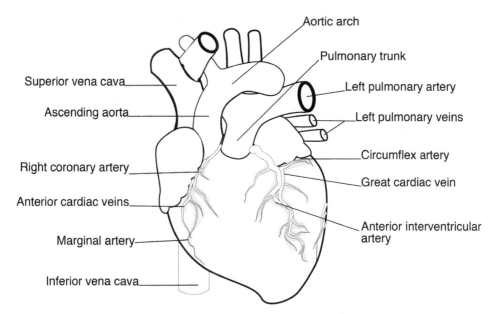

Figure 10.2 The heart. The blood vessels lying on the outside of the heart (as opposed to those entering and exiting it) are those implicated in ischemic heart disease.

Source: Boore et al. (2016), *Essentials of Anatomy and Physiology for Nursing Practice*, Sage

attack. Muscle damage in the heart is very difficult to repair, so heart attacks can cause very serious problems for long-term health, and can be fatal. Another CVD that can be caused by clots is *pulmonary embolism*, where lung tissue is damaged due to lack of oxygen supply from a clot that has occurred elsewhere (**embolus**) and has travelled to the lungs. This condition can also be fatal. Treatment for IHD is very similar to that of atherosclerosis, as atherosclerosis is a key predisposing factor. Improved diet, increased mobility and exercise, and decreased engagement in exacerbating health behaviours (such as smoking and drinking alcohol) are recommended alongside medical treatment.

Congestive Heart Failure

Heart failure is as serious as the name would suggest. It is the state of your heart failing – where it is not able to keep your blood pumping around your body. This can be the result of the muscles in your heart weakening or becoming too stiff (in the case of scarring from heart attacks), and usually takes a long time to develop but can onset quite quickly in some cases. There are a few different types of heart failure, and they have different causes (some due to congenital heart defects, for example). **Congestive heart failure** (CHF), however, is characterised by the backlogging of fluid in the body due to insufficient **ejection fraction** (i.e., the amount of blood pushed out of the heart with each beat), which can cause swelling (**oedema**) around the body. This collecting of fluid is most common in the legs, but can occur elsewhere in the body, and can cause very serious problems when it occurs around the lungs. It is a problem that can also be made worse by the effects it has on the kidneys, where they start to have their own function impaired and are unable to clear sodium and water from our system, making the oedema worse and putting more pressure on an already under-pressure heart. Those with CHF often have severe shortness of breath and will find physical exertion very difficult if not impossible. As with atherosclerosis and IHD, the treatments for CHF are both behavioural (diet, activity, good health behaviours) and medical, but surgery may also be needed.

Warning

There are many books and resources written on specialist diets, mindfulness or meditation techniques to avoid, deter, or reverse heart disease. Be wary of anything that promises 'everything you were ever told is wrong'. As always, there will usually be a grain of truth in them (a good diet is an important component of preventing CVD), but often they will be more about selling something than genuinely helping.

Unfortunately, as with other types of illness that wreak emotional, physical, and financial havoc on people (particularly cancer), there are people who claim that you are having the truth about the illness (or its cure) withheld from you, that this person is going to reveal. Most of the time, those that wish to pedal these 'alternative' cures or therapies will do so under the guise of being 'more honest' than pharmaceutical companies, who are portrayed as evil corporations hell-bent on world domination through the exploitation of illness. Whilst I am not entirely convinced all the motives of pharmaceutical companies are beneficent, the portrayal of these companies as being wholly motivated by domination and population control is both illogical and impractical. I have included some further reading from Professor Luke O'Neill at the end of this chapter who provides an excellent and well-balanced summary of this particular issue.

THE CELL-TO-SOCIETY OF CARDIOVASCULAR DISEASE

Cellular Factors

The question of whether oxidative stress has been involved in the pathogenesis of CVDs has been debated for at least a decade. We know now that certain conditions such as atherosclerosis, which are heavily involved in the pathophysiology of other CVDs, are very much associated with oxidative stress processes (Alfarisi et al., 2020). Specifically, high levels of reactive oxygen species (ROS) through oxidative stress can cause one of the types of cholesterol (**low-density lipoprotein**, known as LDL – the 'bad' cholesterol) to become oxidated as well. The transport of this oxidated LDL across the **endothelium** of the blood vessel can cause **endothelial dysfunction**, a condition characterised by the narrowing of blood vessels due to inflammation – sometimes referred to as *non-obstructive* coronary artery disease because it is not caused by a blockage. So, oxidative stress here can narrow the blood vessels independently of deposits of plaque, and if we add atherosclerosis or hypertension (or both) to that mix, then this causes further stress to our blood vessels (Urso & Caimi, 2011).

There is an entire field of study relating to the genetic associations with CVD, called cardiovascular genetics, which has evolved rapidly over the last few decades to not just help us understand the underlying causes of CVD, but also identify distinct types of CVDs. One of the key factors in the pathogenesis of CVDs is the increase in serum (blood) cholesterol levels. There have been four 'monogenic' (i.e., single gene) diseases identified that cause elevation in plasma cholesterol, thereby predisposing someone to future CVDs (Nabel, 2003). As for epigenetics, if you cast your minds back to Chapter 1 and the Dutch Hunger Winter, there is an excellent example there in how the gene × environment interaction can predispose not just individuals, but generations, to CVD. There is evidence for exposure to tobacco smoke *in utero*, in early life, and throughout life in the onset of CVD (Ordovás & Smith, 2010). Histone acetylation and DNA methylation (two epigenetic processes) have also been associated with **atherogenesis**, which is the creation and formulation of atheroma (Khyzha et al., 2017), as well as the regulation of cholesterol homeostasis (Meaney, 2014), which is the maintenance of cholesterol balance within cells in the body. Another cellular factor not yet mentioned in this book is that of 'microparticles'. Microparticles are by-products of cellular processes such as cell activation and cell death (apoptosis). The role of microparticles in standard physiology is still being explored, but there is also growing evidence for their role in pathology, particularly CVD as they seem to be related to vascular functioning, coagulation (clotting), and inflammatory processes (VanWijk et al., 2003; Voukalis et al., 2019).

System Factors

When it comes to systems involved in the development of CVD, the cardiovascular system is the obvious place to start. As we have seen so far, one of the factors associated with the onset of CVD pathways (particularly **cholesterolaemia** – having a high amount of cholesterol in the blood, and atherosclerosis) is endothelial dysfunction. As mentioned above, cellular processes can increase the likelihood of endothelial dysfunction, but behaviours can as well. A factor that has gained a lot of attention in recent years is that of sedentary behaviour. Being sedentary is not about failing to do sufficient exercise, it is simply about not moving enough. In fact, even for those who do exercise a lot, being sedentary can still be extremely damaging to cardiovascular health (Owen et al., 2010). Sitting is something many cultures tend to do a lot of. We spend a lot of our time at work sitting, a lot of our leisure time sitting as well, and it is extremely bad for us. Prolonged sitting has been shown to disrupt the proper functioning of lower limb arteries as well as putting extra effort on the heart, raising systolic blood pressure and arterial pressure (Paterson et al., 2020, 2022). All is not lost though, as these authors also assessed the impact of frequent interruptions to sitting and found that this can be protective against some of the more harmful effects of being still (and seated) for too long.

The immune system is also heavily implicated in the development of various types of CVD. Atherosclerosis, one of the types of CVD that leads to the development of further, more serious cardiovascular illnesses, is an inflammatory illness as much as a cardio-vascular one. There has been quite a bit of controversy around the immune processes involved with atherosclerosis, with much of the evidence being through animal models as observing a progressive illness over time in humans is very costly and takes a great deal of time. However, there is now the consensus that atherosclerosis most definitely does have an inflammatory component, and anti-inflammatory medications have been shown to be effective in treatment (Libby, 2020). High levels of cholesterol are also asso-ciated with the initiation of several other inflammatory cellular processes in the immune system, and the cells these processes mobilise invade the blood vessel walls increasing endothelial dysfunction (Wolf & Ley, 2019). There are some important cells in the pro-cess of atherosclerosis called **foam cells**, which are immune cells called **macrophages** that are specialised to deal with fatty deposits in places in our bodies. These cells absorb some of the fats, which then makes them look foamy – hence the name. Despite being there to help, these foam cells secrete various signalling molecules that can make inflam-mation worse, so they are increased through the presence of fat deposits and exacerbate the problems caused by those deposits too (Poznyak et al., 2021).

For hormones and the endocrine system, there is a wealth of evidence for their involvement in CVD pathogenesis. **Environmental endocrine disruptors**, chemicals encountered in our environment that mimic our endogenous (i.e., home-made) hor-mones like oestrogen and testosterone, have been reliably associated with both the development and progression of a variety of CVDs (Fu et al., 2020). These chemicals are present in a huge number of different products that are used in the household and in industry, and are not well regulated internationally as yet. Hormone functioning and the functioning of endocrine glands are strongly associated with the functioning of the cardiovascular system, and endocrine dysfunctions (both hypo- and hyper-function) in glands like the thyroid and adrenal glands are strongly associated with hypertension, atherosclerosis, and congestive heart failure (Rhee & Pearce, 2011). An interesting link between the endocrine and cardiovascular systems comes from the supposition that **adipose tissue** (fat) can almost be considered an endocrine gland itself and may serve as an important 'relay point' between the endocrine and cardiovascular systems during the development of cardiovascular diseases, which are often accompanied by the laying down of adipose tissue throughout the body. **Adipocytes**, one of the types of cells that make up adipose tissues, can use hormone signalling in response to physiological cues and have an impact on a variety of other functions important in CVD pathology, such as inflammation, cellular metabolism, and glucose sensitivity (Scheja & Heeren, 2019). One variety of the 'physiological cues' that can instigate the endocrine signalling from these cells comes from the cardiovascular system itself (Oikonomou & Antoniades, 2019), meaning that the interplay between these systems can lead to a self-perpetuating and ever-increasing degree of risk in the development of CVDs, much like that seen with the inflammatory exacerbation from foam cells.

Another important endocrine (and wider system) factor for CVD comes from the gut microbiota. Our diet has a strong influence on the microbiome (along with our adiposity and cardiovascular health), and as much as this can impact a variety of neurological and immunological factors (see Chapter 2) related to the microbiome, there is also evidence that it has a role to play for our cardiovascular system and the diseases that are developed within it. Once more (as with adipose tissue) the perspective here is that the gut microbiota operates as part of the endocrine system, as it is able to communicate with other tissues and organs in the body through complex signalling involving both endocrine and immune molecules. An atypical distribution of the various species of bacteria that make up the gut microbiome in humans has been associated with vulnerability to the development of a variety of chronic illnesses that are mediated by the immune and endocrine systems, such as metabolic syndrome (a key influence on CVD) and inflammatory bowel disease, as well as having direct links to atherosclerosis and other cardiovascular risk factors such as liver function (Busnelli et al., 2020).

Population Factors

The link between psychosocial states and CVD risk of both morbidity and mortality was established a long time ago, and there is a wealth of evidence to support the strong associations between stress (in all its origins and manifestations) and cardiovascular health (Everson-Rose & Lewis, 2005). Populations of people that experience high levels of social and environmental stress are known to be more vulnerable to CVD, including those who are lonely (Hodgson et al., 2020), the unemployed (Dupre et al., 2012), refugees and asylum seekers (Al-Rousan et al., 2022), the bereaved (Buckley et al., 2010), and familial carers (Capistrant et al., 2012). The experience of catastrophic environmental events that cause profound stress are also important in the development of CVD, meaning we have populations of 'types' of people (such as those who are lonely or the unemployed) as well as populations of geographic clusters of people that are at increased vulnerability. There is emerging evidence that the experience of armed conflict amongst civilians is associated with the mortality risk from IHD (Jawad et al., 2019). Those subject to catastrophic events like 9/11, both civilians (Feng et al., 2006) and first responders (Smith et al., 2019), have been demonstrated to be at higher risk of cardiac events following the traumatic event. Similarly, those who have experienced natural disasters such as earthquakes (Ohira et al., 2017) and extreme weather events like typhoons and hurricanes (Babaie et al., 2021) are at increased risk of CVD morbidity and mortality due to the stress and trauma of the situation, but also to the resultant impact on the accessibility of healthcare thereafter. Environmental factors such as air pollution are also known to have strong associations with the incidence and severity of a whole host of CVDs (Cosselman et al., 2015). On the largest scale of population we can possibly imagine, it also seems that there are associations between Covid-19 infection and CVD (Pepera et al., 2022). Covid-19 infection itself appears to put a large amount of stress on the cardiovascular system (along with the immune system), increasing the risk of cardiac injury during acute infection (Bansal, 2020). Moreover, we are seeing longer-term implications of Covid-19 infection on the cardiovascular system too. Whilst we won't know the true consequences of this for a long time to come, this could mean that humanity as a whole may now be more vulnerable to this large collection of cardiovascular diseases due to the impact of a globally uncontained infectious disease. More on this in Chapter 11.

Racism and Cardiovascular Disease

There has been an association between ethnicity and CVD for some time, leading many to think that perhaps this may be associated with genetics. However, as I hope you will have learned so far through this book, the issue of ethnicity is very complicated when it comes to health. There are of course some genetic differences between peoples across the world, but the factors that are associated with health in general that are a product of social and structural injustices far outnumber the potential associations explained by ethnicity-related genetics. Racism is an important and complicated issue for health, and affects both indigenous populations and global majority peoples – particularly when they are considered to be a minority within their social context. There are the effects of interpersonal racism that create stress, fear, loneliness, and many other emotional and psychological vulnerabilities when it comes to health. There are also effects of structural racism, where social contexts and systems that are inherently racist and exclusionary create suffering because those discriminated against are not included in legislation, considered in good practice (for health or any other factors that impact health), or are otherwise excluded from having the same standard or degree of care and support that the more privileged in our societies do. There have been efforts to understand which 'level' of racism may be more impactful for CVD outcomes, and so far it seems that structural effects may be more profound than the stress experienced by interpersonal racism, certainly as evidenced in the case of hypertension (Brondolo et al., 2011).

Structural effects of racism arguably pervade every area of someone's existence; however, some researchers have attempted to adequately list and describe some of the administration-level domains of structural racism in terms of their relationship to CVD outcomes like myocardial infarction (heart attack). Lukachko and colleagues (2014) describe four main domains: 1) political participation, or the degree to which people are able to vote; 2) employment status, including the type of employment and rate of pay; 3) educational attainment, or the degree to which participation in education is supported; and 4) judicial treatment, or rather the over-representation of minority peoples in prison populations. Further than this, I would say that racism also fundamentally impacts access to and quality of healthcare. From medical guidance relevant to certain cultures, and being available in appropriate depth in the language that the person is most conversant in, to having medications and treatments that are both suitable and appropriate across cultural and genetic spectra, and to simply having an inclusive and accessible environment for all people to physically access adequate healthcare, racism is centrally relevant to health outcomes. If you cast back to Chapter 9 where we looked at the social determinants of public health and used the case studies of transport, housing, and education – each of these structural determinants will also be impacted by racist values, ideals, or exclusions. This is relevant for almost all dimensions of health and is not exclusively related to one type of health outcome.

There has been renewed effort and energy for uncovering the depths of the social determinants of health that are rooted specifically in racism, and there has been some excellent work to explore the various mechanisms these have in leading to CVD pathologies. Structural racism, evidenced from neighbourhood-level racial segregation, socioeconomic status, quality of the neighbourhood built and social environment, and 'food environment' (i.e., accessibility of good quality food in locale) have all been shown to be associated longitudinally with incidence of IHD, incidence of CVD risk factors such as Type 2 diabetes and increased body mass index, hypertension, incidence of heart failure, and mortality after heart attack (Powell-Wiley et al., 2022). There are also strong associations between psychosocial indicators of racism such as the higher incidences of adverse childhood experiences (ACEs), depression, lower self-appraised social status, job strain, general stress, loneliness and isolation and perceived discrimination (Powell-Wiley et al., 2022). These factors operate through the cellular and system-level factors described earlier in this chapter but operate at a population scale because they impact entire groups of people, and they can be passed on through generations. Not only this, but people already subject to racist institutions that lead them to being more likely to develop CVD are then subject to bias in treatment by healthcare institutions as well, with racialised groups experiencing less bystander heroic measures (such as cardiac resuscitation or the use of defibrillators), being recommended less frequently for implanted cardiac devices, waiting longer in emergency rooms for care, and being more frequently recommended for less sophisticated medical and surgical intervention (Banerjee et al., 2021). So, here we have structural racism increasing the likelihood of CVD, and also ultimately harming the outcomes of these diseases through the mechanism of inadequate treatment. Much as we have seen with internal contexts (such as foam cells and the presence of adipose tissue), external contexts can increase both risk and negative outcomes in a self-perpetuating manner, but in this case, it is an entirely socially derived context that is arguably easier to reverse than those cellular factors, if only there was a commitment and will to do so.

Key Questions

Using the knowledge you have accumulated throughout this book, have a look at the health onion and see if you can make sense of how racism may affect outcomes in another non-communicable disease. How much do you think that racism affects both the likelihood of developing the illness and how badly someone may suffer from it?

- Think about their likelihood of developing the disease. What social and environmental systems and structures may be stacked against racialised peoples?
- Think about the lifestyles and behaviours that may be associated with the development of the disease. How much control do you think individuals within these racialised groups really have in managing these factors in a system of racism?
- Think about their likelihood of suffering badly with it once it has developed. How might racism impact disease outcomes in terms of medical treatment, psychosocial support, or individual experiences of being able to cope with the disease?

Learning Outcomes Summary

- Apply the knowledge gained throughout the book to the example of cardiovascular disease.

We have looked at cell-, system-, and population-level factors of cardiovascular disease.

- Understand how we can make sense of aetiology and susceptibility through the cell-to-society perspective.

We have identified some groups that have been at higher risk for developing CVD, and from suffering its worst effects.

- Discuss the interaction between the levels of cell-to-society health and its contribution to public health issues in non-communicable disease.

Using the case study of racism and health, we have looked at how social and structural systems influence the vulnerability of racialised groups from the cell-to-society levels to cardiovascular diseases.

FURTHER READING

Gaziano, T., Reddy, K. S., Paccaud, F., Horton, S., & Chaturvedi, V. (2006). Cardiovascular disease. *Disease Control Priorities in Developing Countries* (2nd edition). The World Bank: Oxford University Press.

This chapter provides an overview of various types of cardio- and cerebrovascular diseases.

Javed, Z., Haisum Maqsood, M., Yahya, T., Amin, Z., Acquah, I., Valero-Elizondo, J., ... & Nasir, K. (2022). Race, racism, and cardiovascular health: Applying a social determinants of health framework to racial/ethnic disparities in cardiovascular disease. *Circulation: Cardiovascular Quality and Outcomes, 15*(1), e007917.

This paper provides a very comprehensive overview of the impact of structural racism on cardiovascular disease outcomes. Arguably, these factors can apply to all manner of health outcomes, but this is a particularly well-written and thorough paper that goes into great detail on the mechanisms and impacts of racist institutions on health. I would also recommend reading the paper from Dr Tiffany Powell-Wiley and her colleagues referenced in this chapter.

Lilly, L. S. (2012). *Pathophysiology of heart disease: A collaborative project of medical students and faculty.* Lippincott Williams & Wilkins.

For any of you considering working in the field of heart disease or psychocardiology, this textbook provides an in-depth and comprehensive overview of heart disease.

O'Neill, L. (2020). *Never Mind the B#ll*cks, Here's the Science: A scientist's guide to the biggest challenges facing our species today.* Gill & Macmillan Ltd.
This is a great book full of many levels of myth-busting science, written brilliantly. I can thoroughly recommend Chapters 2 and 3, looking at both vaccines and medicine costs.

Prather, C., Fuller, T. R., Marshall, K. J., & Jeffries IV, W. L. (2016). The impact of racism on the sexual and reproductive health of African American women. *Journal of Women's Health, 25*(7), 664–71.
This article discusses another aspect of institutional racism and its impact on health outcomes. The article is very well constructed, adopting a socioecological approach to understanding the various layers of influence that racism can have on racialised groups and their health.

REFERENCES

Al-Rousan, T., AlHeresh, R., Saadi, A., El-Sabrout, H., Young, M., Benmarhnia, T., … Alshawabkeh, L. (2022). Epidemiology of cardiovascular disease and its risk factors among refugees and asylum seekers: Systematic review and meta-analysis. *International Journal of Cardiology Cardiovascular Risk and Prevention, 12*, 200126. https://doi.org/https://doi.org/10.1016/j.ijcrp.2022.200126

Alfarisi, H. A. H., Mohamed, Z. B. H., & Ibrahim, M. B. (2020). Basic pathogenic mechanisms of atherosclerosis. *Egyptian Journal of Basic and Applied Sciences, 7*(1), 116–25. https://doi.org/10.1080/2314808X.2020.1769913

Babaie, J., Pashaei Asl, Y., Naghipour, B., & Faridaalaee, G. (2021). Cardiovascular diseases in natural disasters; A systematic review. *Archives of Academic Emergency Medicine, 9*(1), e36. https://doi.org/10.22037/aaem.v9i1.1208

Banerjee, S., Aaysha Cader, F., Gulati, M., & Capers, Q. (2021). Racism and cardiology: A global call to action. *CJC Open, 3*(12, Supplement), S165–S173. https://doi.org/https://doi.org/10.1016/j.cjco.2021.09.014

Bansal, M. (2020). Cardiovascular disease and COVID-19. *Diabetes & Metabolic Syndrome: Clinical Research & Reviews, 14*(3), 247–50. https://doi.org/https://doi.org/10.1016/j.dsx.2020.03.013

Brondolo, E., Love, E. E., Pencille, M., Schoenthaler, A., & Ogedegbe, G. (2011). Racism and hypertension: A review of the empirical evidence and implications for clinical practice. *American Journal of Hypertension, 24*(5), 518–29. https://doi.org/10.1038/ajh.2011.9

Buckley, T., McKinley, S., Tofler, G., & Bartrop, R. (2010). Cardiovascular risk in early bereavement: A literature review and proposed mechanisms. *International Journal of Nursing Studies, 47*(2), 229–38. https://doi.org/https://doi.org/10.1016/j.ijnurstu.2009.06.010

Busnelli, M., Manzini, S., & Chiesa, G. (2020). The gut microbiota affects host pathophysiology as an endocrine organ: A focus on cardiovascular disease. *Nutrients, 12*(1), 79. https://www.mdpi.com/2072-6643/12/1/79

Capistrant, B. D., Moon, J. R., Berkman, L. F., & Glymour, M. M. (2012). Current and long-term spousal caregiving and onset of cardiovascular disease. *Journal of Epidemiology and Community Health, 66*(10), 951–56. http://dx.doi.org/10.1136/jech-2011-200040

Cosselman, K. E., Navas-Acien, A., & Kaufman, J. D. (2015). Environmental factors in cardiovascular disease. *Nature Reviews Cardiology, 12*(11), 627–42. https://doi.org/10.1038/nrcardio.2015.152

Dupre, M. E., George, L. K., Liu, G., & Peterson, E. D. (2012). The cumulative effect of unemployment on risks for acute myocardial infarction. *Archives of Internal Medicine, 172*(22), 1731–37. https://doi.org/10.1001/2013.jamainternmed.447

Everson-Rose, S. A., & Lewis, T. T. (2005). Psychosocial factors and cardiovascular diseases. *Annual Review of Public Health, 26*, 469–500.

Feng, J., Lenihanx, D. J., Johnson, M. M., Karri, V., & Reddy, C. V. R. (2006). Cardiac sequelae in Brooklyn after the September 11 terrorist attacks. *Clinical Cardiology, 29*(1), 13–17. https://doi.org/https://doi.org/10.1002/clc.4960290105

Fu, X., Xu, J., Zhang, R., & Yu, J. (2020). The association between environmental endocrine disruptors and cardiovascular diseases: A systematic review and meta-analysis. *Environmental Research, 187*, 109464. https://doi.org/https://doi.org/10.1016/j.envres.2020.109464

Hodgson, S., Watts, I., Fraser, S., Roderick, P., & Dambha-Miller, H. (2020). Loneliness, social isolation, cardiovascular disease and mortality: A synthesis of the literature and conceptual framework. *Journal of the Royal Society of Medicine, 113*(5), 185–92. https://doi.org/10.1177/0141076820918236

Jawad, M., Vamos, E. P., Najim, M., Roberts, B., & Millett, C. (2019). Impact of armed conflict on cardiovascular disease risk: A systematic review. *Heart, 105*(18), 1388–94. https://doi.org/10.1136/heartjnl-2018-314459

Khyzha, N., Alizada, A., Wilson, M. D., & Fish, J. E. (2017). Epigenetics of atherosclerosis: Emerging mechanisms and methods. *Trends in Molecular Medicine, 23*(4), 332–47. https://doi.org/https://doi.org/10.1016/j.molmed.2017.02.004

Libby, P. (2020). Inflammation in atherosclerosis – no longer a theory. *Clinical Chemistry, 67*(1), 131–42. https://doi.org/10.1093/clinchem/hvaa275

Lukachko, A., Hatzenbuehler, M. L., & Keyes, K. M. (2014). Structural racism and myocardial infarction in the United States. *Social Science & Medicine, 103*, 42–50. https://doi.org/10.1016/j.socscimed.2013.07.021

Meaney, S. (2014). Epigenetic regulation of cholesterol homeostasis. *Frontiers in Genetics, 5*, 311. www.ncbi.nlm.nih.gov/pmc/articles/PMC4174035/pdf/fgene-05-00311.pdf

Nabel, E. G. (2003). Cardiovascular disease. *New England Journal of Medicine, 349*(1), 60–72. https://doi.org/10.1056/NEJMra035098

Ohira, T., Nakano, H., Nagai, M., Yumiya, Y., Zhang, W., Uemura, M., … Hashimoto, S. (2017). Changes in cardiovascular risk factors after the great East Japan earthquake: A review of the comprehensive health check in the Fukushima health management survey. *Asia Pacific Journal of Public Health, 29*(2_suppl), 47S–55S. https://doi.org/10.1177/1010539517695436

Oikonomou, E. K., & Antoniades, C. (2019). The role of adipose tissue in cardiovascular health and disease. *Nature Reviews Cardiology, 16*(2), 83–99. https://doi.org/10.1038/s41569-018-0097-6

Ordovás, J. M., & Smith, C. E. (2010). Epigenetics and cardiovascular disease. *Nature Reviews Cardiology, 7*(9), 510–19. https://doi.org/10.1038/nrcardio.2010.104

Owen, N., Healy, G. N., Matthews, C. E., & Dunstan, D. W. (2010). Too much sitting: The population health science of sedentary behavior. *Exercise and Sport Sciences Reviews, 38*(3), 105–13. https://doi.org/10.1097/JES.0b013e3181e373a2

Paterson, C., Fryer, S., Stone, K., Zieff, G., Turner, L., & Stoner, L. (2022). The effects of acute exposure to prolonged sitting, with and without interruption, on peripheral blood pressure among adults: A systematic review and meta-analysis. *Sports Medicine, 52*(6), 1369–83. https://doi.org/10.1007/s40279-021-01614-7

Paterson, C., Fryer, S., Zieff, G., Stone, K., Credeur, D. P., Barone Gibbs, B., … Stoner, L. (2020). The effects of acute exposure to prolonged sitting, with and without interruption, on vascular function among adults: A meta-analysis. *Sports Medicine, 50*(11), 1929–42. https://doi.org/10.1007/s40279-020-01325-5

Pepera, G., Tribali, M.-S., Batalik, L., Petrov, I., & Papathanasiou, J. (2022). Epidemiology, risk factors and prognosis of cardiovascular disease in the Coronavirus Disease 2019 (COVID-19) pandemic era: A systematic review. *RCM, 23*(1), 28. https://doi.org/10.31083/j.rcm2301028

Powell-Wiley, T. M., Baumer, Y., Baah, F. O., Baez, A. S., Farmer, N., Mahlobo, C. T., … Wallen, G. R. (2022). Social determinants of cardiovascular disease. *Circulation Research, 130*(5), 782–99. https://doi.org/doi:10.1161/CIRCRESAHA.121.319811

Poznyak, A. V., Nikiforov, N. G., Starodubova, A. V., Popkova, T. V., & Orekhov, A. N. (2021). Macrophages and foam cells: Brief overview of their role, linkage, and targeting potential in atherosclerosis. *Biomedicines, 9*(9), 1221.

Rhee, S. S., & Pearce, E. N. (2011). The endocrine system and the heart: A review. *Revista Española de Cardiología* (English edition), *64*(3), 220–31. https://doi.org/https://doi.org/10.1016/j.rec.2010.10.016

Roth, G. A., Abate, D., Abate, K. H., Abay, S. M., Abbafati, C., Abbasi, N., … Murray, C. J. L. (2018). Global, regional, and national age-sex-specific mortality for 282 causes of death in 195 countries and territories, 1980–2017: A systematic analysis for the Global Burden of Disease Study 2017. *The Lancet, 392*(10159), 1736–88. https://doi.org/https://doi.org/10.1016/S0140-6736(18)32203-7

Scheja, L., & Heeren, J. (2019). The endocrine function of adipose tissues in health and cardiometabolic disease. *Nature Reviews Endocrinology, 15*(9), 507–24. https://doi.org/10.1038/s41574-019-0230-6

Smith, E. C., Holmes, L., & Burkle, F. M. (2019). The physical and mental health challenges experienced by 9/11 first responders and recovery workers: A review of the literature. *Prehospital and Disaster Medicine, 34*(6), 625–31. https://doi.org/10.1017/S1049023X19004989

Urso, C., & Caimi, G. (2011). Oxidative stress and endothelial dysfunction. *Minerva Medica, 102*(1), 59–77. http://europepmc.org/abstract/MED/21317849

VanWijk, M. J., VanBavel, E., Sturk, A., & Nieuwland, R. (2003). Microparticles in cardiovascular diseases. *Cardiovascular Research*, *59*(2), 277–87. https://doi.org/10.1016/s0008-6363(03)00367-5

Voukalis, C., Shantsila, E., & Lip, G. Y. H. (2019). Microparticles and cardiovascular diseases. *Annals of Medicine*, *51*(3-4), 193–223. https://doi.org/10.1016/S0008-6363(03)00367-5

Wolf, D., & Ley, K. (2019). Immunity and inflammation in atherosclerosis. *Circulation Research*, *124*(2), 315–27. https://doi.org/doi:10.1161/CIRCRESAHA.118.313591

11

APPLYING INTERDISCIPLINARY KNOWLEDGE TO COMMUNICABLE DISEASE:
THE CELL-TO-SOCIETY OF COVID-19

INTRODUCTION

To bring together the learning from the book, this chapter focuses on applying the cell-to-society perspective to an example of a **communicable disease** (i.e., something you can catch from someone else). This chapter focuses on Covid-19, but can easily be applied to other public health priorities, and you will be encouraged to try this yourself with activities throughout the chapter. We will start with an overview of Covid-19, and its relevance as a public health priority, and then we will go through the cellular-, systems-, and population-level approaches to the disease. Cellular- and system-level pathology is explored, along with biopsychosocial determinants at each of those levels. For the population-level approach, socio-economic status and ethnicity are discussed as unique biopsychosocial modifiers of morbidity and mortality. Demographics and lifestyles associated with Covid-19 are discussed with reference to group level influence, and in terms of social gradients.

Learning Outcomes

- Apply the knowledge gained throughout the book to the example of Covid-19.
- Understand how we can make sense of disease spread and susceptibility through the cell-to-society perspective.
- Discuss the interaction between the levels of cell-to-society health and its contribution to public health issues in communicable disease.

WHAT IS COVID-19?

At the time of writing this chapter, Covid-19 has infected 623,573,805 people and killed 6,551,001 globally. Chances are you will all unfortunately know what Covid-19 is, and sadly many of you will have had it at least once already. I started teaching the lecture this chapter is based on in the Autumn of 2020 when the pandemic was in full swing with no available vaccines and few available treatments. It was a worrying time, and although we have developed many different vaccines and treatments at the time of writing this chapter, Covid-19 is still killing many people across the world. I very much hope that we will be rid of it at some point in the future; however, it looks as though for now it may be here to stay. This chapter will focus on the acute infection of Covid-19, but it is also important to note that the virus is now known to cause longer-term consequences that we still do not fully understand. From **post-Covid syndrome** (sometimes referred to as Long Covid) to the lingering damage to the heart that is caused by the virus (Abbasi, 2022), to the central nervous system (Hampshire et al., 2022) and the vascular system (Zanoli et al., 2022), there is much about this virus that goes beyond acute infection. We still do not understand or fully appreciate the devastation that this virus has caused at this stage, or the longer-term legacy that will be left in its wake in terms of consequential disease or vulnerability to disease. We are at a point now where most nations have abandoned attempts to contain the virus and are now trying to 'live with Covid', which is a term I find very difficult for a variety of reasons, particularly with recent news that this tactic in the UK has seen a 95% increase in deaths over the summer period compared with the same period of time last year (García & Duncan, 2022), when efforts were still being made to prevent infections. Whatever happens now, the impact of this pandemic will be felt for generations.

Covid-19 (**CO**rona**VI**rus **D**isease **2019**) is an infection caused by the novel coronavirus (species *coronaviridae*) in the same family as the common cold. It is caused by the **severe acute respiratory syndrome** (SARS) coronavirus SARS-CoV-2, and is typified by severe inflammation of lung tissue.

This novel coronavirus emerged in China in late 2019, and spread rapidly around the world in the early part of 2020. Similar to the first SARS outbreak in 2003, SARS-CoV-2 was shown to cause severe respiratory symptoms, characterised by inflammation and scarring in the lungs, preventing breathing. Initially, it was thought that only those with underlying health conditions would be susceptible to complicated infection, and most would experience very mild symptoms if any at all. Very quickly, the virus started to spread around the world, reaching Europe and other continents in January 2020. What made Covid-19 such a difficult disease to contain was a combination of a few factors. One key factor in the intial spreading of the virus was a long incubation period was required, thought to be 9–14 days for the initial strain of the virus, in which time those infected would start infecting others before symptoms presented themselves. Compare this to the average incubation period of influenza, another coronavirus that has been used as a parallel to SARS-CoV-2 (incorrectly in my opinion, for a variety of reasons), which is around two days. This meant that those who contracted the virus were able to spread it unknowingly for many days before the onset of symptoms, which would instigate them to avoid contact with others. Alongside this, in the earlier days of the pandemic, some that contracted SARS-CoV-2 had **asymptomatic presentation**, meaning they would spend the entirety of their infected time with no symptoms at all. This massively facilitated spread as the person carrying it was unaware they were infectious. Another influential factor in the success (if you can call it that) of the spread of SARS-CoV-2 was the virus's rapid mutation. Viruses are by their nature very mutable, which means they are much more likely to mutate with their rapid replication. This makes them difficult to contain and can change their pathogenesis and presentation in those infected, and allow them to evade treatments and preventive measures such as vaccinations. Since the onset of the pandemic, very many new viral subtypes have emerged and taken over as dominant strains. Not only this, but the mutations that have occurred have made Covid-19 infection hard to identify and definitively diagnose – with changing symptoms, sometimes no symptoms at all, and variable sensitivity of the rapid antigen tests used to carry out home screening and diagnoses to the variants of SARS-CoV-2 that have developed. There have been other, more human, factors associated with the spread of the virus across the world as well. The lack of apparent severity for most of the population has meant some consider it to be no worse than flu, and not really a problem for them, making the adherence to contagion mitigation measures (such as the wearing of masks, distancing from others, and remaining at home when infected) highly variable. The lack of symptoms for some, and the lack of severity for most, led to very far-reaching misinformation about the pandemic as well, creating further rallying against containment measures and safeguards.

One of the factors that makes Covid-19 deadly is its ability to induce **cytokine storm**. Cytokines are those molecular messengers used by the immune system that we encountered in Chapter 5. They tell other cells and tissues that we are under attack, and can mobilise cells and instigate patterns of immune response as a result. Cytokine storm is a massive cascade of pro-inflammatory messages, causing systemic inflammation, and – in the case of Covid-19 – hugely inflaming lung tissue that ultimately prevents breathing (Hu et al., 2021). This constitutes a dual attack for the lungs of a patient with Covid-19, as their cells are being attacked by the virus and by their own cytokines. Cytokine storm is not unique to Covid-19 infection, and can be caused by other coronaviruses (such as the virus that caused the first SARS outbreak), and was first noticed in graft-versus-host disease, a condition that occurs in those with tissue or organ transplants (Tisoncik et al., 2012). It is essentially a widespread over-activation of the inflammatory response that involves a vast number of types of pro-inflammatory cytokines (Channappanavar & Perlman, 2017). The potential to trigger cytokine storm may be why SARS-CoV-2 was more deadly in older people, whose immune systems had encountered many more pathogens previously (Ragab et al., 2020), and may also be why it was less lethal in children, who have less advanced immune systems. The mortality rate of Covid-19 varies between 0.3% and 10% across different populations in the world (Al-Rohaimi & Al Otaibi, 2020), so there is a great deal of variation in individual response to the disease.

THE CELL-TO-SOCIETY OF COVID-19

Cellular Factors

SARS-CoV-2 infects cells that line the airways, and we now know that it is both airborne and transmissible through microdroplets. Early efforts to contain spread focused on distancing people, with the idea that exhaled or projected microdroplets were the principal vector of transmission – the further we were apart, the harder it would be for a microdroplet to land on us. In order to infect cells, SARS-CoV-2 requires certain cellular hardware on host cells to gain entry and then replicate. The term *coronavirus* comes from the fact the **virions** (viral cells) resemble crowns, with spikes protruding from their surface. The virions use the spikes to lock onto cells and then fuse with them. They exploit surface enzymes on the cells that line our airways, particularly ACE2 (**angiotensin-converting enzyme 2**), which serves a variety of functions that help to support our health in the longer term. When SARS-CoV-2 binds to these cells, ACE2 is effectively lost, which may be an important part of the lethality of the disease following infection as ACE2 also functions in an anti-inflammatory capacity (Sharma et al., 2020).

ACE2 is thought to be found in higher levels in the plasma of males, providing more opportunities for SARS-CoV-2 to infect cells throughout the body (Gagliardi et al., 2020; Martínez-Gómez et al., 2022). There is somewhat of a paradox with ACE2 in that SARS-CoV-2 needs more of it to be able to create an overwhelming infection, so having more of it means more opportunities for infection, but if it is also anti-inflammatory then having more should be protective. As the virus infects the cells, it destroys ACE2, meaning we lose the benefit of its anti-inflammatory effects, so it is somewhat of a double whammy that SARS-CoV-2 uses and depletes one of the very things that we need in order to survive the infection. This is not the only instance of this happening in the world of viruses, HIV being another good example of viral capacity to infect and depopulate defences through its selective infection of T-cells (Douek et al., 2002). We also know that like some other viral infections (such as HIV), early **viral load** is likely to be a factor in the severity of disease, and we have seen that higher viral loads are consistently associated with more severe disease and higher mortality (Tsukagoshi et al., 2021).

It has also been suggested that there may be a role for oxidative stress in the development of more serious disease in Covid-19. Many of the factors that are associated with more severe disease from SARS-CoV-2 are also factors associated with higher oxidative stress: being male, older age, lower socio-economic status, and obesity being a few (Chernyak et al., 2020). This is also suggested to be a feed-forward cycle because infection with SARS-CoV-2 also induces more oxidative stress as infected cells are destroyed, thereby weakening the ability to fight off infection. There have been various genetic factors associated with susceptibility and severity of SARS-CoV-2 infection, from genes that encode for ACE2 to other types of cell surface protein that may facilitate infection or worsen immune responses and the associated cytokine storm that can accompany it (Fricke-Galindo & Falfán-Valencia, 2021). Epigenetic factors have also been highlighted, including the gene that encodes ACE2, which certain cancers can enhance the expression of, potentially explaining some of the differences in severity rates seen in patients with comorbidities (Chlamydas et al., 2021).

System Factors

Once infection has started, it is up to the immune system to fight off the infection as best it can. Of key importance in Covid morbidity and mortality is the ability to breathe (supported by the hardware of the pulmonary system) – a function massively impacted by the swelling caused in the lungs. Patients with existing lung conditions, such as chronic obstructive pulmonary disease (COPD: Singh et al., 2022), rheumatoid arthritis with lung involvement (D'Silva & Wallace, 2021), and those who smoke (Reddy et al.,

2021) all seem to be more susceptible to more severe disease. Interestingly, those with asthma do not seem (at this stage) to be at higher risk for more severe disease, and asthmatics are under-represented within Covid patients compared to their prevalence in general populations (Sunjaya et al., 2022). For the cardiovascular system, conditions associated with this system are also thought to confer significant vulnerabilities to more severe Covid infection, and Covid itself is also a risk factor in cardiovascular disease (Pepera et al., 2022). Those with **metabolic syndrome** (a combination of diabetes, hypertension, and obesity) are much more likely to suffer complications with Covid-19 due to the dysfunction and dysregulation of endocrine-immune-vascular communication (Bansal et al., 2020). Patients with autoimmune disorders (particularly rheumatologic autoimmune disorders) also seem to be at greater risk of Covid-associated complications and are at a higher risk of death (Arachchillage et al., 2022). Because it is a viral infection, the immune system has clearly been a very important component of defence or vulnerability to SARS-CoV-2. Covid has been particularly dangerous for those people taking immunosuppressing drugs (Nørgård et al., 2021), who have had bone marrow transplants (Malard et al., 2020), and those with HIV (Danwang et al., 2022), particularly before vaccines were developed. There have been associations made between certain neurological disorders and Covid pathogenesis as well, with both Covid and the neurological disorder symptoms being made worse by comorbidity (Kubota & Kuroda, 2021). Other endocrine dysfunctions have also been associated with the higher likelihood of cytokine storm, meaning any of those factors that may influence healthy endocrine functioning (include chronic stress) may worsen disease outcomes from SARS-CoV-2 infection (Marazuela et al., 2020).

Population Factors

Socio-Economic Status

Socio-economic status has played a huge part in whether people catch SARS-CoV-2 in many countries across the world. The outcomes of this increased likelihood to catch the virus operate through a variety of mechanisms – including access to safe outdoor space to exercise, housing conditions (particularly when housing is crowded and occupants cannot safely distance from an infected other), accessible good-quality food (particularly in the early days of the pandemic when there was a great deal of panic buying in many nations) – and their employment (Rollston & Galea, 2020). The latter point of employment is a particularly important mechanism in Covid, as it operated across several groups with multiple social vulnerabilities (intersecting identities). Those from lower socio-economic status groups and those with ethnic minority status were particularly vulnerable to the harsh effects of the pandemic. Many of these people were working in frontline service roles, and therefore were less able to avoid infection, and many were unable to sustain self-isolation in the case of being infected due to employment precarity, and lack of adequate financial support or sick pay (Burström & Tao, 2020). The scale of the problem was so significant in the UK, Prof Sir Michael Marmot (who you will remember from Chapters 9 and 10) compiled a special report on how to build back fairer after the pandemic, citing the catastrophic and unjust burden of disease and mortality from Covid faced by those in poverty and those underserved[1] by health and social policies (Marmot, 2020). The scale of the problem was so bad in the UK, that if you were in the most deprived areas in the nation, your risk of dying from Covid-19 was twice that of those in the least deprived areas. The story of this social gradient to Covid was the same in the worst-hit countries across the world (in terms of number of deaths relative to population), including Brazil (Figueiredo et al., 2020), Italy (Consolazio et al., 2021), the Russian Federation (Zemtsov & Baburin, 2020), and the United States (Little et al., 2021). Social exclusion and loneliness may also play a huge part in some vulnerabilities – particularly with older people who have had to shield or shelter in place (Seifert et al., 2020).

Ethnic Minority Status

A consistent finding observed in studies around the world has been that white people have borne less of the Covid-19 burden than people of other ethnic (global majority[2]) groups, particularly when those ethnic groups happen to be a minority in the nation they reside in. In the UK, death rates for those from Bangladeshi communities from Covid were twice as high, and those from all ethnic minority groups together were

---

1 A phrase that is often used here is 'hard to reach', but that implies that the groups in question are in some way aloof and uncontactable, and that perhaps some of the responsibility lies with those groups. The truth is that institutions do not work hard enough to reach them, which is why I prefer the term 'underserved'.

2 Global majority groups are often lumped together in clunky phrases such as BAME (Black, Asian, and Minority Ethnic). I choose not to use this phrase for a few reasons, but mostly because it inadequately describes a huge spectrum of groups of people with different cultures, social experiences, and biologies. The use of 'ethnic minority' in this section is similarly clumping people together, but is used accurately as it seems the source of these differences is due to their minority status (and the social fallout from that) rather than their ethnicity per se.

10–50% higher than those from white groups, even when accounting for sex, age, and socio-economic status (Patel et al., 2020). In order to unpick whether these are biological or social factors (or a combination of them both, perhaps) it is helpful to understand 'minority status' and what that means for health. We discussed some of these factors in Chapter 3 and Chapter 10, where we looked at social marginalisation, discrimination, and inequality of opportunity being rooted in the context of being in a minority group. If we are to understand whether non-white populations are more vulnerable to both infection and disease severity with Covid-19, we need to establish whether this is because those individuals are made vulnerable by their environment or by their biology. This is hard though, because we then need to look across countries to understand incidence and mortality rates, but in doing so we cannot control for country-to-country variations in poverty and health service provision, alongside the varying policies associated with controlling (or not controlling) Covid spread, which are also then social factors that impress upon entire nations rather than unequally across groups within one nation. This is perhaps more straightforward with non-communicable diseases because we can take the infection context out of the equation. What evidence there is so far suggests that in countries where non-white populations are the majority (therefore removing the social elements from the equation), the case and fatality rate of Covid-19 has been comparatively lower at points during the pandemic despite sometimes having more fragile health infrastructures (El-Khatib et al., 2020). This suggests that many of the discrepancies observed between ethnic groups are more socially and systemically imposed than biologically rooted. Before we go through some of the evidence that has been gathered so far on this issue, have a go at the exercise to put your cell-to-society learning to the test in the context of this infectious disease.

Key Questions

Using the knowledge you have accumulated throughout this book, have a look at the health onion and see if you can make sense of why ethnic minority groups in many Western nations have been so disproportionately affected by Covid-19. Why is it that these groups may be particularly vulnerable?

- Think about their likelihood of being infected with it (e.g., level of exposure).
- Think about their likelihood of suffering badly with it once infected.

A great deal of research has been conducted so far in an attempt to unpack why people from non-white groups appear to be more vulnerable to the most harmful effects of Covid-19. Perhaps the most comprehensive overview comes from a study that examined the structural inequalities relevant to minority groups in white-majority nations such as the UK and the US, where inequalities relevant to socio-economic determinants of health as well as those associated with developmental and life course vulnerabilities have been identified (Bentley, 2020). In short, in these very unequal societies, those who are not white are more likely to be subject to socio-economic deprivation, impacting housing, employment, education, and community-level health determinants – from disproportionately lower access to health-improving factors (e.g., green space, healthcare facilities, leisure and exercise facilities, transport, and quality housing) and disproportionately higher exposure to health-degrading factors (e.g., environmental stressors such as overcrowding, pollution, and unemployment), to financial restraints that impact on abilities to work from home and to self-isolate when exposed to the virus. In the UK, the poverty rate is twice as high in ethnic minority groups as in white people (Otu et al., 2020), so all the health predictors associated with material deprivation are more prevalent in these groups. Further, the minority status of these groups also impacts other factors across the life course that heighten vulnerability to infectious disease, from higher incidences of diseases such as diabetes and hypertension that increase risk (Ravi, 2020), to higher and deeper exposure to stress that then impacts biological markers of health as well as health behaviours. There is a disproportionate mental health burden in ethnic minority communities that existed before the pandemic, and that has been made worse by the safeguards implemented to prevent the spread of the virus, and the impact of the burden of the number of infections on the health service overall, decreasing access to vital mental health services (Smith et al., 2020). These impacts on minority groups through just being who they are can result in some of the very stark differences observed in mortality, where black individuals in England and Wales have been almost three times as likely to die from Covid-19 than white individuals (Office for National Statistics, 2022).

The working and living conditions of ethnic minorities in countries like the UK have also increased the exposure of individuals and these groups to SARS-CoV-2. Many cultural groups live in multi-generational housing, either because there is a cultural precedent for it or because it is necessitated by the relative poverty they may be subject to in the nation they live in. Living in multi-generational housing means that the likelihood of exposure is greatly increased for all involved, particularly when there are children in the household, who have been mostly left to be freely exposed to SARS-CoV-2 throughout the pandemic and have therefore been open exposure lines to households that were otherwise remaining at home. On the surface, this is no different from other types of family household; however, in multigenerational households, those who are older (the grandparent tier) have been more frequently exposed to SARS-CoV-2 in the household if they have been living with children who may be working out of the house, or grandchildren who have been continuing education in settings with minimal safeguards. Further, those in ethnic minority groups are more likely to have been deemed 'essential workers' (or 'key workers'), whose roles could not be undertaken from the safety of their homes, and who as a group have also had higher incidences of Covid-19 (Topriceanu et al., 2021). This has been another factor associated with the higher infection rate seen in ethnic minority groups in white majority nations, and has also disproportionately affected ethnic minority individuals working in health service roles who have been more highly exposed to SARS-CoV-2 (Moorthy & Sankar, 2020).

On top of all of this, minority status and the deeply rooted social issues that this entails, such as being disenfranchised, underserved, marginalised, racialised, and stigmatised, results in well-established barriers to healthcare access, under-consideration in healthcare guidelines and recommendations, and an entirely reasonable lower trust in government and central institutions (Iacobucci, 2020). An illustration of this comes from the public health guidance around Covid-19 symptomology, which in the UK has been very centred around white skin. Any illness that is not yet fully understood, or any that is known to have relevant symptom presentation in the skin, requires adequate examination and assessment to understand different presentation across different skins. Sadly, this was not the case to begin with in the UK, and as a result many people of colour died due to this oversight as a result of not being able to identify a key 'red flag' in breathing problems: cyanosis, or blue lips. Cyanotic lips suggest a fundamental lack of oxygen that is life threatening, and was listed by most emergency medical contact points as being a red flag for urgent hospitalisation in Covid. However, the observation of cyanosis is much harder in darker skin tones, and this information was not rolled out to those working on health and emergency helplines. Incidences like this only go to entrench feelings of marginalisation and disenfranchisement, which – in turn – continue to support a lack of trust and confidence in the institutions responsible for your public healthcare. An unfortunate example of this comes from Covid vaccination, where ethnic minority groups have once more been underserved in white majority nations (Razai et al., 2021). Qualitative work that has been conducted to understand more about this has highlighted some of the long-standing issues in institutional trust, which has been harmed for decades by racial injustices in healthcare research and development, including vaccine development (Woodhead et al., 2021). To understand more about the historical abuses of global majority people in healthcare research and testing, I have included a reference to a book about Henrietta Lacks, simultaneously a hero of medicine and a victim of phenomenally profound racial injustice, who was involved (in ways you probably don't realise) in the development of Covid vaccines.

Learning Outcomes Summary

This chapter has hopefully demonstrated to you that infectious diseases are much more than just chains of communication. Social, political, and environmental factors are all important to understand spread and vulnerability. Vulnerability to Covid starts at the cellular level, with some groups disadvantaged at this very basic level of consideration. The social and political factors around Covid have made handling the pandemic even more complicated for many nations. For some populations, the effect of Covid has been devastating - and there are virtually no pathways behind this that those populations could control.

- Apply the knowledge gained throughout the book to the example of Covid-19.

We have looked at cell-, system-, and population-level factors of Covid-19.

- Understand how we can make sense of disease spread and susceptibility through the cell-to-society perspective.

We have identified some groups that have been at higher risk for contracting Covid, and for suffering from its worse effects.

- Discuss the interaction between the levels of cell-to-society health and its contribution to public health issues in communicable disease.

Using the case study of ethnic minority peoples, we have looked at how social and structural systems influence their vulnerability from the cell-to-society levels, as well as broader public health outcomes.

FURTHER READING

Platto, S., Xue, T., & Carafoli, E. (2020). COVID19: An announced pandemic. *Cell Death & Disease, 11*(9), 1–13.
This paper provides a good overview of the emergence of the Covid-19 pandemic.

The Health Foundation Covid-19 Impact Inquiry has a variety of resources from work carried out in the UK to understand the inequalities highlighted by the disease and mortality burden of the pandemic. www.health.org.uk/what-we-do/a-healthier-uk-population/mobilising-action-for-healthy-lives/covid-19-impact-inquiry

Skloot, R. (2017). *The immortal life of Henrietta Lacks*. Broadway Paperbacks.
This is a very important book to understand some of the origins of the profoundly harmful injustices in healthcare against people of colour.

REFERENCES

Abbasi, J. (2022). The COVID Heart – One year after SARS-CoV-2 infection, patients have an array of increased cardiovascular risks. *JAMA, 327*(12), 1113–14. https://doi.org/10.1001/jama.2022.2411

Al-Rohaimi, A. H., & Al Otaibi, F. (2020). Novel SARS-CoV-2 outbreak and COVID19 disease; A systemic review on the global pandemic. *Genes & Diseases, 7*(4), 491–501. https://doi.org/https://doi.org/10.1016/j.gendis.2020.06.004

Arachchillage, D. J., Rajakaruna, I., Pericleous, C., Nicolson, P. L. R., Makris, M., Laffan, M., & Study Group, CA-COVID-19. (2022). Autoimmune disease and COVID-19: A multicentre observational study in the United Kingdom. *Rheumatology, 61*(12), 4643–55. https://doi.org/10.1093/rheumatology/keac209

Bansal, R., Gubbi, S., & Muniyappa, R. (2020). Metabolic syndrome and COVID 19: Endocrine-immune-vascular interactions shapes clinical course. *Endocrinology, 161*(10), bqaa112. https://doi.org/10.1210/endocr/bqaa112

Bentley, G. R. (2020). Don't blame the BAME: Ethnic and structural inequalities in susceptibilities to COVID-19. *American Journal of Human Biology, 32*(5), e23478. https://doi.org/https://doi.org/10.1002/ajhb.23478

Burström, B., & Tao, W. (2020). Social determinants of health and inequalities in COVID-19. *European Journal of Public Health, 30*(4), 617–18. https://doi.org/10.1093/eurpub/ckaa095

Channappanavar, R., & Perlman, S. (2017). Pathogenic human coronavirus infections: Causes and consequences of cytokine storm and immunopathology. *Seminars in Immunopathology, 39*(5), 529–39. https://doi.org/10.1007/s00281-017-0629-x

Chernyak, B. V., Popova, E. N., Prikhodko, A. S., Grebenchikov, O. A., Zinovkina, L. A., & Zinovkin, R. A. (2020). COVID-19 and oxidative stress. *Biochemistry (Moscow), 85*(12), 1543–53. https://doi.org/10.1134/S0006297920120068

Chlamydas, S., Papavassiliou, A. G., & Piperi, C. (2021). Epigenetic mechanisms regulating COVID-19 infection. *Epigenetics, 16*(3), 263–70. https://doi.org/10.1080/15592294.2020.1796896

Consolazio, D., Murtas, R., Tunesi, S., Gervasi, F., Benassi, D., & Russo, A. G. (2021). Assessing the impact of individual characteristics and neighborhood socioeconomic status during the COVID-19 pandemic in the provinces of Milan and Lodi. *International Journal of Health Services, 51*(3), 311–24. https://doi.org/10.1177/0020731421994842

D'Silva, K. M., & Wallace, Z. S. (2021). COVID-19 and rheumatoid arthritis. *Current Opinion in Rheumatology, 33*(3), 255.

Danwang, C., Noubiap, J. J., Robert, A., & Yombi, J. C. (2022). Outcomes of patients with HIV and COVID-19 co-infection: A systematic review and meta-analysis. *AIDS Research and Therapy, 19*(1), 3. https://doi.org/10.1186/s12981-021-00427-y

Douek, D. C., Brenchley, J. M., Betts, M. R., Ambrozak, D. R., Hill, B. J., Okamoto, Y., ... Koup, R. A. (2002). HIV preferentially infects HIV-specific CD4+ T cells. *Nature, 417*(6884), 95–8. https://doi.org/10.1038/417095a

El-Khatib, Z., Jacobs, G. B., Ikomey, G. M., & Neogi, U. (2020). The disproportionate effect of COVID-19 mortality on ethnic minorities: Genetics or health inequalities? *eClinicalMedicine, 23*. https://doi.org/10.1016/j.eclinm.2020.100430

Figueiredo, A. M. d., Figueiredo, D. C. M. M. d., Gomes, L. B., Massuda, A., Gil-García, E., Vianna, R. P. d. T., & Daponte, A. (2020). Social determinants of health and COVID-19 infection in Brazil: An analysis of the pandemic. *Revista Brasileira de Enfermagem, 73*(2).

Fricke-Galindo, I., & Falfán-Valencia, R. (2021). Genetics insight for COVID-19 susceptibility and severity: A review. *Frontiers in Immunology, 12*, 622176. https://doi.org/10.3389/fimmu.2021.622176

Gagliardi, M. C., Tieri, P., Ortona, E., & Ruggieri, A. (2020). ACE2 expression and sex disparity in COVID-19. *Cell Death Discovery, 6*(1), 37. https://doi.org/10.1038/s41420-020-0276-1

García, C. A., & Duncan, P. (23 Aug 2022). Twice as many people died with Covid in UK this summer compared with 2021. *The Guardian.* https://www.theguardian.com/world/2022/aug/23/twice-as-many-people-died-with-covid-in-uk-this-summer-compared-with-2021#:~:text=The%20fact%20that%20more%20people,of%20the%20deaths%20in%202021.

Hampshire, A., Chatfield, D. A., Mphil, A. M., Jolly, A., Trender, W., Hellyer, P. J., … Menon, D. K. (2022). Multivariate profile and acute-phase correlates of cognitive deficits in a COVID-19 hospitalised cohort. *eClinicalMedicine, 47*. https://doi.org/10.1016/j.eclinm.2022.101417

Hu, B., Huang, S., & Yin, L. (2021). The cytokine storm and COVID-19. *Journal of Medical Virology, 93*(1), 250–56. https://doi.org/https://doi.org/10.1002/jmv.26232

Iacobucci, G. (2020). Covid-19: Racism may be linked to ethnic minorities' raised death risk, says PHE. *BMJ, 369*, m2421. https://doi.org/10.1136/bmj.m2421

Kubota, T., & Kuroda, N. (2021). Exacerbation of neurological symptoms and COVID-19 severity in patients with preexisting neurological disorders and COVID-19: A systematic review. *Clinical Neurology and Neurosurgery, 200*, 106349. https://doi.org/https://doi.org/10.1016/j.clineuro.2020.106349

Little, C., Alsen, M., Barlow, J., Naymagon, L., Tremblay, D., Genden, E., … van Gerwen, M. (2021). The impact of socioeconomic status on the clinical outcomes of COVID-19: A retrospective cohort study. *Journal of Community Health, 46*(4), 794–802. https://doi.org/10.1007/s10900-020-00944-3

Malard, F., Genthon, A., Brissot, E., van de Wyngaert, Z., Marjanovic, Z., Ikhlef, S., … Mohty, M. (2020). COVID-19 outcomes in patients with hematologic disease. *Bone Marrow Transplantation, 55*(11), 2180–84. https://doi.org/10.1038/s41409-020-0931-4

Marazuela, M., Giustina, A., & Puig-Domingo, M. (2020). Endocrine and metabolic aspects of the COVID-19 pandemic. *Reviews in Endocrine and Metabolic Disorders, 21*(4), 495–507. https://doi.org/10.1007/s11154-020-09569-2

Marmot, M. (2020). Build Back Fairer: The COVID-19 Marmot Review.

Martínez-Gómez, L. E., Herrera-López, B., Martinez-Armenta, C., Ortega-Peña, S., Camacho-Rea, M. d. C., Suarez-Ahedo, C., … Fragoso, J. M. (2022). ACE and ACE2 Gene Variants Are Associated with Severe Outcomes of COVID-19 in Men. *Frontiers in Immunology, 13*(1), 450.

Moorthy, A., & Sankar, T. K. (2020). Emerging public health challenge in UK: Perception and belief on increased COVID19 death among BAME healthcare workers. *Journal of Public Health, 42*(3), 486–92. https://doi.org/10.1093/pubmed/fdaa096

Nørgård, B. M., Nielsen, J., Knudsen, T., Nielsen, R. G., Larsen, M. D., Jølving, L. R., & Kjeldsen, J. (2021). Hospitalization for COVID-19 in patients treated with selected immunosuppressant and immunomodulating agents, compared to the general population: A Danish cohort study. *British Journal of Clinical Pharmacology, 87*(4), 2111–20. https://doi.org/https://doi.org/10.1111/bcp.14622

Office for National Statistics. (7 Apr 2022). *Updating ethnic contrasts in deaths involving the coronavirus (COVID-19), England.* Retrieved 31 Aug 2022 from https://www.ons. gov.uk/peoplepopulationandcommunity/birthsdeathsandmarriages/deaths/articles/ updatingethniccontrastsindeathsinvolvingthecoronaviruscovid19englandandwales/ 24january2020to31march2021

Otu, A., Ahinkorah, B. O., Ameyaw, E. K., Seidu, A.-A., & Yaya, S. (2020). One country, two crises: What Covid-19 reveals about health inequalities among BAME communities in the United Kingdom and the sustainability of its health system? *International Journal for Equity in Health, 19*(1), 189. https://doi.org/10.1186/s12939-020-01307-z

Patel, P., Hiam, L., Sowemimo, A., Devakumar, D., & McKee, M. (2020). Ethnicity and covid-19. *BMJ, 369*, m2282. https://doi.org/10.1136/bmj.m2282

Pepera, G., Tribali, M.-S., Batalik, L., Petrov, I., & Papathanasiou, J. (2022). Epidemiology, risk factors and prognosis of cardiovascular disease in the Coronavirus Disease 2019 (COVID-19) pandemic era: A systematic review. *RCM, 23*(1). https://doi.org/10.31083/ j.rcm2301028

Ragab, D., Salah Eldin, H., Taeimah, M., Khattab, R., & Salem, R. (2020). The COVID-19 cytokine storm: What we know so far. *Frontiers in Immunology, 11*, 1446.

Ravi, K. (2020). Ethnic disparities in COVID-19 mortality: Are comorbidities to blame? *The Lancet, 396*(10243), 22. https://doi.org/https://doi.org/10.1016/S0140-6736(20)31423-9

Razai, M. S., Osama, T., McKechnie, D. G. J., & Majeed, A. (2021). Covid-19 vaccine hesitancy among ethnic minority groups. *BMJ, 372*, n513. https://doi.org/10.1136/bmj.n513

Reddy, R. K., Charles, W. N., Sklavounos, A., Dutt, A., Seed, P. T., & Khajuria, A. (2021). The effect of smoking on COVID-19 severity: A systematic review and meta-analysis. *Journal of Medical Virology, 93*(2), 1045–56. https://doi.org/https://doi.org/10.1002/jmv.26389

Rollston, R., & Galea, S. (2020). COVID-19 and the social determinants of health. *American Journal of Health Promotion, 34*(6), 687–9. https://doi.org/10.1177/ 0890117120930536

Seifert, A., Cotten, S. R., & Xie, B. (2020). A double burden of exclusion? Digital and social exclusion of older adults in times of COVID-19. *The Journals of Gerontology: Series B, 76*(3), e99–e103. https://doi.org/10.1093/geronb/gbaa098

Sharma, G., Volgman, A. S., & Michos, E. D. (2020). Sex differences in mortality from COVID-19 pandemic. *JACC: Case Reports, 2*(9), 1407–10. https://doi.org/10.1016/ j.jaccas.2020.04.027

Singh, D., Mathioudakis, A. G., & Higham, A. (2022). Chronic obstructive pulmonary disease and COVID-19: Interrelationships. *Current Opinion in Pulmonary Medicine, 28*(2), 76. www.ncbi.nlm.nih.gov/pmc/articles/PMC8815646/pdf/copme-28-76.pdf

Smith, K., Bhui, K., & Cipriani, A. (2020). COVID-19, mental health and ethnic minorities. *Evidence-Based Mental Health*, *23*(3), 89–90. https://doi.org/10.1136/ebmental-2020-300174

Sunjaya, A. P., Allida, S. M., Di Tanna, G. L., & Jenkins, C. R. (2022). Asthma and COVID-19 risk: A systematic review and meta-analysis. *European Respiratory Journal*, *59*(3), 2101209. doi: 10.1183/13993003.01209-2021.

Tisoncik, J. R., Korth, M. J., Simmons, C. P., Farrar, J., Martin, T. R., & Katze, M. G. (2012). Into the eye of the cytokine storm. *Microbiology and Molecular Biology Reviews*, *76*(1), 16–32. https://doi.org/doi:10.1128/MMBR.05015-11

Topriceanu, C.-C., Wong, A., Moon, J. C., Hughes, A. D., Chaturvedi, N., Conti, G., … Captur, G. (2021). Impact of lockdown on key workers: Findings from the COVID-19 survey in four UK national longitudinal studies. *Journal of Epidemiology and Community Health*, *75*(10), 955–62. https://doi.org/10.1136/jech-2020-215889

Tsukagoshi, H., Shinoda, D., Saito, M., Okayama, K., Sada, M., Kimura, H., & Saruki, N. (2021). Relationships between viral load and the clinical course of COVID-19. *Viruses*, *13*(2), 304.

Woodhead, C., Onwumere, J., Rhead, R., Bora-White, M., Chui, Z., Clifford, N., … Hatch, S. L. (2021). Race, ethnicity and COVID-19 vaccination: A qualitative study of UK healthcare staff. *Ethnicity & Health*, *27*(7), 1–20. https://doi.org/10.1080/13557858.2021.1936464

Zanoli, L., Gaudio, A., Mikhailidis, D. P., Katsiki, N., Castellino, N., Cicero, L. L., … Zocco, S. (2022). Vascular dysfunction of COVID-19 is partially reverted in the long-term. *Circulation Research*, *130*(9), 1276–85. https://doi.org/10.1161/CIRCRESAHA.121.320460

Zemtsov, S. P., & Baburin, V. L. (2020). Risks of morbidity and mortality during the COVID-19 pandemic in Russian regions. *Population and Economics*, *4*(2), 158–81.

GLOSSARY

Acquired Immune Deficiency Syndrome (AIDS)   AIDS is the condition caused by Human Immunodeficiency Virus (HIV). It is characterised by clinically important markers that indicate the immune system has been compromised to a very severe degree.

Acute stress   Short-lived or otherwise episodic stress. Something stressful with a foreseeable end point, as opposed to chronic stress which has no end point and continues for a long time. Acute stress can play out over a few months and be substantial, like a period of exams, or it can be small and trivial, like a daily hassle.

Adaptive immunity   This 'branch' of your immune system is the one that learns (adapts) over time. Within this part of the immune system are your antibodies, those proteins that recognise patterns of invading pathogens like viruses and bacteria.

Adipocytes   Fat cells within the body. Also sometimes called lipocytes.

Adipose tissue   Fatty tissue throughout the body, usually laid down in specific sites. The term adiposity refers to how much fat someone may have (and where, as in the case of *central adipsosity*). Adipocytes are some of the main cells in adipose tissue.

Adrenal glands   Two glands located above the kidneys. They make up part of the hypothalamic-pituitary-adrenal (HPA) axis, and are responsible for releasing hormones such as adrenaline, noradrenaline, and cortisol (amongst others) when our physiological stress response is initiated.

Adrenaline   A hormone utilised in the fight-or-flight response of the the sympathetic nervous system. Also referred to as epinephrine.

Adverse Childhood Experiences (ACEs)   Particular childhood events that are known to cause long term psychological, social, and sometimes physiological consequences throughout the life course. Examples of this may be childhood neglect, abuse, or deprivation due to poverty.

Aetiology   The cause or set of causes that underlie a medical condition.

Allostatic load   The wear and tear caused by chronic or repeated stress on the various systems within the body. To measure or otherwise identify allostatic load, you need to assess the function of multiple systems.

Amino acids   The molecular building blocks of proteins. These are found in your diet, and are used to create a variety of different signalling molecules and cells in your body.

Angina   A condition associated with very sharp chest pain (*angina pectoris*), this is often a hallmark of reduced blood flow to the muscles of the heart and can serve as an indicator for more severe cardiovascular disease in the future.

Angiotensin-converting enzyme 2 (ACE2)   A cell-surface molecule that is expressed on various tissues in your body, particularly membrane tissues. It is used as an entry point into cells by SARS-CoV-2 and other coronaviruses.

Antibodies   Small proteins that are part of your adaptive immune system. They seek out invading microbes and attach to them, effectively marking them for destruction by other cells of the immune system.

Antioxidants   Molecules in your body that neutralise free radicals that are created in the oxidation process. Some antioxidants can be found through your diet, but you also create your own.

Apoptosis   Programmed cell death – the in-built process of cells to die before they become malfunctional.

Asymptomatic presentation   Of an illness, whether that is an infection or a chronic condition, where there are no apparent symptoms.

Atherogenesis   The creation of atherosclerotic plaque (atheroma) and its deposition within blood vessels such as arteries. This is usually a long process that occurs over time.

Atheroma   Atherosclerotic plaque that is laid down in your blood vessels. It is made up of fats, dead cells, and proteins that circulate in your blood.

Atherosclerosis   A condition characterised by the laying down of atherosclerotic plaques within the blood vessels. It is a condition that also indicates the likelihood of developing further cardiovascular disease.

Autonomic nervous system (ANS)   The division of the nervous system that works automatically to initiate a response for stress, or to de-escalate that response. The two 'arms' of the ANS are the sympathetic nervous system and the parasympathetic nervous system.

Axial and appendicular   Axial bones are those located in your central mass (rib cage, pelvis etc.), and appendicular bones are those in your appendages (i.e., your arms, legs).

Basophils   A type of white blood cell (leukocyte) called a granulocyte. They work in a pro-inflammatory action, signalling to other cells in the immune system to increase inflammation.

B-cells   Also referred to as B lymphocytes, these are types of white blood cells that are created within the bone marrow in humans. They produce antibodies to seek out pathogens and also produce cytokines to signal to other cells in the body.

Biomarkers   A biomarker is any type of cell or substance that the body produces that we can use to understand health. Stress hormones, neurotransmitters, and immune cells can all be types of biomarkers. Biomarkers can be used diagnostically as a means to understand the likelihood of having or developing a disease, and can also be used in research to understand bodily functioning.

Blastocyst   A fertilised egg, capable of developing to be a future embryo.

Blood pressure   A measure of the pressure within your cardiovascular system. It is made up of the pressure within your blood vessels when your heart pumps blood out (systolic blood pressure) and when your heart relaxes to let blood back in (diastolic blood pressure). It is usually expressed in SBP/DBP in milligrams of mercury mmHG.

C-reactive protein   A protein in the blood that correlates with inflammation. It is released by the liver in response to circulating inflammatory factors in the blood, and can bind to certain pathogens to mark them for destruction (in a similar way to antibodies, but less specific). As a biomarker it is also often used to indicate cardiovascular disease.

Cancer   A vast family of conditions that are characterised by abnormal cell growth. There are over 100 different types of cancer currently known to medicine, and we are differentiating new types of cancer all the time. Cancers are said to be *neoplastic* diseases, meaning that they are characterised by the growth of new cells.

Capillaries   Small vessels throughout the body that are most commonly associated with carrying blood. They are the very finest blood vessels we have, and are smaller in diameter than a cotton fibre. Similarly small and fine vessels within the lymphatic system are also referred to as capillaries.

Cardiac output   Literally how much blood your heart pumps out over time. It is calculated by using your heart rate (the frequency of the heartbeat) and stroke volume (the volume of blood pumped out). It is used as a means to understand how strong your heart is, and therefore how healthy it is.

Cardiovascular disease   Diseases of the cardiovascular system (the heart and the blood vessels).

Cardiovascular system   The system within your body made up of your heart (cardio) and the huge network of all of your blood vessels (vascular). Your vasculature includes arteries (very large), veins (medium), and capillaries (very fine) that transport your blood around your body.

Catabolism   The breakdown of complex molecules into smaller particles, usually for the purpose of releasing energy.

Central nervous system (CNS)   The brain and the spinal cord. All other neural tissue beyond this is referred to as the peripheral nervous system.

Cerebrovascular disease   Diseases of the vascular system that are found within the brain.

Chemical species   A group of identical atoms. A bottle of water contains one chemical species: H_2O.

Cholesterol   A type of fat (lipoprotein) that circulates in our bloodstream. Two important types are high density (HDL) and low density (LDL). Cholesterol is an important indicator of cardiovascular health as it is associated with atherosclerosis. When we have too much in our bloodstream, this is referred to as cholesterolaemia.

Cholesterolaemia   Having very high levels of cholesterol in the blood.

Chromosomes   A long thread-like structure within our cells that contains our DNA. In humans, chromosomes are aligned in pairs in all cells but our reproductive cells and have telomeres capping the ends of their structures.

Colony-stimulating factors (CSFs)   Types of proteins that interact with the cell surface proteins of stem cells in your haematopoietic (blood cell creation) system. CSFs serve to help differentiate the stem cells into mature blood cells, usually types of immune cells, and to proliferate through the body.

Communicable disease   A type of disease that can be transmitted from person to person. This can be through a variety of mechanisms, such as through close physical contact, through exposure to blood, through aerosolised particles, microdroplets, and also fomites (inanimate objects capable of sustaining pathogens, such as door handles, tables etc.).

Congestive heart failure   A type of cardiovascular disease characterised by the heart's inability to effectively pump blood around the body.

Coping   Any type of psychological or behavioural mechanism adopted to deal with the effects of stress. There are a variety of different coping styles, both positive and negative, and they can be associated with dealing with the stressor itself, or dealing with the psychological and emotional consequences of that stressor.

Corticotropin-releasing hormone (CRH)   A peptide (i.e., complex amino acid chain) hormone used in the physiological stress response. It is released from the hypothalamus to signal to the pituitary to release adrenocorticotropic hormone, which – in turn – stimulates the release of other stress hormones from the adrenal glands.

Cortisol   A type of glucocorticoid in the family of steroid hormones. It is released from the cortex (outer part) of the adrenal gland as part of the physiological stress response. Its role is to support the prioritisation of brain and muscles receiving energy during the fight-or-flight response by selectively enhancing some processes (such as the release of glucose from the liver into the bloodstream) and selectively inhibiting others (such as inhibiting bone growth and remodelling). It is a common biomarker used in stress research to understand the physiological experience of stress and how this will impact health.

Covid-19   The disease caused by the coronavirus SARS-CoV-2, originally discovered in China in 2019. The disease reached pandemic status in early 2020, meaning that it had reached multiple countries across the globe and was being transmitted through the community and not just from those who had travelled to infected areas.

Cytokine storm   A massive inflammatory reaction mediated by cytokines, the chemical messengers of the immune system. Thought to be one of the key mechanisms underpinning the lethality of Covid-19, other SARS-like conditions, and some other respiratory tract infections. It is responsible for the severe inflammation of the lung tissue that is characteristic of SARS.

Cytokines   Chemical messengers used by the immune system to relay information. Some cytokines may be pro-inflammatory, some may be anti-inflammatory, and others may be in some other way immunomodulatory by enhancing or inhibiting the activity or function of other cytokines or cells. They are produced by a wide range of cells, both cells of the immune system and cells found in tissues (particularly endothelial cells that make up the linings of larger structures such as blood vessels and organs).

Dehydroepiandrosterone (DHEA)   A steroid hormone made by your adrenal glands, but also other endocrine tissues in your body. It is a precursor hormone, and can be converted into other steroid hormones such as sex hormones (like testosterone). It is also released in times of stress, and can be used (both DHEA and its sulphur-bound form DHEA Sulphate [DHEAS]) as a biomarker for stress. It works in opposition to cortisol, however, and can buffer against some of the harmful effects of cortisol. Because of this, sometimes the ratio between cortisol and DHEA (or DHEAS) is used to understand the health impacts of stress.

Differentiation   Of neurons – as the central nervous system develops, new neurons that are 'naïve' or multi-purpose differentiate into specific types of neurons that serve specific functions.

Disability-adjusted life years   A metric of burden of disease. It is calculated by looking at the number of years lost due to premature death, and years spent in less than good health.

DNA damage   An impact of oxidative stress. It is the damage to any of the normal properties or functions of DNA, such as its ability to transcribe and replicate.

Ejection fraction   A metric of heart health, it specifically captures the percentage of your heart volume of blood being ejected with each beat.

Embolus   A mass (sometimes this could be an air bubble as well) that moves through your blood vessels, unattached to the vessel wall, that is capable of obstructing the blood vessel. When this happens it is referred to as an embolism.

Embryo   A developing future human – classified as an embryo up to 11 weeks, gestation.

Endocrine   Referring to the hormonal systems within the body. Endocrine glands are tissues that create hormones. Endocrinology is the scientific study of this system, its tissues, cells, and functions.

Endocrinosenescence   The ageing of the endocrine system that occurs naturally over time.

Endogenous   Coming from inside the body. We have endogenous opioids, which are opioids that are created inside the body (e.g., enkephalins). The opposite of this is exogenous, meaning originating from outside the body. Exogenous opioids are substances found in opium poppies. The prefix endo- means coming from inside, with exo- meaning outside. See also endocrine, exocrine.

Endothelial dysfunction   A characterisations of cardiovascular diseases, particularly coronary artery disease, where restricted or interrupted blood flow is caused by the constriction of the blood vessel rather than anything obstructing the blood vessels.

Endothelium   The fine membrane that lines the inside of the heart and blood vessels, endo- again meaning inside. You also have an epithelium (epi- meaning 'on'), which is your skin and the external surface of your internal organs and blood vessels.

Enteric nervous system (ENS)   A subdivision of your nervous system that exists in your gut. This nervous system is said to be more or less autonomous from the brain, and sends similar chemical messengers to the brain to carry out its motor functions that support digestion.

Environmental endocrine disruptors   Chemicals found in the environment that are capable of altering your natural hormonal responses and functions. Can be found in foods, but most commonly in personal care products like toiletries, and in agents used during manufacture. Examples of these are lead, phthalates, and parabens.

Eosinophils   A type of white blood cell (leukocyte) called a granulocyte. Like basophils, they are largely pro-inflammatory, but can also produce a variety of different molecules used by the immune system such as growth factors. They can also destroy molecules or other foreign substances that have been marked for destruction, and are particularly important in our defences against parasites and bacteria.

Epidemiology   The study of how, where, and why diseases develop across populations.

Epigenetics   The study of how our behaviours and environmental experiences or exposures can change the function of our genes. Epigenetics is not about the mutation of genes, but rather the switching on, or off, of certain gene activities in response to our activities and experiences. Some key mechanisms in epigenetics include histone regulation/acetylation and methylation.

Erythrocytes   Red blood cells. Principally involved in transporting oxygen to and carbon dioxide away from tissues. Erythrocytes are created in the bone marrow as part of the haematopoietic system.

Eustress   A type of 'positive' stress, that is more commonly appraised to be a challenge rather than a threat. Eustress has a beneficial effect on our emotions and attitudes, and is also associated with more positive physiological processes such as the release of endorphins.

Ex vivo   A term used for laboratory work that is conducted outside of the living thing. This may be looking at how immune cells function *in vitro* (in glass) by taking a sample of blood and adding something to it to observe the reaction under a microscope. The opposite is *in vivo*, where we observe physiological processes naturally within the person or animal. An example of this may be administering a routine vaccination and then assessing the antibody response to it over time.

Exogenous   Originating or being located outside the body. Opposite to endogenous.

Fibrinogen   A protein complex from the blood (also referred to as a 'factor') that is involved in clotting and some inflammatory processes, particularly in response to tissue injury or systemic inflammation resulting from infection or from stress.

Foam cells   A specific type of macrophage (a white blood cell that destroys infected cells and invading pathogens) that contains cholesterol, giving them a foamy appearance. They are often found in atherosclerotic plaque (atheroma) that characterises atherosclerosis.

Foetal Alcohol Spectrum Disorder (FASD)   A condition caused by *in utero* exposure to alcohol. A variety of developmental conditions can result from this.

Foetus   A developing future human – classified as a foetus after 11 weeks' gestation. US English: fetus.

Free radicals   An unstable atom or chemical, usually with an odd number of electrons. The requirement to stabilise, and therefore gain an electron or lose an electron to be gained by another atom in the body, can damage tissues and cells.

Glands   Glands are tissue structures in our bodies responsible for synthesising and releasing hormones. We have glands that secrete hormones and substances to work internally (endocrine glands, like the adrenal glands) and glands that secrete hormones and substances that work on our external bodies (exocrine glands, like sweat glands).

Glia   Supporting cells in the central nervous system. There are lots of different types of glia, and one of their roles is to create myelin to insulate neurons.

Glucocorticoids   A class of steroid hormones strongly associated with the stress response, but that are also involved in some of the regulatory processes of the immune system.

Gut–brain axis   The communication axis between the gut (enteric nervous system) and the brain. The bacteria in your gut 'talk' to your brain using cellular messengers, which are also messengers used by the brain and the immune system.

Haematopoietic system   Technically the lymphohaematopoeitic system that is involved with the creation and management of your blood cells (both red and white).

Haemorrhage   The fancy term for bleeding. Used in this book in the context of cardiovascular disease, where blockages of the blood vessels may cause those vessels to rupture, resulting in internal bleeding. US English: hemorrhage.

Hayflick limit   The number of times a cell can reproduce before apoptosis occurs. This is mediated by telomeres, and helps to ensure we have a good stock of well-functioning cells in use.

Health inequalities   Social and environmental injustices that result in unfairness and inequality in regard to mental or physical health.

Heart rate variability (HRV)   The beat-to-beat variation of your heartbeat. Everyone's heart will vary in its frequency of beat, and the time between each beat, at rest and during activity. HRV can be used as an index of future cardiovascular health risk, and is also a useful biomarker for stress (high HRV indicating a greater ability to tolerate physiological changes due to stress).

High-density lipoprotein   A type of cholesterol, sometimes referred to as 'good' cholesterol because it can absorb LDL in the blood and transport it back to the liver, where it can be broken down. Also referred to as HDL cholesterol.

Human Immunodeficiency Virus (HIV)   The virus (and its condition) that is responsible for immune degradation leading to AIDS. The HIV virus infects types of white blood cells called T-cells. These T-cells are important for your immune system to function properly, and as the virus infects them they gradually deplete, leading to vulnerability to opportunistic infections and an overall depleting level of health.

Hypertension   A clinical condition of having blood pressure that is considered to be too high.

Hypotension   A clinical condition of having blood pressure that is considered to be too low.

Hypothalamic-pituitary-adrenal (HPA) axis   The communication axis between the hypothalamus and pituitary in the brain, and the adrenal glands. This is your 'stress axis', and is what is set in motion when we encounter something threatening or stressful.

Hypothalamic-pituitary-gonadal axis   The communication axis between the hypothalamus and pituitary in the brain and the gonads.

Immunosenescence   The ageing of the immune system that occurs naturally as we get older.

In utero   The phrase used when describing a foetus that is still gestating, or still in the womb.

Inflammation   Both a clinical characteristic and a pattern of immunity. You will be able to recognise inflammation as a clinical characteristic or symptom if you graze your skin, or get bitten by an insect – the skin becomes swollen, red, and sore. Inflammation as an immune response (sometimes referred to as sytemic inflammation) is a pattern of proinflammatory immune behaviour to mobilise immune cells when we are under attack by a pathogen.

Innate immunity   The immune system that you are born with. Sometimes referred to as cellular or cell-mediated immunity, it is the parts of your immune system that rely on multi-purpose killing cells to destroy foreign invaders and clean up dead cells in your body.

Integumentary system   This is the skin basically, and the various immune and endocrine properties it has. It keeps outside bits out and inside bits in, but also allows some inside bits out (like sweat) and some outside bits in (like UV radiation from the sun). It is a complicated and very sophisticated system that most of us don't really give a second thought to, but saves our lives day in and day out. The next time you get a scratch or a bite, watch your skin repair itself and marvel at how incredible your integumentary system is.

Interferons   Proteins in your immune system that 'interfere' with the cellular processes of invading pathogens, in part preventing them from mobilising or replicating. They are also important conductors of your immune system, informing other cells of threat (from pathogens or cancer), and can mobilise some white blood cells to seek and destroy.

Interleukins   Interleukins are types of cytokines, the chemical messengers of the immune system. We know now that interleukins don't just talk to the cells of the immune system, they can also speak to our brains and endocrine tissues. They are made by white blood cells and some other cells in the body, and they have recently begun to be used as therapy for some conditions such as cancer.

Intersectionality   The combination of any number of social identities that can confer either privilege or inequality. Usually used in terms of those identities that result in discrimination and various layers of social and personal inequalities such as our 'race', gender, sexuality, disability status, ethnicity, or social class.

Ischemia   The loss of blood flow to an organ or tissue that may be caused by a blockage.

Ischemic heart disease   The condition characterised by restricted and inconsistent blood flow to the muscles of the heart. If blood flow is cut off, this can cause tissue death in the heart muscle and can also cause a heart attack. Also referred to as coronary heart disease (CHD) and coronary artery disease (CAD).

Leukocytes   White blood cells, the immune cells that are responsible for identifying and neutralising invaders as well as 'cleaning up' dead cells and other cellular waste.

Loneliness   The condition of having a discrepancy between desired and actual social contact with others, in terms of both frequency and quality. Someone can be surrounded by people but still feel lonely if they are not experiencing the type of connection with others that they wish to. Similarly, some can be completely alone but not feel lonely because their desired social connections are being fulfilled.

Long bones   Any bone in your body that is longer than it is wide. They have bone marrow within, which is where some of your blood cells are made. These are bones like your collar bone (clavical), your leg bones (femur, tibia, fibula), bones in your arms (humerus, radius, ulna), and some of the bones in your hands and feet too (metacarpals, metatarsals, and phalanges).

Low-density lipoprotein   A type of cholesterol, sometimes referred to as 'bad' cholesterol because having high levels of this type of cholesterol is associated with heart disease. Also referred to as LDL cholesterol.

Lymph   A clear fluid created in your body that is pushed around your lymphatic system with your bodily movements. It is mostly made up of immune cells such as white blood cells.

Lymph nodes   Junction points in your lymphatic system where lymph is filtered by specialised cells to clear you of harmful microbes and molecules. Lymph nodes in certain areas may swell whilst you are fighting a local infection, such as the nodes in your neck when you have an upper respiratory tract infection like a cold.

Lymphatic organs   The larger organ structures associated with your lymphatic system like your thymus and your spleen. These tissues are responsible for creating some of the immune cells in your body that you rely on to maintain your internal health and defend you from invasion.

Lymphatic system   The system responsible for creating, mobilising, and maintaining the cells of your immune system. It runs parallel to your vasculature, but has specialised structures to support its working such as organs that create cells and nodes to filter out harmful cells.

Lymphocytes   Types of white blood cells that are created in either the thymus (T-lymphocytes, or T-cells) or the bone marrow (B-lymphocytes, or B-cells). T-cells have a lot of different properties and functions, but are very good at killing malfunctioning cells (such as the beginnings of tumours) and in maintaining appropriate immune responses. B-cells similarly have a lot of different properties and functions, but one of their most important jobs is creating our antibodies.

Macrophages   A type of white blood cell that surrounds and engulfs infected cells, microbes, dead cells, or anything else that is flagged as being dangerous or not needed. They also play a part in initiating certain immune responses in times of attack.

Memory T-cells   Types of T-cells (usually classed as part of our innate immunity) that respond to specific pathogens (so technically part of our adaptive immune response). The 'memory' they have of the pathogen allows them to mount an aggressive and specific response if we encounter that pathogen again in the future.

Menarche   The initiation of menstrual periods in puberty.

Menopause   An endocrinological change point in the bodies of people with uteruses and ovaries. Characterised by the ceasing of menstrual periods.

Metabolic syndrome   The name given when someone has both high blood pressure and diabetes and is obese. It is a condition in itself, but is also a risk factor for other chronic conditions such as cardiovascular and cerebrovascular disease.

Metabolism   Chemical reactions that underlie our very existence. There are three main properties of metabolism: 1) the breaking down of food and nutrients into basic molecular blocks to use for the creation of proteins, fats, and acids needed for cellular processes; 2) the conversion of energy from foods into energy needed by cells; and 3) the clearing up of cellular waste. Can be catabolic (breaking down) or anabolic (creation or synthesis).

Metastases   The secondary cancer growths characteristic of more advanced stages of cancer, where it spreads to another organ or structure within the body. Used as a clinical marker for cancer staging as well as prognosis and treatment.

Microbiome   Your very own zoo of bacteria (helpful and harmful) that exist both within you and on your skin; the literally billions of microbes that your body sustains in various places. We are discovering more about how our microbiome actually supports our health, and how it can communicate with various systems in our bodies.

Migration   Of neurons – as the central nervous system develops, new neurons migrate to specific areas in the brain.

Monocytes   The largest class of white blood cells. Macrophages are types of monocytes, and there are also dendritic cells that are types of monocytes. They are very useful in tissue repair, and can play a part in the development of our adaptive immunity too.

Morphology   The characteristic shape or appearance of something.

Myelination   The process of glial cells producing myelin to insulate neurons. Myelin protects the delicate projections of the neuron (the axons) and facilitates electrical conduction to make the signal faster. Not all neurons myelinate.

Myocardial infarction (MI)   A heart attack. Occurs when the blood supply to the heart muscle is blocked, usually by a clot, either significantly decreasing flow or stopping it altogether, triggering the death of cells.

Natural Killer (NK) cells Another type of lymphocyte, thought to originate in the bone marrow, that works in a similar function to some of the killer types of T-cells. As their name suggests, they kill cells. Unlike macrophages, NK cells release substances to trigger the death of the cell they are targeting. They are most effective at killing cells that have been infected by viruses and in killing tumour cells as well.

Neuroendocrine Refers to any endocrine tissue that is also part of the nervous system, such as the pituitary or hypothalamus. Can also refer to neuroendocrine hormones (also called neurohormones), which are hormones that originate in these neuroendocrine tissues like corticotropin-releasing factor or vasopressin, or hormones created elsewhere in the body that can have an affect on neural tissue such as noradrenaline.

Neurogenesis The creation of new neurons, particularly as the brain and central nervous system are being created during gestation.

Neuropeptides Chemical messengers used in the nervous system. 'Peptide' means they are a complex chain of proteins, and they can operate both directly and indirectly in the nervous system. Some examples are neuropeptide Y, oxytocin, and insulin.

Neurotransmitters The main means of neuron-to-neuron communication in the nervous system to make your brains and bodies function. Examples are serotonin, dopamine, acetylcholine and histamine.

Neutrophils These are white blood cells that are some of your first lines of defence when you are infected by something. Along with eosinophils and basophils, they are granulocytes, but they are the most abundant in your bloodstream, making up about 40–70% of your white blood cells. They are important in the early stages of infection, and (like macrophages) engulf invading microbes when they are encountered.

Non-communicable disease Any type of disease that cannot be transmitted from person to person like an infection. Diseases like cardiovascular disease, cancer, diabetes, and Alzheimer's are non-communicable.

Noradrenaline A hormone utilised in the fight-or-flight response of the sympathetic nervous system. Also referred to as norepinephrine.

Oedema A build up of fluid in the body that characterises swelling. When you are bitten by an insect, this creates a small and very localised oedema. Larger and more general types of oedema can happen as a result of poor circulation or lymphatic drainage, or because of more serious conditions like congestive heart failure. US English: edema.

Oestrogen   A steroid hormone that is important in puberty and for the functioning of the ovaries, as well as pregnancy. It also has some immune-modulatory impacts and is associated with bone integrity. US English: Estrogen.

Optimism   A psychological perspective, sometimes considered to be a relatively stable trait characteristic, typified by having a positive outlook on life.

Osteoblasts   Cells that form bone tissue.

Osteoclasts   Cells that break down bone tissue.

Oxidation   The loss of electrons in an unstable atom or chemical (a free radical).

Oxidative stress   The status of imbalance between free radicals and the anti-oxidants that can neutralise them. When there are too many free radicals in the body, they will stabilise by electron exchange with other atoms in cells and tissues, potentially damaging them and resulting in DNA damage.

Parasympathetic nervous system (PNS)   A subdivision of the autonomic nervous system. The opposite 'arm' to the sympathetic, it serves to *rest and digest*, and de-escalate the stress response created by the sympathetic.

Pathogens   A micro-organism or agent that causes disease. Can be a virus, fungus, bacteria, or parasite.

Peptide hormones   Like neuropeptides, these types of hormones are chains of amino acids. If they work in the brain (which most do), they can be referred to as neuropeptides. Examples are glucagon, parathyroid hormone, ghrelin, and growth hormone.

Peripheral nervous system   Any other part of your nervous system that is not your brain or spinal cord. All of the nerves you have throughout the rest of your body can be considered to be your peripheral nervous system. The word 'periphery' is often used in science to denote anything in your body that is not your brain or spinal cord.

Peripheral resistance   The resistance of your arteries to the internal pressure of blood flow. Your autonomic nervous system can increase (sympathetic) or decrease (parasympathetic) your peripheral resistance, and so can drugs, and the viscosity of your blood. Some drugs given for hypo- or hypertension work to increase or decrease your peripheral resistance, mimicking your autonomic nervous system.

Phagocytosis   The engulfing of cells by other cells. Macrophages use this technique to surround and consume cells they need to target.

Post-Covid syndrome   The name given to long-lasting symptoms after acute Covid-19 infection. We are still trying to understand more about what it is and why it happens in some and not others. Also referred to as 'Long Covid'.

Progesterone   A steroid hormone that is important in puberty, and for menstruation and pregnancy.

Proliferation   Of neurons – as the central nervous system develops, new neurons are created. Sometimes also referred to as neurogenesis. New neurons are created throughout our lifetime, but most are created in the very earliest stages of development.

Pruning   Of neurons – as the central nervous system develops, connections between some neurons are pruned away if they are less important so that connections that are more important can be prioritised.

Psychobiology   The interdisciplinary study of psychology and biology, encompassing a variety of subdisciplines that all examine and incorporate an understanding of how the brain and body communicate with each other.

Psychobiotics   The name given to probiotics (and some prebiotics – the things that support probiotics) that are intended to have an impact on the gut–brain axis communication.

Psychoneuroendocrinoimmunology (PNEI)   The combined study of PNI and PNE. This field seeks to understand psychological factors (behaviour, emotional, environmental, and social) and how they influence the working of the immune and endocrine systems.

Psychoneuroendocrinology (PNE)   An interdisciplinary field that seeks to understand psychological factors (behaviour, emotional, environmental, and social) and how they influence the working of the endocrine system.

Psychoneuroimmunology (PNI)   An interdisciplinary field that seeks to understand psychological factors (behaviour, emotional, environmental, and social) and how they influence the working of the immune system.

Psychophysiology   The interdisciplinary field that looks at physiology in regard to psychological processes and experiences. Often uses measures of physiological activity (for example from the heart or brain) to understand more about how psychological factors influence the physical operation of the body.

Puberty   The process of physical and hormonal changes experienced in the transition between childhood and adulthood.

Public health   The field of preventing ill health and promoting good health in large populations of people.

Public health psychology   A branch of health psychology that focuses on using health psychology in public health modalities and settings (i.e., in population health).

Pulmonary embolism An interruption or blockage of blood flow in the lungs, often caused by a clot.

Pulmonary vascular disease Like cardiovascular disease or cerebrovascular disease, this is a disease that affects the vasculature, but in this case is specifically oriented around the lungs.

Quality-adjusted life years A metric used in population health that estimates how many years a patient will have after a diagnosis of an illness that would be equivalent to one year in good health.

Quality of life (QoL) Quality of life (QoL) is a metric used to understand the subjective appraisal of the standard of someone's life with relevance to their social and cultural context. This may be measured in terms of someone's subjective financial status, their employment, and the standard of their living environment. A related concept is Health-Related QoL (HRQoL), which is a similar idea but applied with specific relevance to someone's health.

Reactive oxygen species Also referred to as *free radicals*.

Redox Reduction-oxidation reaction in cellular processes. Comprised of oxidation, a loss of an electron, and reduction, where there is a gain of electrons in an unstable atom or chemical.

Remodelling A biological process that effectively repairs or otherwise re-configures the way something operates in the body. Neural pruning, the process of trimming away less-used pathways to prioritise much more important pathways, is a type of remodelling. Remodelling in bone is the process of scaffolding and regrowing bone material in the case of fractures.

Respiration The chemical reaction that allows the transmission of oxygen into cells, and the transmission of carbon dioxide outside cells.

Self-perpetuation Self-perpetuation refers to a situation that keeps itself going consistently, that cannot change without meaningful and purposeful intervention.

Severe acute respiratory syndrome (SARS) The syndrome associated with Covid-19 and other coronaviruses. It is characterised by the rapid inflammation of lung tissue, compromising the ability to breathe.

Sickness behaviour A pattern of behavioural and emotional responses when the body is under attack by a pathogen. This usually begins before we even know we are ill, with our immune systems sending signals that are received by our brain to initiate those behaviours that seek to preserve us whilst we are vulnerable, and maximise our ability to fight off infection.

Sinoatrial node   Our in-built pacemaker that sets our heartbeat.

Social epigenetics   The field associated with social conditions and circumstances and how they can create cellular-level changes within the body to affect health.

Social gradient of health   The all-too-common phenomenon of a linear relationship between social circumstance and health, where the more prosperous and socially advantaged you are, the better your health will be, and vice versa.

Social support   The concept of emotional, instrumental, or informational support from others in our lives to assist when we are stressed. Social support can come from anyone – human or animal – and is only really reliably determined by the person receiving it. As with loneliness, the number of people in our support network is not as important as the quality of those relationships, and the ability we have to be able to glean the type of support we need in certain circumstances from that network.

Steroid hormones   Types of hormones made from steroids (derived from cholesterols), mostly those hormones created by the adrenals (e.g., cortisol, adrenaline) and the gonads (e.g., testosterone, oestrogen).

Stress   A word commonly used, but often poorly defined. We can talk about stress as being a psychological phenomenon, where we experience an emotional and behavioural response in reaction to a situation that puts us under some sort of pressure or threat. Stress is also a physiological phenomenon, where our bodies mount a response that will prepare us to fight or to run away. Stress is extremely subjective, and will be experienced differently by everyone from person to person, but also within people, with stressful situations being appraised differently when experienced again, or after having experienced other stressful situations. We can have acute stress, which is usually short lived with a determinable end point, or chronic stress, which lasts a long time, impacts a number of aspects of our lives, and may be uncertain in its ending.

Sustainable Development Goals (SDGs)   A collection of 17 interlinked and comprehensive goals set out by the United Nations to be adopted by all nations, regardless of their development status, that form a 'shared blueprint for peace and prosperity for people and the planet, now and into the future'.

Sympathetic nervous system (SNS)   A subdivision of the autonomic nervous system. The opposite 'arm' to the parasympathetic, it serves to initiate the state of *fight or flight* (or sometimes freeze). It mobilises the body for action, prioritising those systems and processes that will allow us to fight or run away, and slowing or shutting down any other processes to enable that prioritisation.

Synaptogenesis   The creation of synapses, or communication junctions between neurons.

T-cells   White blood cells that originate in the thymus. There are many different types of T-cells, such as helper, cytotoxic, and memory T-cells. They play an important role in the overall functioning of your immune system, both in terms of its defence against pathogens and in regulatory functions.

Telomeres   The cap on the end of your chromosomes. They work as a reproduction counter, and get shorter each time your chromosomes are replicated. After getting to a certain point, your telomeres will be so short that your cell will die. This ensures you usually have a good stock of healthy well-functioning cells in your body. Telomerase is a biomarker used to understand the status of your telomeres.

Testosterone   A steroid hormone that is important in puberty and for the functioning of the testes. It also has some impacts on bone integrity and muscle development.

Th1/Th2 immunity   A pattern of immune response based on T-helper (Th) cells. The balance between Th1 and Th2 is supposed to be kept in order in healthy individuals, but the balance can be swayed one way or another by stress, by certain health behaviours, and by disease.

Thymic involution   Age-related degeneration of the thymus.

Thyroid   A gland in your neck that creates hormones that regulate the metabolic processes in your body. Several autoimmune conditions can impact the thyroid, causing it to go into overdrive (hyperthyroidism) or to slow down (hypothyroidism). Thyroid hormones also impact your behaviour and emotions, so thyroid diseases can often mimic mental health conditions.

Trabecular bone   Bones with a matrix-like infrastructure. The matrix means the bones are lighter than they would be if the bone was completely solid, and the trabeculae absorb shock, helping to maintain the strength of the bones.

Translational research   A field of research that seeks to provide evidence that can be turned into effective strategies and interventions to benefit human health and wellbeing.

Tumour necrosis factor (TNF)   A type of cytokine, or immune signalling molecule, that plays a role in various immune functions, and also has some processes in endocrine function. As it sounds, it was originally thought to be key to attacking tumours; however, we now know that some tumours can actually create TNF.

Vagus nerve   A cranial nerve that projects right down to the abdomen. A primarily parasympathetic conduit, it provides motor control to the heart, lungs, and gut. It is also a key pathway for brain-to-immune communication as well. It is the longest nerve in the ANS.

Vasculature   The networks of blood vessels in your body, comprised of arteries, veins, and capillaries.

Vertebrae   The bones in your spine.

Viral load   The amount of virus that is present in your bloodstream or in infected tissue.

Virions   Viral cells.

White blood cells   The main cells of your immune system.

Zika virus   A virus that is relatively mild in adults, but that can cause devastating damage to an embryo or foetus.

INDEX